A NEW LOOK AT A WORLD PLAGUE

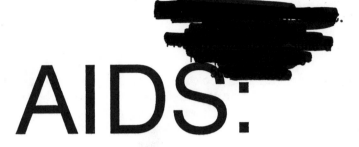

AIDS:

HOPE

HOAX

and

HOOPLA

Michael L. Culbert, D.Sc.

with an introduction by

Bruce W. Halstead, M.D.

The Bradford Foundation

THE ROBERT W. BRADFORD FOUNDATION,
A TRUST
Chula Vista, California

First Printing 1989
Second printing May 1990

LIBRARY OF CONGRESS CATALOGUE CARD NUMBER 88-93058

ISBN: 0-934740-15-1

PRINTED IN THE UNITED STATES OF AMERICA

Lovingly dedicated

to the memory

of

DEAN BURK, Ph.D., 1904 - 1988

friend — mentor — original thinker

ACKNOWLEDGMENTS

While it is impossible to acknowledge each and every contributor to the research which went into the current book (and its predecessor monograph, AIDS:TERROR, TRUTH, TRIUMPH), I would particularly like to cite the help, guidance and sharing of their time of Robert Cathcart, M.D.; Robert Strecker, M.D.; Laurence Badgley, M.D.; Steve Caiazza, M.D.; Eva Lea Snead, M.D.; Emanuel Revici, M.D.; Robert Atkins, M.D.; Bruce Halstead, M.D.; and Henry W. Allen, biochemist. And there is no complete way to express my heartfelt thanks to the HIV/AIDS patients themselves with whom—by the hundreds—I have spoken, including those who entered the experimental treatment program in Mexico. This work could not have come to fruition, of course, without the insights, innovation and support of Dr. Robert Bradford and Rodrigo Rodriguez, M.D., of the Bradford Research Institutes. Nor could the constantly altered manuscript have survived without the dedicated word-processing input of my good friend Dante Camino.

PLEASE NOTE

TABLE OF CONTENTS

INTRODUCTION

By Bruce W. Halstead, M.D.
World Life Research Institute
Colton, CA 92324

The "AIDS virus" is incredible, but hardly more incredible than the research that is going on in the investigation of the beast. It is generally accepted in the most stilted medical circles that AIDS is not only the medical plague of the century, but is a disease pandemic that has few equals in the medical history of mankind.

By a strange quirk of virological biology the AIDS organism, whatever it might be, has challenged the thinking of the communicable disease community to a superlative degree that no medical expert of this century ever thought possible.

AIDS has in many respects taken the entire field of medicine on a gruesome trip back into the Dark Ages and stands in the side wings challenging the technological drama that is rapidly unfolding -- and thus far without a very impressive therapeutic showing. The Surgeon General's Office honestly admits we don't have a cure for AIDS!

The amount of research effort by some of the finest minds in the fields of pharmaceutical chemistry, virology, molecular biology, immunology, biochemistry and every other related scientific discipline have vented their frustrations in attempting to deal with AIDS and their quest for a cure.

In looking beyond AIDS there are some very interesting similarities in two other disease categories, *viz*: cancer and radiation sickness. Carcinogenesis may play a role in each of these disease categories. If one were to place a statistical priority on each of these disorders, the mortality potential of radiation sickness outranks all of the rest of the medical problems of this planet put together.

Strange to say, the treatment of radiation sickness is a topic that has attracted a relatively minor amount of attention by the scientific medical community compared to AIDS, cancer, and for that matter most other disorders.

It is noteworthy, however, that the United States Government openly admits that in the event of a nuclear disaster we have neither a preventive nor a therapeutic solution as to how to adequately handle the mass casualties of radiation sickness. The Chernobyl accident made it clearly evident that Russia doesn't have a quick fix available for radiation sickness, either.

Cancer is the next mortality-statistic runner-up. Despite the triumphant furor in the media about the wonderful cancer "cures" via the cancer establishment, the findings by Harvard University statisticians Bailar and Smith (1986): "we are losing the cancer war", and the United States General Accounting Office, are quite to the contrary.

Note the following statement from GAO's report (1987): "GAO has also determined that the improvements in patient survival have been most dramatic for the rarer forms of cancer and least dramatic for the most prevalent cancers. As a result, even though the absolute number of lives extended is considerable, this number remains small relative to all cancer patients."

For the year 1989 the number of cancer deaths will be about 500,000, a mortality rate that has been steadily increasing over the last several decades -- all of which raises the ugly question: WHY?

THERAPEUTIC RESEARCH STRATEGIES

The diseases AIDS, cancer and radiation sickness have one thing in common in that they all present a complex of pathophysiological conditions which must be addressed if therapeutic success is to be achieved. Moreover, each of these disorders is involved with the immune system to a significant degree.

It is becoming increasingly evident that a multifactorial therapeutic approach may be required if medicine is to conquer these disorders. However, in the past multifactorial therapeutics has been frowned upon and glibly dismissed as "polypharmacy". It is the contention of this writer and the author of this book, Michael L. Culbert, that it is time to take a fresh look.

In the development of modern pharmaceuticals there has been a steady evolution in the direction of the "magic bullet" approach accompanied by the Pasteurian or Cartesian mentality, to wit: one disease -- one drug -- one patient -- and a drug monopoly. This is the story of monopharmacy. An approach that is beginning to spell medical catastrophe.

THE TREATMENT OF AIDS

The AIDS experts have generally agreed that there is no satisfactory treatment for AIDS even though an enormous amount of effort has been directed in quest of the "magic bullet". Many medical scientists formerly engaged in cancer research have now become "AIDS experts". Unfortunately, some of the same thinking prevalent in the cancer approach has inseminated the AIDS field. The prevalent use of AZT is an example of this cross fertilization.

In cancer therapy, cytotoxicity, radiation and surgery are the therapeutic hallmarks of oncologists. A cancer victim suffers from the inroads of carcinogenesis and immunoincompetence and is sold a therapy that is carcinogenic and lowers the immune system. This line of molecular illogic has been successfully sold to both the medical professional and layman alike -- all at a cost of millions of lives.

In AIDS the victim is suffering from an acquired immune deficiency disorder and is sold AZT, a highly toxic immune depressant. The merits of AZT (3'-azido-3'-deoxythymidine) have been loudly proclaimed as a "safe, effective therapeutic agent" (within the narrow context of FDA's thinking) for use in the treatment of AIDS.

However, the scientific evidence clearly attests to the fact that AZT, like many cancer chemotherapeutic agents, is neither safe nor effective despite the endorsement by the United States Food and Drug Administration. Sommadossi and Carlisle (1987) have correctly pointed out: "Surprisingly, little attention has been give thus far to the effects of these antiviral drugs on such 'host' cells as those of bone marrow." This comment appeared after the approval by the Food and Drug Administration.

As of 1987 detailed knowledge of the toxicity of AZT was nonexistent. It has since been determined that AZT tends to depress the bone marrow. The temporary benefits of "improvement of quality of life and increase in survival time" is turning out to be a short-term delusion all at the expense of the wishful patient and to the long-term benefit of the pharmaceutical industry.

Aside from the vaccine and monoclonal antibody routes which are being vigorously explored in conventional pharmaceutical circles there are other modalities which need to be examined -- which is the subject matter of this book.

The AIDS virus is a complex packet of genetic materials, in this case RNA cloaked in glycoproteins and lipids. The AIDS virus cannot replicate itself without the use of the infected cell's genetic machinery and the use of the vital reverse transcriptase enzyme. Because of the intimate involvement of viral proteins with those of the host cell it is difficult to develop a therapeutic agent which is capable of destroying the virus without injuring the host cell.

Unfortunately, in modern pharmaceutical therapeutic strategy there is used all too often a Sherman tank approach using highly toxic agents which end up killing the disease and the patient. If the truth were known there are probably more people dying of the treatment than the disease. All of which brings up the subject of the "therapeutic index", which is the relationship between therapeutic effectiveness and toxicity, or the ratio of the toxic dose to the effective dose.

An interesting dichotomy exists in the pharmaceutical mentality within the United States which is becoming increasingly nonsensical. Simply stated, in minor illness the therapeutic index is generally required to be high, but in life-threatening illness the pharmaceutical industry and the FDA have been willing to accept a wide variety of extremely toxic substances having a very low therapeutic index.

Again, the classical example of this therapeutic compromise is the extensive use of cancer chemotherapeutic agents and radiation which are both carcinogenic and lower the immune system. The more serious the disease, the more poisonous the substance that is used and approved by regulatory agencies.

There is another side to this therapeutic coin which becomes frightening and may ultimately be seen as a form of self-imposed genocide.

Consider the following concept. If one attempts to review even a modicum of the vast sea of molecular, biochemical, bioorganic, immunochemical, biophysical and physiological literature dealing with the human body, one is forced to conclude that a human being is in essence a biochemical symphony. It is a complex of vastly intricate chemical and physical components fearfully and wonderfully made, orchestrated by a variety of poorly understood delicate mechanisms.

If this system is to operate effectively there must be a finely tuned balance of nutrients which operate in conjunction with the mental faculties, incorporating adequate amounts of pure air, clean water, a reasonable amount of sunshine and adequate rest.

This concept is not too profound but is quite basic. It deals with the elementary concepts of cellular homeostasis and immunocompetence. These basic concepts appear to be poorly understood by the pharmaceutical industry at large.

The frightening aspect of this matter is the danger of executing these basic principles in the clinical arena by the practicing physician. To be more specific: In the state of California under California Health and Safety Code 1707.1 we find the following: "The sale, offering for sale, delivering, giving away, prescribing or administering any drug, medicine, compound or device to be used in the diagnosis, treatment, alleviation or cure of cancer is unlawful and prohibited unless" .... it is approved by the State or Federal Food and Drug authorities.

Under the legal "Validity" of this law is included "foods as well as drugs". Moreover, any time a licensed physician or layperson makes a scientifically valid claim that a particular food is useful in preventing or treating a disease, that food automatically becomes a drug.

Furthermore, this legal principle is followed throughout the United States backed by the heavy hands of a host of regulatory and prosecutorial agencies. Keep in mind that AIDS, cancer and radiation sickness may all involve carcinogenesis.

The continual love affair with the toxic approach to drug therapy in critical illness has led to a neglect of more rational, nontoxic synergistic approaches to health care such as are employed in traditional medicine worldwide, including the United States.

The use of natural products that have been safely used for thousands of years is generally suppressed by the U.S. Food and Drug Administration, criminalized by other regulatory agencies, and scorned by the pharmaceutical industry at large.

This is the epicenter of a progressively worsening health care situation dealing with chronic degenerative disease; an ever spiraling national health bill exceeding $500 billion a year (in excess of 11 percent of our gross national product), a loss of the cancer war, no cure for AIDS in sight, and no way of protecting our citizenry from radiation exposure. All of which suggests that it is high time that we come in line with some of the thinking of the World Health Organization.

In 1977, the Thirtieth World Health Assembly adopted a resolution (WHA 30.49) urging governments to place adequate emphasis on the utilization of traditional health systems. This was done in recognition of the fact that global health goals, particularly in the area of chronic degenerative disease control, were not going to be achieved by the year 2000 utilizing only the current medical modalities.

TRADITIONAL MEDICINE

There is a distinct difference in the rationale of Western medicine and that employed in the Orient. Western-trained physicians generally employ a medicinal agent consisting of a single synthetic chemical ingredient or a single natural extractive. Most of these drugs have a high degree of toxicity and an alarming number of carcinogenic, mutagenic, teratogenic or immune suppressive properties.

In contradistinction, Oriental traditional physicians employ a combination of herbs which have had centuries of use in humans and do not produce significant side effects. In fact, to the contrary, a large number of the these herbs have been found to have antimicrobial, anticancer, antiradiation, and immunomodulating properties to a highly significant degree.

Furthermore, there is a substantial body of well documented scientific data which supports these traditional claims. Moreover, these herbal products are used as a synergism of nutrients rather than as individual drugs.

vi

The specific herbs and other natural products used in the prevention and treatment of AIDS will be discussed in a forthcoming publication entitled *AIDS: Immunity and Chinese Medicine Symposium, Proceedings,* Oriental Healing Arts Institute, 1989 (In Press).

AIDS: HOPE, HOAX AND HOOPLA

Michael L. Culbert has now embarked on a difficult mission with the writing of this book. To the more conventional, this book may at first blush appear to be unacceptable and a matter worthy only of scorn. On the other hand, if conventional clinicians had achieved their lofty therapeutic goals, this book would not have been written.

There is now a vast avalanche of scientific data dealing with the subject of AIDS. It is estimated that there is presently in excess of 100,000 technical articles written about this topic. The library at the World Life Research Institute houses more than 16,000 articles and about 50 books on the single subject of AIDS. For the most part the research dealing with AIDS follows only the conventional approaches and fails to discuss any alternatives.

There is a growing amount of good quality scientific peer review research which clearly documents that there are marine and terrestrial natural products that exhibit antiviral activity, have the ability to suppress reverse transcriptase, have anticancer properties and act as positive immunomodulators. Unfortunately, many of these compounds and their potential analogs are being neglected or completely ignored, and much of this scientific data is not infiltrating mainstream scientific literature.

Yes, the AIDS story is incredible, but so is western medicine's approach to the treatment of chronic degenerative disease. In the light of the death-dealing scourges of AIDS, cancer and radiation sickness, modern medicine can no longer afford the luxury of ignorance of man's empirical achievements of the past.

Mike Culbert's approach is one that is deserving of serious examination. He has attempted to examine the other side of the coin and we are in his debt for this significant contribution.

LITERATURE CITED

Bailar, J.C., and E.M. Smith
      1986   Progress Against Cancer? New Eng. J. Med.
              314:1226-1232.

Sommadossi, J.P., and R. Carlisle
      1987   Toxicity of 3'-Azido-3'-Deoxythymidine and
              9-(1,3-Dihydroxy-2-Propoxymethyl) Guanine for
              Normal Human Hematopoietic Progenitor Cells in
              Vitro. Antimicrobial Agents and Chemo.
              31(3):452-454.

U.S. General Accounting Office (GAO)
      1987   Cancer Patient Survival: What Progress Has Been
              Made? Report to the Chairman, Subcommittee on
              Intergovermental Relations and Human Resources,
              Committee on Government Operations, House of
              Representatives, March 1987.

AUTHOR'S FOREWORD
To the second version

Going into the last decade of this century, AIDS has left its mark on the United States and the world -- and this is only the beginning, many fear.

A watershed of sorts was reached in the U.S.A. in 1989: the number of AIDS cases (if there can be full agreement as to what "AIDS" really is) reached and passed 100,000 -- still over half the officially reported cases in the world.

The 1989 version of this book was written as an extension of an earlier monograph published in 1986. The 1989 update had to be revised again for this 1990 version because of the onrush of information about AIDS -- the good, the bad, the unexpected.

While figures may change and new disclosures be reported almost daily in the multiple puzzles of AIDS, the primary concepts we published in 1986 remain not only true but, we believe, reinforced:

AIDS is not a guaranteed death sentence; it has not been shown that the intriguing "new" virus HIV is the sole cause of the syndrome (or, as some would have it, any cause at all), and, happily, the ranks of the long-term survivors are expanding at a rapid pace. Now, as in 1986, these long-termers have two things in common: a positive mental attitude and either the abandonment of "orthodox" medicine altogether or a mingling of such approaches with "alternative" therapy.

The complexion of the syndrome has changed as well:

It is no longer a quick-death malady but increasingly presents as a long, lingering, up-and-down series of medical events. The sum total of "orthodox" therapy at this time is geared to managing or slowing down the syndrome, with no actual "cure" in sight, either from a drug or a vaccine.

This reality buys time both for a payoff in the billions of dollars now committed to research (while allowing AIDS to become a vast new industry, profit-taking from which may bypass cancer in general in a short period of time) and for the development of new information which may help save or prolong the lives of AIDS victims.

At this period in the Age of AIDS, there are three schools of thought:

The doomsayers on the one hand, convinced that a killer disease, probably manufactured by man, has been let loose on the planet and virtually assures the death of, or substantial diminution in, the human race; the optimists, who believe the syndrome will be mostly limited to its original target groups, despite the gradual encroachment -- though not yet the rush -- into the general world population; and those in between who see -- as do we -- both threat and opportunity for new knowledge.

This revised printing of AIDS: HOPE, HOAX AND HOOPLA retains the original concepts, if an altered title, because the message remains the same:

This writer, and the research efforts with which he has been associated, continues to see hope in the overall picture, in terms of prevention, treatment and eventual cure/control. We continue to point to the misinformation and disinformation aspects of the AIDS paradigm (which is as much sociocultural, economic and political as it is medical) as encompassed by "hoax" and "hoopla."

We continue to note that the allopathic medical paradigm, the information-processing/thought-control system of Western medicine, as nurtured and sustained by pharmaceutical interests, has never been more shaken than by the AIDS disaster -- and that this shaking is good for us all.

There is yin and yang, threat and opportunity, in all of this. Due directly to the AIDS threat, more knowledge about human immunity has been assembled and learned in the past decade than in all foregoing human history.

And vastly more knowledge of how the human mind (and indeed all aspects of "the X-quality") is involved with both ease and dis-ease is developing over the single subject of AIDS.

In the U.S.A., due directly to the lack of effective response to AIDS by the entrenched allopathic industrial establishment, more citizens are more aware than ever before of the central political issues involved in the fight for medical freedom of choice.

It may be, as a poetic twist of fate, that the great killer disease of the final years of the 20th century brought with it a gift of political liberty: the restoration of medical freedom of choice in America.

And it will be up to all of us, with unswerving faith in Divine Providence, to nurture that freedom. -- MLC

x

PROLOGUE: A SURVIVOR FROM 'THE GRAND, GAY TIME'

"It was a grand, gay time, and in a certain way, since I enjoyed it all so much, it's hard to say I regret it -- certainly I am paying for it now. Yet it has all been a learning experience, an evolution, a transformation. Life has, in the main, been a pleasant experience, even if practically everything I am now doing is involved in just staying alive."

The words tumble effortlessly from the mouth of Stanley R. The one thing he cannot reveal is his true identity. He came to terms with confessing his sexual orientation many years ago; he is matter-of-factly "gay" and in no way crushed by that reality, if only because, from the earliest awareness, he had understanding parents who did not believe he was a bad seed of Cain somehow dropped into their genetic pool. He has full medical insurance -- something he fears might be yanked from him in the state where he currently resides if his true condition were known.

Stanley R. is in his early 50s -- yet he looks several years younger and, at first blush, is the picture of health. Sophisticated, urbane, intelligent, holder of a PhD in a certain scientific discipline (and former professor at a noted East Coast university), he works a full shift 5 days a week at an art-oriented store which returns him an income far below what he once had, particularly during the "grand, gay" times in San Francisco.

Stanley R.'s other job is more deeply humane -- he voluntarily spends hours on the phone, or in letter-writing, or in attending public and private meetings of people afflicted with AIDS or AIDS-related diseases, or other medical calamities which the Six O'Clock News assures us are incurable.

He shares and learns. Because Stanley R., as of 1990, had survived well over a decade (possibly a decade and a half) with "HIV disease" -- to some, AIDS, though he never had, as far as he can remember, the single combination of ingredients which would make the Centers for Disease Control's current case definition of "full-blown AIDS."

Of more than a thousand patients I have interviewed or been in contact with over the AIDS years, quite aside from those processed through our Bradford Research Institute program, Stanley R. is the survival champion.

Stanley R., who once had a lot of money, admits to being "flamingly" and promiscuously gay since his teen-age years. He knew the bushes of New York's Fire Island, the massive, opulent bathhouses of 1970s San Francisco. A self-described "anal erotic" who admits countless penetrative sexual intercourse episodes in trips around the world, he told me in April 1990 that "I could have picked this up anywhere. I certainly was the right profile for it. But I suppose it was San Francisco."

The Midwest native recalls that, before 1978, his only medical complaints were yearly bouts of pneumonia which he usually got in November of every year. His only really abused drugs were the antibiotics -- "legal" drugs -- which he wolfed down in great quantities year after year, primarily to stave off lung infections.

"I wasn't the picture of health, but I was basically a well person," he said.

"But around 1978 it began -- I mean, all these symptoms, coming and going. A stiff neck, swollen glands, on and off, ear aches--terrible, horrible ear aches -- splitting headaches, all kinds of paints in the joints, and night sweats -- unbelievable, drenching night sweats.

"I was also not eating right at the time, but I didn't know about such things then. I was still having a wonderful time. The doctors kept looking for all kinds of things -- syphilis, hepatitis, meningitis, advanced pneumonia -- but they couldn't find them. They treated me for all these things anyway."

More antibiotics, more drugs, more inexplicable, un-explainable, unrelenting symptoms.

At the time, a handful of San Francisco physicians, some of them gay themselves, were seeing, among their mostly gay clientele, increasing numbers of young men with just such a panoply of complaints. Across the continent, New York doctors were seeing "gay bowel syndrome," a puzzling array of parasites, diarrhea, gastroenterological complaints, sometimes accompanied by fever and weight loss.

"I knew, we knew, something was wrong, but just what, we couldn't be sure," Stanley R. remembers. "Since this all began around 1978, it is pretty sure, on retrospect, that I was infected well before, maybe the mid-1970s, who knows? We didn't have the blood test then, and no other test could show what was really going on.

"These things came and went, from 1978 to 1979 to 1980. Then by 1981 I was among the patients the doctors agreed fit the case definition for what was being called AIDS, although they had several other names for it first. It hit me hard. All these years, all these symptoms -- and suddenly there was the panic.

"Those of who lived through it remember it well. Suddenly we were looked at as if we had 'the mark of the Beast.' There was talk about 'rounding up all those awful people.' We were scared. I was scared. Everybody knew AIDS was instant death. People around us were dying. We could die at any time. The good, gay times were over."

Stanley R. was caught up in the early AIDS panic -- he avidly consumed every shred of news, every film clip, every snippet from an underground paper or the open press dealing with the strange new killer disease. His ever-active mind turned toward an open-throttle, all-out fight for survival.

"Those were the days we all smuggled in drugs -- from Mexico, Japan, Germany. You name it. A lot of airline stewards and stewardesses got rich off me, a lot of them ripped me off. But I would follow any lead, get any drug. Little by little, the money was running out. Buy this, get that. And it all cost."

A voracious reader and student with an academic background, Stanley's obsession became survival and new knowledge. Just as soon as "the virus" -- or rather, antibodies to it -- was said to have been found, and "the AIDS test" developed, he took it. As expected, he had antibodies to what was then called HTLV-III. With symptoms going back to 1978, it was obvious to him he had been in the AIDS loop, as of 1983, for at least 5 years, perhaps more.

But he was also aware he was neither dead nor dying, though each new symptom was terrifying and the media kept informing AIDS-infected male homosexuals they were doomed.

"The more I read, the more I studied, I came to doubt a lot of things I had been told by the doctors," he recalled 7 years later. "I began to understand that there certainly weren't any cures from drugs, and that what was going on must have something to do with total lifestyle, even food. I began to see that AIDS patients were basically immune-depressed, both physically and mentally. It began to make

sense when I read books that said that overhauling the immune system or detoxifying the body and/or thinking positively could all help overcome anything."

The other thing about "going natural" he said, was economic -- "I found I could afford this approach."

From the mid-1980s on, there is very little of a holistic/metabolic nature that Stanley R. has not done, or does not continue to do.

"I'm just constantly adding things as I go. There is no magic bullet, no cure, there is no one thing that is working."

From a hematological standpoint, Stanley R's "T-cell tests" (immune panels) have reflected absolute T4 cell ("helper") numbers -- the alleged immunological guidepost to HIV/ARC/AIDS -- ranging from between 450 to 30, or moderately low to very low. When we spoke with him in April 1990 they were 108, and he recalled a fairly recent herpes outbreak -- a sign of ongoing immune dysfunction. Yet he was healthy, active, and could not recall an actual "sick" day in years. At the time he was negative for P24 antigen--a suggestion HIV was inactive, if that meant anything.

Vitamins, minerals, enzymes, amino acids, antioxidants, oxidants, hydrogen peroxide, Dioxychlor, Chinese herbs, experimental foreign drugs and substances, workouts with a "frequency machine" (bioelectrical therapy attributed to the ideas of the late Royal Rife), "color therapy," exercise, and some things too bizarre to mention -- he has done, or does, all of these.

He learned early about the importance of diet -- the need to reduce or eliminate refined carbohydrates, stimulants, drugs in general, most meat and dairy products, and replace them with natural fruits and vegetables, sprouts and natural grains, natural juices and roots. He is a confirmed vegetarian.

His AIDS-era life has been one of learning. "I am constantly on the phone, asking questions, answering questions, following up leads, talking to science writers [that's how I found you], writing letters. This is a learning curve, and there's no end."

A veteran survivor from the AIDS years, Stanley R. does not believe a single virus causes AIDS any more than a single vitamin pill or meditation technique will cure it.

"One thing I have learned, and that is that probably the biggest survival factor is attitude. Thank God I have had love and joy in my life.

"If you look back, and life has not been a pleasant experience, you're going to be sicker. Whatever else has happened, life to me has been a pleasant experience, and it still is. I am a joyous person. I have incentives."

One of the incentives is his total involvement in sharing knowledge and selflessly helping others. He has not taken a dime in this personal crusade -- by being involved with others he has also greatly helped himself. He is not being mawkish or banal when he says, "There is something cosmic in all this. I'm a changed person."

He believes there are many others who have followed his same path, but have never gone public. For reasons either of protecting sexual orientation or the terror AIDS still has for many, they quietly revolutionize their lives.

Self-effacing to a fault, he says, almost disturbed, "Look, I haven't done anything unique. I've read and learned and followed the leads of others. I'm not exceptional."

I believe he is exceptional, and that there are other exceptional people out there.

This book is offered in the spirit of Stanley R. and many faceless heroes, who came very close to the visage of the Almighty and did not blink.

They represent the finer side of human nature -- and hope for us all.

Michael L. Culbert
San Diego, California
Spring 1990

Chapter One

WHAT GOES ON HERE?

In 1990, the World Health Organization (WHO) estimated that between 5 and 10 million people in the world had been infected by the virus said to cause this century's most feared new killer -- Acquired Immune Deficiency (or Acquired Immunodeficiency) Syndrome (AIDS). WHO's spokesmen added that within five years the numbers might go up tenfold -- to 50 to 100 million infected.

ITEM: WHO had made virtually the same assessment in 1988 and 1987. By 1990 WHO estimated that there were anywhere from 350,000 to 480,000 cases of "full-blown" AIDS. As WHO's Jonathan M. Mann said: "The pandemic is still in its early stages and its ultimate dimensions are difficult to gauge, but by now it is apparent that AIDS is an unprecedented threat to global health."[1] Biophysicist John Platt, PhD., writing in *The Futurist* in 1987, estimated[2] that within 10 years the worldwide death toll from AIDS could exceed that of the Black Death in the Middle Ages.

ITEM: By early 1990, there were just over 204,000 actual AIDS cases officially reported (in distinction to estimated) from 152 countries. The parameters defining just what AIDS is had so changed (12 "indicator diseases" in the absence of laboratory evidence [i.e., blood work] of AIDS; 12 "indicator diseases" definitively diagnosed and with laboratory evidence of infection; 7 "indicator diseases" that were "diagnosed presumptively" and with laboratory evidence of infection) that a vast array of symptoms, conditions and diseases and combinations thereof may now be classed as "AIDS." (See Appendix I.)

Africa is thought to be the continent of highest infection with "the AIDS virus," with some unofficial estimates suggesting that vast sectors of the African population will be wiped out. It is broadly held that AIDS originated in that continent.

ITEM: Despite estimates by WHO in 1989 of

1

"more than 100,000" actual AIDS cases in Africa, actual reporting of figures country by country is far behind that estimate. Somewhere between 50 and 60 percent of actual AIDS cases are reported from the United States alone, rather than Africa. Some observers in AIDS-afflicted African countries (which together account for about 10 percent of the Dark Continent's population) have failed to find evidence of wholesale slaughter by the new killer. Nor is there any firm evidence AIDS originated there.

ITEM: If by 1990 there were something over 204,000 actual cases of AIDS from an estimated 5 to 10 million people infected with the alleged "AIDS virus" even under new definitions of what constitutes AIDS, the indication was that only between 1 and 6 percent of all persons thought to be harboring "the AIDS virus" actually had AIDS.

In the United States, which at this time has the majority of actual AIDS cases in the world (120,000 as of 1990), the condition primarily affects male homosexuals and intravenous drug users (although there are now increases in the general heterosexual population primarily due to IV drug abuse, contaminated blood transfusions and sexual acts with "high risk" people and mother-to-infant transmission.)

ITEM: In Africa, the presumed locus of the largest area of mass infection by "the AIDS virus," neither homosexuality nor drug addiction has anything to do with AIDS. It is a disease of sexually active heterosexuals, divides almost exactly 1:1 between men and women and overlaps with U.S. AIDS primarily in the statistical correlate of promiscuity.

ITEM: In some countries, particularly southern Europe, AIDS statistically correlates more with intravenous drug abuse than sexuality -- either hetero- or homo-.

ITEM: Statistical evidence over the years has found that U.S. AIDS relates not to the population subgroup identifying itself as homosexual but to a specific sex act (passive anal intercourse) which, while probably more common among male homosexuals than heterosexuals, is by no means restricted to the former. U.S. AIDS also correlates as strongly with drug abuse *in general* as it does with sexual practices.

In the United States, revised official figures in 1990 were that between 600,00 and 1.3 people were probably infected by "the AIDS virus."

ITEM: These startling figures indicated a dip of 10 to 15% in case increases annually from earlier predictions and estimates of "AIDS virus" infection and actual AIDS cases.[17] The U.S.' 1989 estimate of between 1 and 1.5 million infectees had also been phased back from earlier predictions, as reality began to seep into the picture of global catastrophe painted earlier.

ITEM: Two non-governmental studies in 1988 claimed the U.S. figures for presumed "AIDS virus" infection might be underestimated by as much as 50 percent.[3,4] A governmental survey by the General Accounting Office (GAO) in 1989 indicated that the official figures might be understated by a third.[14] Yet a private (Hoover Institute) "back calculation" in 1989 suggested the official figures were overstated by half.[16]

ITEM: Even if the official figures are correct, then approximately 5 or 6 percent of persons infected with "the AIDS virus" in the U.S.A. actually have "full-blown" AIDS, as currently defined by the Centers for Disease Control (CDC). Probably many thousands more have preliminary or parallel conditions, but at this time no estimates of alleged infection or actual cases come anywhere near the rate of cases of, and death from, cancer (1.2 million new cases diagnosed per year in the U.S.A., with 550,000 deaths annually), or anywhere near the death rates of the influenza epidemic in the U.S.A. in 1918 or the Black Death and syphilis in Europe in the Middle Ages and the Renaissance.

The AIDS case rate seemed to be doubling yearly in the U.S.A. The government earlier estimated 365,000 cases "will have been diagnosed" by 1992 but added the figure could be anywhere between 205,000 and 440,000 by then. The 1990 revision suggested these figures are far too high.

ITEM: These widely varying projections are widely varying because of the increasing difficulty of

3

predicting (a) how many people are actually infected with "the AIDS virus"; (b) what it really means to be infected with "the AIDS virus"; and (c) what the incubation period of "the AIDS virus" really is.

The official pronouncements concerning AIDS are that it is "inevitably" and "uniformly" fatal. At the present time there is no known cure for AIDS or any vaccine to prevent it. Arguments among the medical orthodoxy are primarily not over whether AIDS will kill the patient, but when and under what circumstances.

ITEM: There are known documented cases of Americans alive, now, for 10,9,8 and 7 years with "full-blown" AIDS. There is, from statistics and records-keeping, evidence that some Americans may have had either AIDS or "HIV infection" as early as 1974 and 1977 and still be alive. The fatality rate of full-blown AIDS has actually tended to stabilize at around 60 percent, suggesting that large numbers of AIDS patients are neither dead nor dying.

The only real defense against AIDS is said to be education, sexual selectiveness (if not outright celibacy), and mass testing of the population with AIDS antibody tests. Indeed, the only screen for safeguarding blood supplies is such a test, we are told.

ITEM: The various antibody tests for "the AIDS virus" may turn in both "false positives" and "false negatives" due either to the nature of the tests or the nature of "the AIDS virus." A negative test cannot prove an individual is not harboring "the AIDS virus"; a positive test cannot prove that he *is*. Nor can a positive test prove if or when an individual will become ill with AIDS. Since a positive test will in fact induce stress and possible paranoia in the testee without providing specific information, the thundering question is: What good is the AIDS test? The muted answer would seem to be: not much.

Even so, political extremists and the general uninformed have called for quarantining people based not only on antibody tests but on the *presumption* they might be "positive." And one country -- Cuba -- has already begun domestic lifetime detention based solely on blood tests for "the AIDS virus." Far more precise "virus culture" and "viral antigen" tests

4

for HIV now exist but have not yet been made generally available.

New information on the lengthy period of time between infection and antibody appearance (which may be up to 3 years) has rendered HIV antibody tests even more unlikely to be reliable defenders of the blood supply or prognosticators of AIDS in recently infected "high-risk" patients.

Medical orthodoxy notes that there are specific perturbations in "immune panels" (among T4 and T8 cells and their ratios, primarily) which suggest, but do not confirm, AIDS or any of its preliminary conditions. Such perturbations and positivity on "AIDS virus" antibody tests indicate laboratory evidence of AIDS, we are told.

ITEM: There are cases of clinical AIDS in which there are no such immune disturbances; there are cases of immune disturbances with no evidence of AIDS; there are immune disturbances without positivity for "the AIDS virus"; there are cases of "AIDS virus" positivity without immune disturbance.

Best evidence currently suggests the "spontaneous" appearance of AIDS in three entirely different geographical areas at or around 1977/78.

ITEM: Aside from a confirmed case of AIDS in the U.S.A. in 1968 (from both retrospective analyses of stored blood and clinical signs/symptoms reported at the time), there are reports of retrospective "AIDS virus" infections occurring in Africa as early as 1959 and 1972 and in South America as early as 1968. It may be argued that positivity for "the AIDS virus" in some of these cases may have been mistaken for some other condition or infection, or that the tests were not done properly -- and virus culturing, particularly from stored blood, is at best a tricky business -- but if this trend of thought is adhered to consistently it would bring into question the relevance of AIDS sampling from stored blood in general.

ITEM: The sudden appearance of an entirely new killer disease in three separate geographical areas at the same time is without precedent in history. (So is its capability, all by itself, of utterly demolishing a human immune system.)

By this time, the reader has every right to ask:

5

What goes on here?

What, indeed ...

Nine years from the naming of the new syndrome and six years from the alleged co-discovery of its alleged or putative single causative agent, what is really known about AIDS and its presumed cause are:

1. There is a vicious new syndrome in the world whose central feature is the obliteration of the human immune system and the invasion of the human central nervous system.

2. The syndrome itself is not a disease and does not kill. But its actions on the immune system in particular cause the body to be left open to a debilitating series of "opportunistic infections" and forms of cancer which *do* kill.

3. None of the "opportunistic infections" or forms of cancer is new. Many are rare, but all are known pathological entities.

4. Routes of transmission of the cause or causes of the syndrome, at this time, appear to be limited to blood and semen.

5. It is extremely doubtful that "full-blown" AIDS will develop in an infected person unless he or she is already immuno-compromised -- already sick -- in some way or ways.

6. "The AIDS virus" -- or, more correctly, viruses -- while statistically highly associated with AIDS, have not been convincingly demonstrated to be the single agents which bring about the extreme debilitation and ultimate death observable in AIDS patients. As controversy over "the AIDS viruses" swirled in 1990, it nonetheless became evident that the primary one, HIV-1, may at least be a "marker" for the AIDS infection curve, the inability of antibodies and even viral antigens to it to be found in many cases attributable both to the peculiar mechanics of HIV and the lack of precision of viral screening tests.

7. HIV-1, while it has many elements in common with other retroviruses, is a unique structure apparently without precedent in the world.

8. The vast amount of people infected with "the AIDS virus", or who at least have antibodies to the virus, are not "sick."

9. The actual outcome of either infection with "the AIDS virus" or the presence of antibodies to "the AIDS

virus" is not known.

10. The period of incubation of "the AIDS virus" is unknown. The time between presumed exposure and onset of symptoms (if any) has been estimated at from six days to a lifetime. Each year that passes, American medical orthodoxy adds 12 more months to the presumed period of incubation, to estimates (now) of 10 to 14 years.

11. Medical orthodoxy has no cure for AIDS or any guaranteed way to inhibit or inoculate against "the AIDS virus." This has led to the assumption of the inevitability of a 100 percent death rate.

12. Many people are surviving either with "full-blown" AIDS or pre-AIDS conditions at levels far beyond the estimates set by medical orthodoxy. Innumerable "AIDS-infected" people have been alive without developing any AIDS-related conditions for years.

13. Just as it cannot be absolutely demonstrated that "the AIDS virus" alone causes AIDS, it cannot be absolutely demonstrated that AIDS inevitably results in death.

14. As this book will show, the infection curve whose final stop is full-blown AIDS is almost certainly manageable and the progression to full-blown AIDS is almost certainly preventable. But it is neither manageable nor preventable through the reliance on medicine as usual, as championed by the U.S.A. and, by implication, most of the Western World.

In the meantime, there is a 15th basic truth that can be stated about AIDS:

It is expensive, and, as such, it is already swiftly forming a global new industry which in a relatively short period of time may eclipse the proliferation of industries and profit-taking which have grown up around cancer.

U.S. health officials in early 1988 estimated[5] that AIDS care was expected to account for from $6 billion to $16 billion of direct medical spending within three years, figures which do not include treatment of preliminary or parallel conditions associated with AIDS. New York City expenditures on AIDS in 1988 were estimated at $475 million for that single city for a single year, with a tag of $1 billion expected in 1991.[6]

By the turn of the century, American life insurance companies estimate, AIDS-related deaths could cost the industry $50 billion.[7] The AIDS-related cost to the nation in terms of lost personal income due to illness and premature death will be $66.4 billion by 1991, economists claim.[8] A University of California-San Francisco Institute for Health Policy Studies survey in 1989 estimated that annual treatment for "AIDS virus"-infected people in the U.S.A. may reach a staggering $5 billion yearly.[15] (The 1990 revision of AIDS and "AIDS virus" infections may reduce these numbers.)

A 1988 analysis of several previous studies of AIDS suggested that the lifetime cost of medical care per patient (in the U.S.A.) would not exceed $80,000 -- an amount similar to that for other major diseases -- and that, if current estimates of projected AIDS incidence hold up, the cumulative lifetime costs of 270,000 patients diagnosed between 1981 and the end of 1991 would not exceed $22 billion. This would be, by American standards, "small" compared with the galloping cost of "health care" (which by 1990 was projected at $600 billion.)

This more sanguine assessment might make the costs seem less staggering in an affluent nation, but for AIDS tracing, diagnosis, treatment and control in central Africa and other impoverished parts of the world, there simply is no iota of good news on the economic front.

At this time, U.S. medical officialdom, assailed from all sides for lassitude in bringing new AIDS drugs to the market, has approved only two new drugs for full-scale use -- the toxic and dangerous azidothymidine (AZT), which can cost $700 per month per patient, and alpha-interferon, almost as expensive, approved for Kaposi's sarcoma. Neither drug is a cure, though AZT is said to slow down progression of disease the earlier it is given, despite its own immune-depleting effects. In 1989 the U.S. approved the aerosol version of pentamidine, an old drug, for Pneumocystis pneumonia, and Ganciclovir for the AIDS visual complication CMV retinitis.

The *Los Angeles Times*, surveying Africa's response to AIDS, quoted a Malawian health official: "It doesn't matter whether the treatment costs $1 million per patient, or $1,000, or even $10. None of these countries can afford an AZT program."[10] In some of Africa's "AIDS zone" countries there is hardly enough cash for new needles let alone expensive blood tests of dubious value. In countries where the median income is $300 per year the cost of a few

8

"diagnostic assays" means the wipeout of annual salaries.

By any dimension, then, AIDS has the potential of becoming another huge medical industry. At a time when U.S. hospitals were beginning to empty (due to a combination of high costs, government oversight, cutbacks in federal programs, reassessment of medical techniques, and even, occasionally, better medicine) AIDS has come along to fill them up again.

With virtually everything from persistent athlete's foot and unexplained night sweats to lengthy flu symptoms suggesting some point of the AIDS infection curve, and a battery of new tests to locate, monitor and capture antibodies to, pieces of, and even the whole "AIDS virus" as laboratory proof of the new killer, and with an ever-growing raft of symptoms and conditions now suggesting AIDS even when presence of "the AIDS virus" cannot be confirmed, there was little likelihood of an early end to a rapidly mushrooming new industry.

In the U.S.A., site of the greatest number of actual, officially reported AIDS cases as this decade began, it was intriguing, exasperating, mystifying and frustrating that only two toxic synthetic "new" drugs had been approved for use against AIDS -- though another drug was approved for limited "compassionate" use and other "old drugs" were allowed for treatments of some forms of full-blown AIDS. The U.S.' legendary slowness in new-drug development was continuing even as useful approaches and modalities were being used in other countries.

Any number of promising new substances were stymied by the giant drug company-favoring and progress-choking red tape of the Food, Drug and Cosmetic Act, a cobbled together political monster responsible for more deaths and suffering in the U.S.A. than any combination of killer diseases. Upwards of 200 drugs, substances and ideas for AIDS were being tested or surveyed or analyzed in the U.S.A., yet clearance, approval or mass use in most instances still seemed years away.

The Food and Drug Administration (FDA), an administrative satrapy and policing office so swift to crush opponents of the drug industry in the medical marketplace and so slow to approve anything developed from outside the confines of a veritable network of major international drug houses, had loosened its regulations three times in the name of AIDS, but these moves were too little too late to stave off a rapidly growing political reaction bordering on revolution. The austere FDA was actually "shut down" by thousands of enraged AIDS activists in October 1988 protesting the obscene lentitude of FDA approval of new drugs.

Part of the Big Business of AIDS surfaced in October 1988 as the U.S. Congress' Committee on Government Operations reported[12] on "AIDS Drugs: Where Are They?"

Among many other matters the document focused on the use and development of AZT and pentamidine -- the prior as an antiviral against HIV, the latter as a treatment for *Pneumocystis carinii* pneumonia (PCP).

The report noted that AZT was tested unsuccessfully in the 1960s as a cancer treatment, but that in 1984 the National Cancer Institute (NCI) discovered antiviral activity in the drug. In 1987 AZT was approved and the manufacturer, Burroughs Wellcome, was granted a use patent for exclusive rights to sell AZT for AIDS treatment for 17 years -- and it was, at the time, the most expensive drug ever marketed.

The report adds that NCI, along with the National Institute of Allergy and Infectious Diseases (NIAID), "not only participated heavily in the development of the drug, but also supplied Burroughs Wellcome with large amounts of thymidine, a scarce and expensive ingredient. However, because the Federal Government has granted the company an exclusive patent on AZT, the Government will not share in profits from its sale, nor is it in a position, under current law, to affect the cost of the drug to the public.

"Burroughs Wellcome has never agreed to make public its portion of the cost of development and producing AZT, nor adequately justified the extremely high price of the drug. Company representatives testified at a Congressional hearing in March 1987 that research and development costs had been $80 million. The cost of AZT to Federal and State governments under the Medicaid Program was $20 million in by 1987 and is estimated to grow to $155 million in by 1990.

"Burroughs Wellcome lowered the price of AZT 20 percent in December 1987. This was possible, according to company spokespersons, because of the decreased production costs. This would certainly suggest that the profit margin on the drug is quite comfortable. In fact, by April 1988, the value of the parent company's shares had quadrupled from the date the company went public in February 1986..."

While AZT was being approved, potentially much less expensive antivirals, such as ribavirin, were getting the runaround -- and potentially useful foreign imports, ranging from dextran sulfate (Japan) and ozone infusion techniques (West Germany) to the Israeli fatty acid combination AL-721, Foscarnet (Sweden) and Imuthiol (France) -- either were not allowed for use officially or were simply in various stages of "investigation."

Pentamidine, one of the two drugs approved for the treatment of PCP, and classed as an "orphan drug" (developed before the updated Food, Drug and Cosmetic Act regulations), was brought back to production by LyphoMed, a small generic drug company, at the request of the Centers for Disease Control (CDC), the congressional report stated.

The report added:

"When it was first marketed under the Orphan Drug Act in October 1984, pentamidine retailed at $24.95 per vial. By August 1987, the cost per vial had reached $95.49. ... LyphoMed seized an opportunity to develop a marketing and sales staff for the company and to resolve its problems at the expense of this one drug. At a cost of at least $100,000 per year to hire, train, and maintain just one physician sales specialist, LyphoMed hired 27. The company plans to expand this sales staff to 40 by the end of 1988."

Rep. Ted Weiss, chairman, Human Resources and Intergovernmental Relations Subcommittee, summarized LyphoMed's problems: "... you saw a good thing which could be used to build your company to a size that you'd never anticipated. And how do you pay for it? You pay for it by soaking the clientele. I think it is really unfortunate that you decided to take this ... approach ... to meet CDC's challenge."

To LyphoMed's credit it should be noted that the company has since made some pentamidine available on a charity basis.

FDA intransigence, medical monopoly obsession with single-cause diseases and the rapid spread of an alleged new "human retrovirus" have been helping bring about actual social dislodgment. Terrified AIDS victims, in the main told to wait-and-see if they "tested positive", faced fear, anguish, discrimination, ostracism, job and status loss.

"Guerrilla clinics" and "shoppers' clubs" for unapproved drugs sprang up in the hardest-hit AIDS communities (particularly the gay sanctuaries of New York, San Francisco and Los Angeles) and an underground industry of unapproved treatments, novel theories as to "AIDS virus" origins and whole new lifestyle approaches began to appear.

By 1990, even while the beleaguered population of male homosexuals remained the statistically highest "reservoir of infection," homosexual communities were busily changing their habits, new infections among gays were levelling off and in some cases declining, but AIDS rates were rising among women, AIDS-infected infants and children and intravenous drug users.

The presumptive high rate of infection in hemophiliacs made it seem that possibly one whole innocent segment of the population might actually come near elimination -- that is, if "the AIDS virus" really caused AIDS, and that was a bigger question in 1990 than ever before. Not only most "AIDS virus"-infected hemophiliacs but most HIV infected people in general were still alive and reasonably well.

The medical orthodoxy's single-minded commitment to "the AIDS virus" theory, compounded by the total impuissance of the medical establishment to do anything *about* "the AIDS virus", were helping fuel social paranoia and mass prejudices on a scale rarely seen. The assumption that "they brought it on themselves" was directed toward male homosexuals and IV drug users as if somehow these groups had actually caused the disease.

A U.S. Spanish-language newspaper in 1987 asked editorially: "Should society help these people who are marked for death to escape victorious from their disease? ... Should a taxpayer pay for the cure of someone who has been the victim of the use, abuse and degeneration of their sexual organs?"[11]

Talk of quarantining had spread from idle chit-chat to actual referendums in several places, particularly California, under the thought that if everyone could be forced into taking "the AIDS test" then the "positives" could be separated out from the rest of the population (the 21st century's scarlet letter) in an ever-growing administrative/policing orgy of quarantining.

So far such efforts have largely been unsuccessful, but with a general frenzy whipped up by compliant media, which almost unquestioningly followed the lead of U.S. medical orthodoxy, the inherent fears of the greater population concerning a mysterious new killer disease converged with subsurface prejudices and pent-up hostility against whole classes of people. The union of fear and loathing gave vent to even more talk of quarantine and persecution.

The outbreak of AIDS on a broad scale neatly jibes with several events in recent scientific and medical history:

The World Health Organization's smallpox eradication vaccine campaign in central Africa, the launching of a hepatitis B vaccine program for male homosexuals first in New York and later elsewhere, and even continued world polio eradication efforts with a possibly contaminated vaccine. The locales and timeframes all match, in general, as does, for example, the presence of AIDS in considerable numbers in Brazil, by the beginning of this decade the number four country in cumulative AIDS cases.

The outbreak also dovetails with government-supported efforts to develop man-made immunosuppressive viruses, perhaps as part of the U.S. "Conquest of Cancer" program's obsessive commitment to seeking the viral causation (and possibly management) of cancer. It also occurred within a decade of rapidly developing knowledge about the genetic code of life itself and the advent of "designer drugs."

(It is an interesting commentary that the U.S. government-level cancer research agency which so thoroughly failed to come up with the answer to the cause and cure of cancer was the same team, in general, to which the conquest of AIDS was handed -- and that the scientist who helped develop AZT for AIDS use became the head of that agency, the National Cancer Institute.)

Some of these overlaps and realities have given rise to the most insidious possibility of all -- "the AIDS virus," whether or not it acts alone, is itself a manufactured structure, its sudden presence in the bloodstream of the human family a gruesome laboratory error or a contrived plot of mind-bending proportions.

13

(And we will ponder the distinct possibility that much of what many believe to be AIDS might turn out to be "the great masquerader" -- syphilis -- in a startling new guise. If this line of reasoning has any merit at all, it would be good news, for it would mean that much of AIDS is "curable" through traditional methods -- and that much energy, time, funds and grief have been misspent on looking for the wrong cause.)

Through it all the incessant drumbeat of death-expectation has resounded with a funereal cadence of gathering momentum: *AIDS is death.*

One of the objectives of this book, quite aside from calling into question the central hypotheses of the AIDS industry, is to stress that there is hope and optimism at this particularly dark hour, and that neither the invincibility of "the AIDS virus" nor the certainty of death from AIDS is a truth chiseled in stone. Both suffer greatly at the hands of logic and truth.

First, there is the growing possibility that HIV -- the so-called "AIDS virus" -- doesn't cause the syndrome at all, and may be only a "co-factor" to something else.

We will demonstrate that methods exist now for the successful control and management of AIDS, that victims are living longer and in some cases actually overcoming the "inevitably fatal" killer, but through routes and methods ignored or damned by the U.S. medical establishment.

In what amounts to the greatest assembly of research, theory, funds and feverish activity ever mounted on a global scale in such short order to combat what is becoming a world pandemic, there are opportunities and challenges:

There is the challenge of collective investigative and therapeutic efforts to head off a population-threatening condition.

There is the opportunity to find new therapeutic models for the medicine of the future -- and to learn more about the human immune system and how it is modulated and influenced than ever before.

As of Fall 1988 Cuba was the only nation in the world to have mandated universal "AIDS virus" testing and enforced isolation of all presumptive carriers of the putative virus -- an ironic twist whereby Cuba, as an ideological arch-enemy of the U.S.A., would slavishly follow the single-agent etiology theory of AIDS so thoroughly promoted by American experts.

Ronald Bayer, associate professor at Columbia University's School of Public Health, was a member of the first U.S. delegation to visit what Cuba calls its "sanitarium" -- a place where carriers of the so-called "AIDS virus" (at the time 171 men and 69 women) are quarantined from society and will spend the rest of their lives.

(In 1990, Cuba claimed that after 75% of its "sexually active" population had been tested, there were 434 HIV carriers and 63 AIDS cases, with 27 deaths.)[18]

Bayer told the *Los Angeles Times*[3] of the complex of modestly furnished apartments: "It was neither barracks-like nor dungeon-like, although I have to assume we were shown the best... But even if it all looked as good as what we saw, it does not resolve the moral justification of incarceration based on supposed future behavior."

The medical ethicist, who spoke to various detainees, noted that so far few of the camp's residents had developed clinical symptoms of AIDS.

That reportorial phrase should reverberate: Cubans had been rounded up and quarantined for life not on the basis of any actual disease but on the presumption they would get one because somehow they were "positive" on a test for "the AIDS virus." This line of logic originated not in Cuba but in the United States.

Is this the fate that awaits the world until the multiple AIDS mysteries are solved?

REFERENCES

(1)   Mann, Jonathan M., et al., "The international epidemiology of AIDS." Scientific American, October 1988.

(2)   "AIDS toll could exceed Black Death, biophysicist predicts." American Medical News. Nov. 20, 1987.

(3)   Lawrence, Mark, "AIDS underestimated by 50%, study says." Los Angeles Times, August 20, 1988.

(4)   "AIDS danger to heterosexuals cited." (United Press International) San Diego Union, March 6, 1988.

(5)   Pinkney, Deborah S., "Dramatic hike forecast for future AIDS care costs." American Medical News, March 11, 1988.

(6)   "NYC AIDS care to top $1 billion." American Medical News, June 5, 1987.

(7)   "Insurance firms fear heavy AIDS impact." (Associated Press) San Diego Union, August 5, 1987.

(8)   "Economists see AIDS costs at $66.4 billion by 1991." American Medical News, March 20, 1987.

(9)   Bloom, David E., and Geoffrey Carliner, "The economic impact of AIDS in the United States." Science, Feb. 5, 1988.

10)   Hiltzik, Michael A., "Africa facing reality of AIDS war amid social changes in urban life." Los Angeles Times, Nov. 14, 1988.

(11)   La Prensa (Washington D.C.) quoted in "The extension of AIDS." Lancet, Oct. 1, 1988.

(12)   "AIDS drugs: where are they?" 73rd report by the Committee on Government Operations, U.S. Govt. Printing Office, Oct. 19, 1988.

(13)   Zonana, Victor F., "Cuba's AIDS quarantine called 'frightening.'" Los Angeles Times, Nov. 4, 1988.

(14)   General Accounting Office, June 1989.

(15)   New York Times News Service, Sept. 15, 1989.

(16)   "A recount of AIDS carriers." Time, Oct. 9, 1989.

(17)   Centers for Disease Control, January 1990.

(18)   Reuter News Service, April 28, 1990.

Chapter Two

TRACKING THE KILLER

From the earliest reports of AIDS, the understanding of the new syndrome and the attempt to trace its natural history developed into biochemical mystery thrillers which paralleled the intense sociopolitical and cultural dimensions of the killer disease.

For Western orthodox medicine, AIDS has represented, for the first time, a condition which is seemingly incurable, at least by the means so far tried. It has posed the gravest historic challenge to the standard medical model (allopathy) dominant in the Western world, and has riveted attention on multifactorial concepts of disease causation and management.

Yet, despite the potential of a disaster of enormous proportions befalling the whole of humanity, nine years after the definition of the syndrome, the killer condition was still essentially limited to its original populations, and they contrasted dizzyingly: male homosexuals and intravenous drug users in the West and the general heterosexual population of parts of Africa remained clearly at risk, the general heterosexual population of most of the rest of the world did not.

No one was taking great comfort in this strange disparity, for AIDS was creeping -- though not rushing -- relentlessly into "non-high risk" groups.

And, just because the means of transmission of whatever agents truly were at the root of the condition (if indeed the agents are more important than the condition of the host, a question very much in doubt) seemed limited to blood and semen, no one could state with total confidence that some other means of transmission does not occur, or could not occur.

The fear of new modes of transmission evolved from the understanding by virology of the nature of transmission of both human and animal viruses -- they need not be restricted to a single common mode of transference.

History had shown the capacity for viruses to mutate over time, and the alleged "etiological agent" of AIDS is, if nothing else, highly regarded in its uncanny ability to mutate, leading some people to suggest that it was never appropriate to speak of a single human "AIDS virus" since the offending structure could mutate so swiftly within a single individual that new mutations might always be occurring.

Yet, during the first nine years of AIDS, the rampant spread of the syndrome through the general population -- a new Plague -- simply had not occurred.

As we shall see it is not at all a demonstrated fact that a single new agent is the "cause" of the spectrum of AIDS (the HIV/LAS/ARC/AIDS infection curve), that there are profound questions as to whether "the AIDS virus" actually causes AIDS, and as to how many people for how long a time have been carrying "the AIDS virus" and what it may mean to be carrying "the AIDS virus." In 1990 these were unanswered questions despite the most rapidly assembled and costly expenditure in research funds and technology ever mounted on an international scale in the name of public health.

The syndrome was not named until 1981, and first in the U.S.A., though retrospective analysis and evaluations showed that actual AIDS cases were occurring in the United States and Europe at least as early as 1977. One U.S. case has been positively identified in 1968.[42] Two others have been identified as infected since 1974.[43] Huminer *et al.* identified 19 probable AIDS cases in the U.S. occurring before the onset of the AIDS epidemic -- if retrospective documentation is reliable and if HIV preservation in stored blood means anything.[73,74]

Early clues something medically novel was occurring came from the sudden appearance in (usually) young males, most of them homosexuals and/or drug users, of usually rare and fatal diseases, particularly a virulent, deadly pneumonia called *Pneumocystis carinii* (though the organism itself is common), and Kaposi's sarcoma, normally thought of as a relatively benign skin cancer in central Africa and other tropical areas, but taking on an aggressive, deadly guise in the West.

Many other "opportunistic infections" following the strange and apparent sudden destruction of AIDS victims' immune systems at comparatively young ages were appearing. These included *Candida albicans* infections and a whole host of influenza-like and mononucleosis-type conditions and the rapid spread of rare viral, bacteriological, fungal and parasitical diseases. Encephalitis, meningitis, tuberculosis and some rare forms of cancer came to be noted as part of the syndrome.

A high correlation between early AIDS cases and later pre-AIDS conditions was noted with unexplained persistent and intermittent swollen glands [lymphadenopathy, later considered on its own as lymphadenopathy syndrome (LAS)].

In Europe, travel between that continent and Africa, and arrivals in Europe of more affluent Africans, seemed to indicate an early AIDS epidemiological factor, as did the presence of a higher-than-normal AIDS outbreak among Haitian refugees in the U.S.A. and also as did travel patterns among AIDS patients between the U.S.A. and the Caribbean.

Even before the delineation of "the AIDS virus" researchers presumed either some new agent must be involved in the seemingly sudden outbreak of a new disease or that something was re-activating latent diseases. The first cases of the HIV/AIDS infection curve were "full-blown", terminal cases, almost all of whom were dead within a few months to two years of diagnosis. As AIDS numbers grew, mortality rates climbed from 40 to 60 percent, and then seemed to stay at about that level -- that is, 60 percent of full-blown AIDS cases are dying over an ever-expanding period of time.

Physicians found they could manage some of the end-state disease conditions, but only temporarily. For a time, death apparently ensued from as early as four months after diagnosis to about two years, and was occurring an average of 224 days after hospitalization.

By 1990, the long-term survival prospects were brighter for full-blown AIDs cases, due both to the experimental uses of certain drugs and to a tremendous increase in knowledge about the syndrome and its "opportunistic" infections, yet death was still considered inevitable -- except for an increasing amount of victims surviving longer periods of time on "unorthodox" therapies.

Phrases such as "turnaround" and "breakthrough" accompanied the announcement[77] Aug. 17, 1989, by the National Institute of Allergy and Infectious Diseases (NIAID) that in a study of 1,900 patients it was found that

AZT could slow down the development of AIDS in asymptomatic patients. What this might mean vis-a-vis AZT-resistant "AIDS virus" strains and the fact that AZT is not a cure remained to be seen. Medical orthodoxy then argued for the use of AZT in pre-AIDS conditions and found it "effective" in lower doses [78,79]

(A New York physician whom we highly respect, noting the possible drug-profit bonanza in elevating the use of AZT from AIDS patients to the possibly millions of HIV-infected asymptomatics, wondered, "Where will this stop? AZT for the whole at-risk population before infection? Pre-natal administration of AZT?" No one knew.

(And the manner in which AZT was literally rushed to the fore on the basis of inconclusive and possibly sloppily performed tests[80,81] has been questioned in detail by probing journalists.)

Indeed, going into the last decade of this century, the unfolding scenario of AIDS is that of long, lingering, debilitating chronic disorder rather than a quick trip to the grave. It is, in a sense, a drug-industry delight: an incurable, unstoppable disease that can seemingly only be "managed" through a lengthening list of toxic synthetic drugs and antibiotics, yet never "cured."

By 1983 a putative "AIDS virus", usually referred to as "closely related to" or "associated with" AIDS (but not, strictly speaking, causing AIDS) or rather three (or more) forms of the alleged etiological agent had been isolated, named and statistically linked to "full-blown" AIDS and to a predecessor or parallel condition.

As propaganda advanced and the media followed the lead of medical orthodoxy, the presumptive agent came to be called"the AIDS virus" and a sometimes nasty dispute over the name of the agent was ultimately resolved, by 1986, as HIV -- Human Immunodeficiency Virus. Since then, at least one similar but different virus, HIV-2 (HTLV-IV), has been found, and there are suggestions of even other viruses, perhaps some mutated from HIV. HIV-2 is found in West Africans who do not appear to be ill, at least from that virus. HIV-2 has now made its appearance in the Western Hemisphere, but seems relatively less lethal than HIV-1, if in fact HIV-1 is acting alone.[53,54]

Adding intriguing new elements, both the American researcher who is credited with co-discovering "the AIDS virus" and an Armed Forces Institute of Pathology scientist have isolated a new virus and another microbe from AIDS patients.

The former, HBLV (or human B-cell leukemia virus) has been changed in nomenclature to HHV-6 (human herpesvirus 6),[44] and is also associated with the "Lake Tahoe Syndrome" infection.

The second, first cautiously identified as a "virus-like infectious agent" (VLIA), was practically overlooked in the flood of papers and presentations at the Fourth International AIDS Conference in Stockholm in 1988.[45,46] But research on the agent continued in 1989, with Shyh-Ching Lo, MD, noting[55,56,57] that he had successfully cloned VLIA from 7 of 10 AIDS patients and that VLIA is pathogenic (disease-producing) in monkeys.

By 1990, though, Dr. Lo's "VLIA" was termed a "mycoplasma" -- or structure between a virus and bacteria in size. Unlike HIV-1, which may be inoculated in animals without making them ill, Dr. Lo's *mycoplasma incognitus* killed all four monkeys into which it was injected within 7 to 9 months.[82,83,84,85,86,87]

Whether these new agents are co-factors, actual AIDS causes or irrelevant fellow travellers remains to be elucidated. It was the *New York Native* publication which more than any other first ferreted out knowledge of these new structures within the HIV/AIDS controversy.[47,48]

By 1984-85, a predecessor or parallel condition was beginning to be referred to on its own as "AIDS-related complex" (ARC), and was said to affect at least six or seven times more patients in the U.S.A. than AIDS itself while fatal in about 10 percent of cases.[1,2]

The geographical distribution of full-blown AIDS vis-a-vis infections by the putative agent or agents presented amazing contrasts: in Africa, where millions of people are thought to be harboring the presumed etiological agent,[3] substantial research indicated that probably the majority of virus carriers were relatively healthy and, of equal importance, did not fit into the "high risk" categories established by the U.S. government's Centers for Disease Control (CDC), in that they were essentially not male homosexuals, intravenous drug users, hemophiliacs or other recipients of transfused blood or blood products.

Yet in the U.S.A., where full-blown AIDS is numerically more concentrated (more than 55% of all cases out of 144 countries reporting in 1990) male homosexuals and/or IV drug users comprise the majority of AIDS patients, even though increasing cases of heterosexual AIDS and pediatric AIDS are being added to the pool of hemophiliac and blood products-recipient patients.

This statistical reality has given rise to some of the most pervasive sociological and political paranoia ever encountered in the U.S.A., with talk of actually quarantining suspected "AIDS carriers" growing in intensity and becoming a fact in Cuba.

Brazil, among "third world" countries, and estimated to be the fourth "AIDS nation" in terms of total cases, presented a pattern similar to that of the U.S.A. -- male homosexuals and drug users predominate, with some 32.4% of the homosexual population of Rio de Janeiro apparently infected by "the AIDS virus", some nurses picking up the infection from healthcare work, and prostitutes increasingly showing signs of the condition.[4,5,6]

Haitians, originally considered a "high risk" group primarily on the basis of refugee and immigrant entrance into the U.S.A. in the 1970s, were dropped by the CDC as a separate risk category for AIDS in light of a reassessment, still controversial, of the earlier classification.[7]

Going into the beginning of the 1990s, the HIV/LAS/ARC/AIDS infection picture also presented these elements:

By 1990, it was apparent that, at least in the U.S.A., the percentage numbers of HIV/AIDS victims in the various "high risk" groups were beginning to change: the rate of new cases of and death from HIV/AIDS among male homosexuals was beginning to plateau out or even decline, but striking rises were occurring among intravenous drug users and children born to AIDS-infected persons. AIDS is already the ninth leading cause of death among children 1 to 4 and by 1991 might constitute a tenth of all pediatric hospital cases, figures suggest.[58]

The statistics/numbers game now clearly has opposite poles. On the one hand, some observers claim that AIDS is of such little impact on the non-drug-using "straight community" as to be virtually no threat[59] and question the raising of huge amounts of federal funds to combat it. They cite an assessment that less than 1 percent of the total population is infected and figures that suggest that monogamous heterosexual couples are essentially free from danger, with a low HIV infection rate in the U.S. military still seeming to hold.[8,9,10] On the other hand, the early optimism that antibody tests largely protect the nation's blood supply continues to be shattered as new evidence mounts that antibodies may not appear in AIDS victims for from many months to years following infection.[60] And devotees of the HIV conspiracy theory continue to stress the likelihood of mass infection in the world population as a whole as part of a biological warfare scenario.[61,62]

One investigator, Michael Fumento, charged in 1990 in a provocative book that the whole issue of AIDS as a threat to the general heterosexual population is overblown hype:

"A middle-class non-IVDA (intravenous-drug-abusing) heterosexual in the Chicago suburbs or Orange County, California -- or, indeed, in almost any area of the country -- has less of a chance of getting AIDS in the next year than of being struck by lightning or drowning in a bathtub," he wrote.[89]

Fumento is a former AIDS analyst for the U.S. Commission on Civil Rights, and his book voiced the deep suspicions of many that the AIDS crisis is overblown. ("The goal of the AIDS industry in general is sheer self-perpetuation," he charged.)

One could take consolation in the fact that "only" 1 of every 250 needlestick injuries by health workers in the U.S.A. working with AIDS patients has resulted in HIV infection[63] or be concerned over a Centers for Disease Control (CDC) finding in 1989 that 2 out of every 1,000 American college students is positive for HIV antibodies.[64]

· Since researchers kept advancing the time of incubation and the natural history of the HIV/AIDS infection curve became more noticeable in the analyses of, by 1990, some 120,000 full-blown AIDS cases in the U.S.A., it was still apparent that the nation was seeing infections that might have occurred anywhere from a few to many years prior; the full extent of infection and its outcome remained unknown.

· While the transmission of an agent or agents through semen and blood remains highly related to AIDS

23

and ARC, other predisposing or co-factors are *almost certainly* necessary for the development of either or both conditions, as ensuing chapters will show. The fact remains that transmission factors so far are almost exclusively sex acts, blood transfusions, and drug injections with contaminated needles.

· It has become clear that AIDS, despite the "rush to judgment" in the U.S.A. on the part of many investigators and the media, is *not* a "gay disease" any more than it is strictly an "IV drug users'" disease. (Though, as we will show, by re-examining even CDC statistics, one can make a case -- in the U.S.A. -- for AIDS being every bit as much a "drug-users' disease" [from IV *and other* drugs] as it is a plague striking a certain segment of male homosexuals.)

· Even utilizing the one-mode theory of AIDS causation, there is major controversy over whether the virus or viruses actually originated in Africa, or actually appeared there at about the same time as they did in the United States and the Caribbean. Until the precise history of AIDS transmission is written, all that was known in 1990 was that AIDS or AIDS-like diseases "spontaneously appeared" in those three areas at or about the same time in the late 1970s. (Reevaluations of sera from patients, however, now make it clear -- see Chapter Three -- that "AIDS virus" or "AIDS-virus-like" viruses were existing in *healthy* Venezuelan aborigines at least as early as 1968 and in *healthy* Ugandan children at least as early as 1959. The African data have been subjected to a good deal of doubt. The Venezuelan data stood intact in 1990.)

· The statistical evidence -- even if researchers agree on the identity of "the AIDS virus" -- makes it extremely unlikely that the virus actually "causes" AIDS by itself. The supporting evidence, as we detail in Chapter Three, is that not all carriers of antibody to HIV advance to AIDS (indeed, statistically, and at least to date, the *great majority* have not), there are cases of AIDS without there being either detectable virus or antibody, cases of AIDS-like immune suppression without HIV virus or antibodies, and considerable samples of multiple exposures to known infected people (be they sexual partners, blood-transfusion donors, recipients of infected sperm for artificial insemination, infected mothers of infants, etc.) where neither antibodies, nor virus, nor AIDS developed -- and other cases in

24

which antibodies appeared and disappeared and in which AIDS was diagnosed as a transitory, non-fatal disease.

· The particular depression in the immune system most frequently correlated with HIV/AIDS (namely, reversal of the T4:T8 lymphocyte ratio) is by no means always associated with AIDS and ARC and has been found to be associated with other viruses, diseases and conditions, forms of malnutrition being among them. That is to say, neither a T4:T8 ratio reversal nor a "positive" antibody test for HIV can confirm AIDS.

· Despite the isolation of the putative "AIDS virus" from an impressive variety of human tissues and excretions, investigators now generally agree that it is difficult to contract "the AIDS virus", far more difficult than, say, becoming infected with hepatitis B (frequently associated with AIDS), and that "casual contact" with assumed carriers of HIV represents virtually no health risk. Moreover, "the AIDS virus", one of amazing biochemical properties, and possessed of almost "Houdini" - like escape mechanisms and immune surveillance-avoidance capability, is itself apparently weak.

· At least in the Western world, about 60 percent of "full-blown" AIDS patients die -- not of AIDS, but any of a number of "opportunistic" infections from other viruses, bacteria, parasites, fungi, etc., especially *Pneumocystis carinii* pneumonia as well as from rare forms of cancer (particularly Kaposi's sarcoma, which may not even *be* cancer, and non-Hodgkin's lymphoma).

· While it is fairly well established that the effect of AIDS infection is the demolition of the immune system (through a virtual wipeout of its T4 or "helper" cell subset) as well as infection of the monocyte/macrophage system, it remains unclear why only *certain* infections and conditions affect, and are ultimately lethal to, full-blown AIDS patients, rather than their being killed (as is often the case with cancer) by any of a wide variety of more common infections which assume deadly dimensions as the patient's immune system collapses. As an enormous information load of information has developed around HIV, it has also become clear that the alleged "AIDS virus" is associated with more than immunological and neurological invasion, and is at least present in a great variety of tissues.[65] But whether, and/or the extent to which it is causative or indicative of pathology, still remain open questions.

· It is also evident that a substantial number of ARC patients remain very much alive and it is not by any means clear that they will advance to AIDS. It is also true that one may advance from infection to AIDS while bypassing ARC. All are simply stops along the HIV/AIDS infection curve.

· It is increasingly recognized that AIDS has cerebrospinal and central nervous system complications and that it may actually strike that system first. "AIDS dementia" is now often diagnosed.

· To date, standard drug treatment approaches to AIDS, and also more novel techniques utilizing alpha-interferon and interleukin-2, have been mixed at best, utter failures at worst. Various anti-viral and immune-enhancing drugs are being used experimentally in several countries. The most politically disturbing element in such experimental therapy is within the home of by far the greatest number of AIDS cases, the U.S.A. itself, primarily because of the highly restrictive and progress-intimidating constraints of the Food, Drug and Cosmetic Act.

· Early in the plague, such pre-existing drugs as suramin and cyclosporine-A were tried, and failed. Azidothymidine (AZT), a highly toxic synthetic "old" drug for cancer, in which it failed, became the first drug approved by the U.S.A. specifically for HIV/AIDS. It was followed by approval of alpha-interferon for Kaposi's sarcoma.

In 1987 and 1988 the Japanese drug dextran sulfate, used for 20 years in arteriosclerosis, was found useful in HIV/AIDS but was not yet available for general use in the U.S.A., nor was ribavirin (Virazole), originally developed in the U.S.A. and used with some success for several years in HIV/AIDS cases.

Evidence gathered that an Israeli-pioneered fatty acid combination, AL-721, was useful in anti-viral and immune enhancement activity, that isoprinosine was active as an immune enhancer, that acyclovir, already used against herpes, could be of benefit in HIV/AIDS. None was "legal" as general AIDS treatment in the U.S.A. in 1989.

At international conferences, new products including Ampligen (mismatched, double-stranded DNA), D-penicillamine, experimental drugs similar to AZT including DDA (dideoxyadenosine), and DDC (dideoxycytidine), DHPG (dehydroxypropoxymethyl-guanine), DNCB (dinitri-

26

chlorobenzene), Foscarnet (phosphonoformate), fusidic acid, Imreg 1, various interferons, pre-existing drugs such as Naltrexone and Dapsone, and Tumor Necrosis Factor were discussed, together with natural substance-derived compounds including Peptide T. All showed some benefit, and most made it to experimental-stage research at U.S. university research centers, to be used alongside existing antibiotics and other drugs against the continually developing series of "opportunistic" infections accompanying the decline of immunity.

Inasmuch as these drugs or combinations of them have at least been anecdotally associated with longer survival rates, some relief of symptoms, etc., it became a growing political issue in the U.S.A. as to why they should not be more readily available. (In Mexico, as we will show, the use of several of these drugs -- most of which have some form of toxic side effects -- in combination with "natural" and non-drug therapies turned in optimistic results).

By 1990, the medical/pharmaceutical establishment was still blissfully ignoring non-drug or "eclectic" approaches to AIDS, if perhaps only because of the philosophical clash between the allopathic paradigm, with its randomized-double-blinded-placebo-controlled testing approach, and the eclectic and holistic treatment paradigms, stressing multifactoriality and individuality in causation and treatment (see Chapter Thirteen).

U.S. orthodoxy, badgered by lobbyists, politicians and gay activists, continued to make it easier to release synthetic drugs for use. Ganciclovir (DHPG, Cytovene) was released for treatment of the blinding CMV retinitis eye disease which strikes some AIDS patients. Recombinant erythropoieten was cleared for use in combating the anemia caused by AZT(!) And, even as some successes in life-extension were being attributed to AZT, development of AZT-resistant HIV strains was reported.[66]

The allopathic community was also agog over the possible viral-inhibiting capabilities of soluble CD4, a genetically altered protein,[67] and Compound Q, also known as tricosanthin and GLQ 223, a highly purified extract of a protein found in Chinese cucumbers and long used in mainland China to induce abortions.[68] And early trials suggested that a less toxic version of an AZT-like drug, DDI

(2',3'-dideoxyinosine), and results of a huge trial of AZT itself, suggested that these drugs would "slow down" the course of AIDS, though not "cure" it.[75,76]

News that AZT also caused cancer in laboratory animals -- nothing really new in the history of toxic cancer-fighting drugs -- did not seem to dim the medical establishment's embrace of AZT (even as manufacturer Burroughs Wellcome kept trying to acquaint the public with its brand name, Retrovir, or zidovudine.)[89]

The establishment,equally atwit over "AZT workalikes" for a time, in 1989-90, had great enthusiasm for DDI -- until six AIDS patients died of pancreatitis, a toxic side effect attributed to the drug.[90] This kept the way open for Burroughs Wellcome against a competing drug company in the mushrooming AIDS market. And early studies of tricosanthin were both confusing and disappointing.[91]

The standard or orthodox approach in the U.S.A. remains attempts at inhibiting "the AIDS virus" itself, or destroying its protective envelope, or inhibiting the enzyme reverse transcriptase which is necessary for the action of retroviruses; and/or bolstering the immune system temporarily, at whatever other cost to the body. Attempts at developing a vaccine, or vaccines, are hampered both by the unusual biochemical characteristics of the putative "AIDS virus" (or viruses) and by the still-unresolved questions as to whether these structures actually *cause* AIDS.

At the Fifth International AIDS Conference in 1989 in Montreal, Dr. Joseph Sonnabend was on hand to place things in their proper perspective:

"The HIV hypothesis has consumed all our resources and yet hasn't saved a single life," he said.[77]

The use of natural metabolic therapies (vitamins, minerals, enzymes, amino acids, herbs, essential fatty acids, dietary manipulation, detoxification, acupuncture, exercise, physical therapy, homeopathy) began to turn in results against HIV/AIDS both in the U.S.A. and abroad.

But such natural approaches by themselves or in conjunction with the standard or orthodox drug modalities remained essentially excluded from the journals of the allopathic medical establishment.

We will point out that a number of vital connections to AIDS have either been overlooked or essentially ignored.

Among them:

    -- The role of dietary factors in depressing the immune system, particularly in the West in general and the United States in particular, through the fullscale alterations in the food chain brought about by food processing. The hydrogenation of polyunsaturated fatty acids and deficiencies in natural essential fatty acids (EFAs), key minerals and vitamins will be discussed.

    -- The intriguing statistical relationship between fluoridated water and the initial clusters of full-blown AIDS cases, particularly in the U.S.A., but with international ramifications as well, with emphasis on the immune depressing effects of this common industrial chemical.

    -- The connection between drugs -- both legal and illegal -- in immune depression to the point where the HIV/AIDS infection curve can just as easily be described as a result of drug intoxication as it can be attributed to specific sexual practices.

    -- The synergism between HIV/AIDS and syphilis, which some see as the missing link in the infection curve.

    -- The possible connections between HIV/AIDS and vaccinations.

    -- The understated role of intestinal and other parasites in helping depress the immune system, and/or further depressing the immune system as parts of either the cause or consequences of AIDS.

    -- The understated role of poor sanitation and hygiene.

    -- The possible biological warfare connection in AIDS by design, error, or misplaced science.

    -- The connection between "the AIDS virus" and animal viral infections.

    -- The usually downplayed reality of multiviral infections in AIDS patients, with particular emphasis on widespread Epstein-Barr Virus (EBV) and cytomegalovirus (CMV), together with concurrent or prior infections with hepatitis B, herpes and venereal disease. (By 1988 and 1989, however, even the most allopathically minded researchers were beginning to speak of viral co-factors to HIV as it became clear, even to them, that "the AIDS virus" -- or viruses -- could not be acting alone. [See Chapter

Five.])

-- More importantly, we will show that therapies based on building host resistance and immune enhancement rather than on synthetic drugs alone hold the best hope of treating and managing AIDS, and that AIDS patients who have opted for "holistic" and "eclectic" treatment modalities are tending to live longer and do better than do AIDS and ARC patients treated with single or multiple synthetic drugs. This is not to eschew the role of anti-viral drugs in a total program. Part of our evidence for this comes from the limited caseload (100 patients by 1990) seen in Mexico under auspices of the Bradford Research Institute, in which holistic/eclectic approaches could be utilized in an environment free from bureaucratic constraints.

-- And, most importantly, we will indicate what seem to be appropriate measures to prevent AIDS even in individuals who may at this time seem to be "high-risk" candidates. The growing evidence from metabolic/nutritional therapy has indicated that, while dealing with life-threatening pathologies is a complicated, uphill struggle, prevention of the same is relatively simple. In terms of AIDS, prevention revolves around lifestyle changes, proper nutrition, immune system enhancement and prudent sex lives.

From the beginning, a number of American scientists were leery of the handling of the AIDS panic in the United States, and their concern largely arose because of the dominance in America of a single school of medical thought -- allopathy, a term usually advanced by homeopaths in the 19th century to distinguish drug-and mineral-using practitioners from themselves[11] but eventually more or less grudgingly accepted by the allopaths themselves.

Given tremendous impetus by the Koch-Pasteur Germ Theory of Disease of a century ago and by the modern international pharmaceutical trusts of the current era, allopathy can loosely be defined as the theory that a disease is caused by a germ, or pathogen, and that all that is required for treatment is to find the antagonist to the pathogen, administer it and cure will result.

In terms of the development of antibiotics against specific infections, this approach has had more than passing merit. As I and other writers have pointed out in other places, allopathic approaches simply do *not* have much merit in resolving the chronic, systemic degenerative disease conditions that characterize the industrialized West, where actual parasitical and bacteriological infections have been replaced by metabolic dysfunctions and deficiency states as the killer diseases of the modern era.[12,13]

With the onset of AIDS, there was a standard allopathic rush to define "the" cause in order to develop "the vaccine" or fashion "the drug" which would kill it, all in accordance with standard (which is to say, allopathic) thinking.

The richness of the controversy is encompassed in such quotations as these:

"The authoritative assertion that HTLV-3 [*the earlier designation of HIV -- ed.*] causes AIDS was made in the absence of adequate information about the prevalence of antibodies of the virus in different populations . . ." -- Dr. Joseph Sonnabend, former scientific director of the AIDS Medical Research Foundation.[14]

The same source also noted that "although many infectious agents do not cause disease in all who are infected, there is little precedent for a pathogenic virus which causes *no* disease in one population and serious illness in others."

It also cited John Martin and Carol Vance, Columbia University School of Public Health researchers, who pointed out that "the dominance of the germ theory model of AIDS has resulted in research that either ignores or only inadequately addresses ... life-style factors believed to have direct consequences (though of unknown magnitude or duration) for immunological functioning."

And Arthur J. Ammann, MD, University of California School of Medicine-San Francisco, noted:[15] "There is no historical precedent for believing that a single infectious agent is capable of abolishing a normal immune system."

He analyzed: "...If a single agent were responsible for AIDS, then the syndrome should have existed prior to the beginning of the epidemic in 1981 (unless HTLV-III is a newly emerged virus). If HTLV-III is a new virus, then one must ask why AIDS is confined to a selected population of persons 'at risk' and has not been reported (*as of 1984-ed.*) in medical workers involved in the management of patients with AIDS. The latter observations suggest that a single agent by itself is not capable of causing AIDS but that other factors, such as additional viral infections or pre-existing immunosuppression, are prerequisites for the development of AIDS."

Sonnabend proposed a "multifactorial model for the development of AIDS in homosexual men"[16] which stressed the interplay of other viruses, plus multiple allogeneic (i.e., non-self) semens plus venereal disease. He appended to his original paper a note which reflected the recent "discovery" of HIV: "It would appear that the vast majority of the individuals in the high-risk groups who become infected with this virus already have immune perturbation prior to infection by the agent ... We ... continue to predict that interaction with Epstein-Barr virus, cytomegalovirus, and other agents contributing to immune perturbation are required to permit the virus to induce AIDS."

As early as mid-1983, San Francisco researchers Jay A. Levy and John L. Ziegler proposed[17] that AIDS disease occurs in "high-risk" people whose immune systems have already been compromised by such immune-depressing conditions as cancer, organ transplants, repeated viral infections, repeated venereal disease, and heavy use of antibiotics.

They also predicted that many people in areas where AIDS diseases were then occurring had probably already been infected by the organism but had been able to fight off the germ because of their normal immunity.

The gradually developing reality that HIV infection is widespread in Africa while AIDS cases themselves are modest, and that there are cases of actual transient AIDS cases among health-care workers and/or otherwise healthy partners or relatives of AIDS-infected people tends to bear out the earlier Levy-Ziegler assumptions.

In 1984, Arthur Berken, MD, a clinical professor of medicine at the State University of New York-Stony Brook,[18] noting the "nearly equal incidence of AIDS in males and females in Zaire in contrast to the overwhelming male incidence" in the U.S.A., wrote that "since I am unaware of any other example of such variability of sexual preference by an infecting organism in different parts of the world, I remain skeptical that AIDS is caused by a transmissible agent. Rather, it is the result of an immunologic paradox in which hyperfunction of humoral immunity results in hypofunction of cellular immunity."

It is illustrative of the allopathic paradigm and the drug/medical business in the U.S.A. that these sober early voices stressing the possible multifactoriality in HIV/AIDS rather than its single cause were gradually drowned out by furor over the discovery of "the AIDS virus" and the massive development of propaganda concerning "the cause of AIDS." The primacy of HIV soared and the allopathic thought process roared ahead at full steam as a new industry sprouted around the virology of AIDS. By the last decade of this century, HIV (and therefore the AIDS infection curve) is becoming the focus of what is already a multi-billion-dollar new industry, with grants, awards and scientific prestige to be meted out to those snapped into line and rallying around the flag. There is, at this time, little financial interest in pursuing "non-HIV-centered" approaches.

By mid-1985 it could not be stated with any certainty that infection with "the AIDS virus" would lead to AIDS. The editorial opinion of the *Journal of the American Medical Assn.* was[19] that "many (but not all) who are exposed to the virus become infected, but only some (perhaps 5% to 10% per year) who become infected ultimately demonstrate symptoms" and "antibody testing of serum samples is a valuable method to determine who has been exposed to the virus but it does not make the diagnosis of AIDS."

After that time, researchers, using various sets of studies, increased the percentages by which HIV "seropositives" might advance to full-blown AIDS -- and such estimates ranged far beyond the 1985 assessments.

So by 1988 a number of large "cohorts" had been studied for enough years that *Lancet* could report:[25] "Surprisingly, perhaps, after several years of close study, questions remain about the natural history of AIDS itself. In none of the large cohort studies have 50% or more of the seropositive individuals got symptoms so far and estimates of the interval from seroconversion to symptomatic disease now range from 8 to 14 years. This observation implies that some infected subjects may remain symptom-free for the whole of their natural lifespan."

Unfortunately, this sanguine view was undercut somewhat by a continuing evaluation of the San Francisco caseload -- by 1989, 77 percent of men in the study (based

33

originally on blood taken for the hepatitis B vaccine project) had developed some level of AIDS symptomatology. This still left a surprising 23 percent who had allegedly been incubating HIV for 11 *years* without symptoms.[69] Whether the AIDS caseload in this study says more about AIDS or the hepatitis B vaccine is open for inquiry (see Chapter Eleven.)

The 1988 *Lancet* review of AIDS also made it quite clear that despite HIV's predilection for T4 "helper" cells, "it remains unclear precisely how T4 cell depletion, the hallmark of disease progression, is mediated."

In a prospective follow-up of 200 homosexual men in Finland, Valle and associates in 1985 indicated[20] a broad spectrum of infection ranging from "transient infection through chronic provirus state, asymptomatic virus producer state, LAS [lymphadenopathy syndrome] or ARC and rarely full-blown AIDS."

They added: "Cofactors probably determine the final outcome of infection in the individual."

While "the AIDS virus", while clearly a retrovirus, is also considered a "lentivirus" because of its capacity for slow incubation, there are nonetheless cases of rapid onset, as was reported in a handful of health-care workers[21] and in the Sydney AIDS Study Group in Australia, in which sudden, acute symptoms occurred as early as six days following probable exposure to the "AIDS-related retrovirus" (ARV).[22]

Subsequent data suggest the sudden onset of flu-like symptoms within a few days of HIV exposure in many people. Indeed, such symptoms may be the only direct effect of HIV-1 infection.

In spring 1985 it was claimed that almost 80% of AIDS patients, quite aside from whatever other manifestations of the syndrome and its attendant diseases they were showing, suffered from some form of central nervous system and brain disorder, ranging from depression and severe headaches to memory loss, speech impairment, blurred vision and paralysis, and that "the AIDS virus" not only attacked the immune system but could directly affect the central nervous system as well.[23]

The degree of cerebrospinal and neurological AIDS involvements and when they appear are matters which have since been subjected to wide-ranging debate. The amount of central nervous system involvement may not be as high as earlier feared.[71,72]

Radding, of New York University Medical center, proposed[24] that HIV infects the nervous system, probably through parasympathetic neurons, and that AIDS becomes manifest "only after the infection travels up the brain stem, and then eventually reaches down to the thymus, where the T cells become infected by virus budding from the neurons..."

He also noted that a nasopharyngeal route of transmission could be involved, particularly in the use ("sniffing") of cocaine (and, by implication, the inhalation of nitrite "poppers" -- see Chapter Six).

Acute encephalopathy was coincident with seroconversion for HIV in patients studied by Carne et al[26] but "neurological signs and symptoms resolved quickly." The disease ranged from prodromal general malaise to epileptic-like seizures and even coma. This particular study reflected the possibility of acute brain symptoms with AIDS in addition to the chronic symptoms noted in earlier cases.

In 1985 researchers began distinguishing "ARC"-level cases from full-blown AIDS since the now-widening span of general malaise seemed to affect the same people who might later develop AIDS but whose symptoms did not fit CDC's parameters for full-blown disease.

AIDS-Related Complex, sometimes preceded by LAS (lymphadenopathy syndrome), presented a pattern of night sweats, intermittent fevers, weight loss, swollen glands, vague generalized muscle, joint and bone pains, diarrhea and yeast infection.

These symptoms, as we note elsewhere, may just as easily be part of the infectious mononucleosis or secondary syphilis presentations as well and may also be seen in what would later be known as "chronic fatigue syndrome" or "universal reactor syndrome." Elevated titers of Epstein-Barr virus were/are frequent participants in the diagnostic picture.

By 1985, then, an ever-expanding group of conditions, disorders and diseases was seen along a route whose terminus was full-blown AIDS. The difference seemed to be that numerous LAS or ARC-level patients were often just holding their own, living through intermittent bouts of sickness, occasionally advancing to terminal disease but otherwise not guaranteed death despite the persistent, continuing media propaganda which continued to equate positivity for AIDS antibodies to AIDS itself, and any component of clinical AIDS to death.

In 1987, the CDC changed the parameters for "full-blown" AIDS to include "AIDS dementia" symptoms, certain opportunistic infections and elements of ARC, together with a lengthening list of immunological disturbances and positivity for HIV antibodies, and also a category of AIDS signs and symptoms *without* positive blood profiles (that is, actual proof of HIV antibodies or antigens or T-cell distortions.)

The new guidelines served to complicate the picture and led many researchers to think of one long curve of infection ranging from exposure to infection by HIV at some point through a process of many months to many years terminating in the destructive features of "full-blown" AIDS.

The CDC case definition change is a critical event in AIDS history, for it so widens the possible definitions of AIDS (see Appendix I) that a clinician might make a diagnosis of the killer condition in the absence of any supporting blood work simply by noting any of various "indicator diseases" in a patient and just guessing at his lifestyle.

The possibilities for misdiagnosis are now considerable, and they have occurred. The situation is analogous to the vast symptomatology of syphilis in an earlier era and to mononucleosis later: there are so many signs and symptoms of presumptive syphilitic infection that it is possible to diagnose a syphilitic without knowledge of his blood tests.

With growing numbers of doctors clamoring for use of "preventive" toxic drugs (particularly AZT) to head off later development of HIV/AIDS and being able to diagnose AIDS without confirmatory blood work (antibody/antigen tests, virus culture, immune panel distortions), pharmaceutical giants are expected to have a field day.

Even *with* blood work, the world is left with at times meaningless and possibly false readings on antibody tests (though one or more positive ELISA -- enzyme-linked immunosorbent assay -- tests followed by a "Western Blot" are essentially confirmatory for HIV).

Far more expensive research antibody, antigen and virus-culture tests have not yet been determined to be absolutely precise for the virus itself so that "seronegativity" might not mean the patient is *not* harboring the virus and "seropositivity" might not mean that he *is.*

Confused or erratic behavior by persons in presumed "high risk" groups can now just as easily be attributed to "AIDS dementia" (or what some now call "AIDS Dementia Complex") as to a hundred other possible things. The unspoken philosophy for clinicians would seem to be: "when in doubt, call it AIDS." (That is, if the patient is anyone but a celibate 80-year-old nun who never had a blood transfusion.)

Whatever the etiology of AIDS, it leads to a multiplicity of rare disorders and infections, with most of them singly being able to kill, and which are even more deadly in combination.

The most common and fast-acting of the deadly AIDS sequelae is *Pneumocystis carinii,* a parasite (now thought to be fungal rather than protozoan) which causes pneumonia. Usually associated only with severely immune depressed people and up to now rare as a disease (but present in a dormant state in many people) in the Western hemisphere, *P. carinii* is the most frequently encountered fatal infection to strike AIDS patients.

It is followed in total number of cases by Kaposi's sarcoma, a kind of cancer-like disease which differs from the "classical" form endemic in parts of central Africa. But other cancers, including non-Hodgkin's lymphoma, immunoblastic lymphoma and B-immunoblastic sarcoma, are increasingly seen.

Also common in AIDS patients is infection by *Toxoplasmosis,* a parasite that can attack the eyes, heart and central nervous system; the parasite *Cryptosporidium,* frequently seen in AIDS patients suffering watery diarrhea; the widely diffused fungus *Candida,* which may be a "marker";[28] and a devastating fungus, *Cryptococcus neoformans,* which attacks the lungs, central nervous system, lymph nodes, bone marrow and intestinal tract.

Common bacteria appearing in AIDS patients are *Mycobacterium avium-intercellulare* (MAI) and *Mycobacterium tuberculosis,* which cause different kinds of tuberculosis.

The proper place of Kaposi's sarcoma in all of this has been a controversy almost from the beginning.

As suspected by the Bradford Research Institute and others, KS may not be cancer at all, and recent evidence[49,50] suggests this. When seen in Africa, the Mediterranean and parts of the Third World over the past few decades, KS is at worst an ugly skin disease of bluish/purplish lesions but the disease is not usually fatal. It is noticeably declining in U.S. AIDS.

It seemed to be associated in the early AIDS epidemic with other aspects of terminal disease and, with immune systems severely depressed, can and did prove fatal. However, KS lesions might occur earlier rather than later in the HIV/AIDS curve, as Redfield and his associates have noted,[27] and the early-lesion, late-disease aspects of KS confused the presumptive theories as to the natural history of AIDS.

Some of the longer-surviving "AIDS patients" are KS patients in whom there simply have been transient skin lesions and little if anything else. If the proponents of the AIDS-as-syphilis school of thought (Chapter Twelve) are correct, KS lesions are only signs of a form of syphilis anyway.

At the outside, KS is another opportunistic infection in the HIV/AIDS infection curve, and whether it should always be considered part of "full-blown" AIDS is problematical. Our own experience has been that a number of well diagnosed KS cases who were HIV-positive do not always have the immune panel distortions common to AIDS and some of them have not been "sick."

A landmark event in AIDS history involved Kaposi's sarcoma:

In January 1990, New York epidemic researchers reported six cases of homosexual men who had KS but did not have evidence of HIV infection.[92] Their suspicion was that KS is caused by some virus or agent other than HIV -- a logical extension of the reality that HIV had not been found in Kaposi's lesions in prior research, and that KS is a very old disease in several parts of the world.

In the earlier AIDS era, KS accounted for 21% of the cases of AIDS seen in homosexual men (yet was seen in only 1% of hemophiliacs with AIDS.) With KS cases declining in the late 1980s as homosexual men moderated their sex lives, the clues became glaring: KS, perhaps not cancer at all, at least in the early phase, is a sexually transmitted opportunistic infection and far less likely to be transmitted through Factor VIII, the blood product characteristically provided hemophiliacs. The presence of KS in men without HIV also undercut the HIV-as-AIDS-cause doctrine. It potentially removed such a bloc of "AIDS patients" away from HIV as to pose a bigger question than ever before as to the single-virus theory of the syndrome.

As we note in Chapter Five, other viruses seem to play major roles in AIDS, either as causes, co-factors or as organisms reactivated some way, the more prominent of these being EBV and CMV. The latter, usually dormant and usually not dangerous in healthy carriers, may itself be a cause of blindness and death in advanced AIDS.

A classical and in a few ways typical (for U.S.A.) AIDS case was presented by Burkes, et al.[29] It involved a 40-year old male homosexual with a prior history of anal fistula repair, syphilis (three times), gonorrhea (10), and hepatitis B. The man also frequently used cocaine, amphetamines, LSD, marijuana, and amyl nitrite (poppers). He described approximately 900 sexual contacts in the past. He presented with simultaneous *P. carinii*, acute cytomegalovirus infection, Kaposi's sarcoma and B-immunoblastic sarcoma.

Severe compromise of both T- and B-cells was noted. He was dead four months from diagnosis, with autopsy revealing organ destruction by widespread cancer.

Earlier, an unseemly political battle raged over claims as to where and when AIDS actually appeared -- and as to who should get credit for initially identifying "the AIDS virus" or viruses, to say nothing of the American dialogue over a possible quarantine of carriers of AIDS.

And the World Health Organization (WHO), monitoring information on AIDS from throughout the world at its Geneva, Switzerland, headquarters, was reported in late 1985 [30] to be keeping a tight lid on information and to be aware of a reluctance on the part of health authorities in parts of Africa and elsewhere to present statistics. The situation had only partly improved by 1989-1990.

The East Bloc, which denied cases of AIDS existed there until late 1985, belatedly admitted a few scattered cases but consistently maintained the line that AIDS is of

U.S. origin. East Bloc propagandists, and some well credentialed African researchers and also other investigators, have strongly questioned the "African genesis" of AIDS.

Indeed, the African genesis theory remained a bigger puzzlement in 1990 than a few years prior, when the trend of "establishment" thought was that somehow HIV had "jumped species" from a simian known as the African green monkey.

The delineation of several HIV-like simian viruses which cause AIDS-like disease in some species (but not in all), and the similarity of one of these to a second strain of HIV now called HIV-2 or HTLV-IV (originally limited to areas of West Africa and apparently *not* causing severe disease in humans) widened speculation that somehow an animal-origin virus had entered the human family via Africa.

With the virtue of hindsight, while virologists can see both similarities and differences between the various animal and human structures, it is logically as appropriate to suggest that AIDS-inducing or AIDS-like viruses originated in man (or were placed there?) and transferred to monkeys as it is to speculate that animal viruses migrated to man!

The similar animal viruses now reported -- and their original descriptions and delineations[37,38,39,40,41] further muddied the HIV/AIDS picture -- are SRV (SAIDS-Related virus, SAIDS being the misnomered "simian AIDS", which, while causing immune deficiency in captive rhesus monkeys and as a relative of another virus which causes immune deficiency in rhesus macaques, is *not* the equivalent of, or even closely related to, HIV); SIV (for simian immune deficiency virus), which is not strongly related to HIV but does "cross-react" with HIV-2, the second "human AIDS" virus which strikes West Africans who remain essentially healthy; SIVmac (isolated from captive rhesus macaque monkeys in the U.S., where it causes immune deficiency); SIVagm (isolated from African green monkeys, in which it does *not* cause illness, and originally thought to be a direct ancestor of HIV); and SIVsm (isolated from African sooty mangabey monkeys, in which it does *not* cause illness.)

There is some question as to how many of these similar viruses exist, how many are the products of experi-

40

ments, and how many, while existing, cause disease in their natural hosts (even though they may in their captive or unnatural hosts.)

In 1988, the Harvard School of Public Health was stunned by a mini-scandal: the AIDS research scientists (Max Essex and Phyllis Kanki) who are pre-eminent in simian AIDS research as well admitted[32] that their isolation of a second AIDS virus apparently was the result of a laboratory accident -- contamination of human blood samples with an AIDS-like virus found in monkeys.

This chilling disclosure only fueled the speculation that HIV itself, somehow, might be a laboratory experiment or accident in which animal viruses served as the base.

The Essex-Kanki research, errors and all, nonetheless is eloquent. The researchers themselves wrote in 1988[33] that "clearly SIV is the closest known animal virus relative of HIV, but it is only about 50 percent related on the basis of sequence analysis -- not close enough to make it likely that SIV was an immediate precursor of HIV in people."

Their work has also shown that people in West Africa have been infected with a far less pathogenic "AIDS virus" distinct from that which has been said to have devastated central Africa (and the central African one is thought to be similar to, if not identical with, HIV in the rest of the world).

In the meantime, HIV has been injected into various species of animals, but it can only successfully be inoculated into chimpanzees -- where it causes only mild disease (lymphadenopathy primarily) and is not lethal. By Fall 1988 it had successfully infected rabbits[51] and, by Winter 1988, test mice.[52] It has so far failed to kill test animals directly.

At the Fifth International AIDS Conference in Montreal in 1989, polio vaccine pioneer Jonas Salk announced that a vaccine-like "HIV immunogen" had been able to "clear" HIV infection in two chimpanzees.[70] This suggested an important step toward the development of an HIV vaccine, yet the obstacles to any such event seemed formidable due to the capability of HIV to create variants of itself and constantly change from person to person.

Confusion in naming and delineating HIV continued because of the insistence by "establishment" researchers in the U.S.A. that "the AIDS virus", originally called HTLV-III in this country, was a lineal descendant of other viruses (HTLV-I, HTLV-II) researched at the same federal laboratories. It is now recognized that HIV is significantly distinct from HTLV-I, a strain of virus said to cause a rare leukemia in humans, and HTLV-II, which may be connected to another rare leukemia -- or may cause nothing at all.

But even there semantics proved confusing and obfuscating: HTLV originally referred to "human T-cell leukemia/lymphoma virus" and later was changed to "human T-lymphotropic virus" as it became clear that leukemia *per se* was not part of the HIV/AIDS picture.

With sequential analysis, researchers can compare viruses -- which are, after all, only submicroscopic particles of protein surrounding bundles of genetic information and which are non-living parasites which depend on living host organisms for their "replication" -- and relate them to each other.

The existing research no longer can prove an African genesis, or even an animal genesis, for HIV, although it can suggest that somehow various species of similar, but distinct, viruses evolved in a parallel manner in various species. None of this speculation, however, can fully account for the explosive appearance of HIV/AIDS in humans in three separate geographical areas at or about the same time.

By reading the Western press and even perusing CDC and WHO statistics, one would get the impression that Africa is about to be totally destroyed by the new disease, often referred to there as "slim."

Some extremist-political assumptions, adducing a sinister plot by certain forces attempting to foist genocide on the planet, have estimated the number of HIV infections and AIDS cases to be higher than even the WHO estimates.

Nonetheless, as of 1990, it was the U.S.A., with more than 100,00 full-blown AIDS cases, or the majority of officially reported full-blown cases, where the big challenge seemed to be. Attempts were made to explain away the persistent lack of a total death march in central Africa on the basis of poor reporting, politics, bad research, and the like.

In 1987, Felix I.D.Konotey-Ahulu of Cromwell Hospital, London, went on an African tour to see first-hand

42

about the "catastrophe" said to be brewing in Africa. He reported his findings in *Lancet*[34] and among them were such observations as these: "Africa has 50 countries. The total population of the African countries with an AIDS problem is less than 10 percent of the population of the entire continent... I met and examined a number of very ill patients but did not find people dying by the dozen with AIDS."

Dr. Konotey-Ahulu was not denying a considerable AIDS problem in the continent, simply noting that what he called "journalistic hyperbole" was doing a disservice to the emerging countries.

With evidence now almost totally ending the African green monkey-to-man transpecies transmission hypothesis,[35] and with African AIDS cases in retrospect generally not older than in the U.S.A., it is honest to speculate not only which came first, an animal virus, a human virus, or a manufactured virus, but also -- where did the first virus appear? (And is any of this truly relevant to AIDS?)

The matter dominated an AIDS meeting in Brussels in November 1985. Dr. D. Serwadda, associated with England's Institute of Cancer Research, said at the Brussels meeting: "There is such an accusing finger pointed at Africa as the cause of AIDS. The evidence is not quite overwhelming... A lot of what is written in medical journals is not true."[31]

San Francisco Chronicle reporter Randy Shilts, who covered the event, also quoted Dr. Akinyele Faibiyi, a professor at the University of Nigeria: "We might as well call this virus U.S. AIDS. We feel victimized by all this talk of AIDS starting in Africa. It is not true." Reporter Shilts also spoke of "a number of scientists [muttering] despondently about a catastrophe brewing in Africa."

Certain political groups in the U.S.A. have accused the Soviet Union and WHO of lying about AIDS cases in Africa[36]. As we note elsewhere, intellectual inquiry on several sides asks whether the "AIDS virus", so new to the world, is not possibly a product of biological warfare.

To the extent that there is a triggering viral connection in AIDS, then what has happened in other animal species as well as man -- development of a "herd immunity" -- could foreseeably occur even with "the AIDS virus."

43

REFERENCES

(1)   Slaff, James I., and John K. Brubaker, The AIDS Epidemic. New York: Warner Books, 1985.

(2)   Shilts, Randy, "A 'hidden' group of victims infected by the AIDS virus." San Francisco Chronicle, May 6, 1985.

(3)   Haseltine, William A., testimony, Special Hearing for Funding for AIDS, Labor, Health and Human Services, and Education Subcommittee, U.S. Congress, September 26, 1985.

(4)   Veronesi, Ricardo, "O governo subestima a AIDS," Veja (Brazil), October 16, 1985.

(5)   "A multiplicacao do mal: a AIDS se espalha." Veja (Brazil), Aug. 14, 1985.

(6)   "Alto indice da AIDS em transvestis e prostitutas." E.S.P. (Brazil), Aug. 23, 1985.

(7)   Frank, Elliott, et. al., "AIDS in Haitian-Americans: a reassessment." Cancer Res. (Suppl.), 45, 4619s-4620s, September 1985.

(8)   Heyward, W.L., and J.W. Curran, "The epidemiology of AIDS in the U.S." Scientific American, October 1988.

(9)   Fourth International Conference on AIDS, American Medical News, July 22, 1988.

(10)   Haverkos, H.W., and Robert Edelman, "The epidemiology of acquired immunodeficiency syndrome among heterosexuals." J. Am. Med. Assn., 260:13, Oct. 7, 1988.

(11)   Coulter, Harris L., Divided Legacy: The Conflict between Homeopathy and the American Medical Association. Richmond, CA: North Atlantic Books, 1973.

(12)   Culbert, Michael L., What the Medical Establishment Won't Tell You That Could Save Your Life. Norfolk, VA.: Donning, 1983.

(13)   Harper, Harold, and M.L. Culbert, How You Can Beat the Killer Diseases. New Rochelle, N.Y.: Arlington House, 1977.

(14)   Freudenberg, Nick, "Health education and the politics of AIDS." Health/PAC Bulletin, 16:3, 29, May-June 1985.

(15)   Amman, Arthur J., "Etiology of AIDS." J. Am. Med Assn., 252:10, 1261-1262, September 14, 1984.

(16)   Sonnabend, Joseph A., et. al., "A multifactorial model for the development of AIDS in homosexual men." Ann. N.Y. Acad. Sci., V. 437, 177-182, 1984.

(17)   Perlman, David, "UC scientists' new theory on AIDS." San Francisco Chronicle, July 29, 1983.

(18)   Berken, Arthur, "AIDS: neither new nor transmissible?" N.Y. State J. Med., September, 1984.

(19)   Lundberg, George D., "The age of AIDS: a great time for defensive living."

J. Am. Med. Assn., 253:23. 3440-3441, June 21, 1985.

(20)   Valle, Sirkka-Liisa, "Diversity of clinical spectrum of HTLV-III infection." Lancet, Feb. 9, 1985.

(21)   Weiss, Stanley H., et al., "HTLV-III infection among health care workers."J. Am. Med. Assn., 254:15, 2089-2093, Oct. 18, 1985.

(22)   Cooper, David A., et al., "Acute AIDS retrovirus infection." Lancet, March 9, 1985.

(23)   Smith, Fran, "AIDS ravages victims' brains, studies find." San Jose CA Mercury, April 23, 1985.

(24)   Radding, Wilson, "Is AIDS caused by a neurotropic virus?" J. Am. Med. Assn., 253:19, 2831, 1985.

(25)   Steel, Michael, "Fourth international AIDS conference". Lancet, July 2, 1988.

(26)   Carne, C.A., et al., "Acute encephalopathy coincident with seroconversion for anti-HTLV-III." Lancet, Nov. 30, 1985.

(27)   Redfield, R.R., and D.S. Burke, "HIV infection: the clinical picture." Scientific American, October 1988.

(28)   Klein, Robert S., et al., "Oral candidiasis in high-risk patients as the initial manifestation of the acquired immune deficiency syndrome." N. Eng. J. Med., August 9, 1984.

(29)   Burkes, Ronald L., "Simultaneous occurrence of Pneumocystis carinii pneumonia, cytomegalovirus infection, Kaposi's sarcoma, and B-immunoblastic sarcoma in a homosexual man." J. Am. Med. Assn., 253:23, 3425-3430, June 21, 1985.

(30)   Dabici, Rita L., "Lid on AIDS at WHO HQ," Medical Tribune, Dec. 25, 1985.

(31)   Shilts, Randy, "AIDS loses out to African politics." San Francisco Chronicle, Nov. 25, 1985.

(32)   Steinbrook, R., "Harvard scientists admit error in AIDS virus report." Los Angels Times, Feb. 18, 1988.

(33)   Essex, M.,and Phyllis J. Kanki, "The orgins of the AIDS virus." Scientific American, October 1988.

(34)   Konotey-Ahulu, F.J., "AIDS in Africa: misinformation and disinformation." Lancet, July 25, 1987.

(35)   Steinbrook, R., "Research refutes idea that human AIDS virus originated in monkeys," Los Angeles Times, June 2,1988.

(36)   Hamerman, Warren J., "World Health Org. lies about AIDS in Africa." Solidarity, XVI:67, Nov. 1, 1985.

(37)   Barin, F., et al., "Serological evidence for virus related to simian T-lymphotropic retrovirus III   in residents of West Africa." Lancet, December 21/28, 1985.

(38)   Kanki, P.J., et al., "Serologic identification and characterization of a macaque T-lymphotropic retrovirus closely related to HTLV-III."

Science 228: 1199-1201, 1985.

(39)   Daniel, M.D., et al., "Isolation of T-cell tropic HTLV-III-like retrovirus from macaques." Science 228: 1202-1204, 1985.

(40)   Kanki, P.J., et al., "Isolation of a T-lymphotropic virus related to HTLV-III/LAV from wild-caught African green monkeys." Science: 230: 951-954, 1985.

(41)   Kanki, P.J.., et al., "High prevalence of antibodies to simian T-lymphotropic virus type III in African green monkeys & recognition of STLV-III viral proteins by AIDS and related sera." Lancet, i: 1330-1332, 1985.

(42)   Garry, R.F., et al., "Documentation of an AIDS virus infection in the United States in 1968." J. Am. Med. Assn. 260:14, Oct. 14, 1988.

(43)   Stein, Rob, "A medical mystery: researchers hunt for the longest surviving AIDS patients." Los Angeles Times, Mar. 28, 1988.

(44)   Gallo, R.C., and Luc Montagnier, "AIDS in 1988." Scientific American, October 1988.

(45)   Lo, S-C, et al., "A newly identified virus-like infectious agent derived from a patient with AIDS." Armed Forces Inst. of Path., Washington DC, 1987.

(46)   Lo, S-C, et al., "Fatal infection of non-human primates with the virus-like infectious agent (VLIA-sb51) derived from a patient with AIDS." American Registry of Pathology, Armed Forces Inst. of Path., 1987.

(47)   Ortleib, C., "Will Gallo change his tune?" New York Native, August 17, 1987.

(48)   "Dr. Shyh-Ching Lo's virus." New York Native, June 6, 1988.

(49)   Chase, Marilyn, "Kaposi's sarcoma not a true cancer, research suggests." Wall Street Journal, Oct. 21, 1988.

(50)   "Progress reported in researching Kaposi's." San Francisco Examiner, Oct. 8, 1988.

(51)   "Poison offers possible AIDS treatment." (Associated Press) Escondido CA Times-Advocate, Sept. 22, 1988.

(52)   CBS News, Dec. 27, 1988.

(53)   Cortes, Eduardo, et al., "HIV-1, HIV-2, and HTLV-I infection in high-risk groups in Brazil." N. Eng. J. Med., April 13, 1989.

(54)   Avanian, John Z., et al., "HIV-2 infection in the United States." J. Am. Med. Assn., May 25, 1989.

(55)   Myers, Beverly, "More details of AIDS-linked, viruslike infectious agent revealed." J.Am. Med. Assn., June 16, 1989.

(56)   Lo, Shyh-Ching, Am. J. Trop. Med. Hyg., 40: 213-226, 1989.

(57)   Lo, Shyh-Ching, Am. J. Trop. Med. Hyg., 40: 399-409, 1989.

(58)   Centers For Disease Control (CDC), March 1989.

(59)   Charen, Mona, "An epidemic that wasn't." (Creators Syndicate) San Diego Union, April 23, 1989.

(60)   Imigawa, David, et al., "Human immunodeficiency virus type 1 infection in homosexual men who remain seronegative for prolonged periods." New Eng. J. Med., June 1, 1989.

(61)   Strecker, Robert R., "The Strecker memorandum." (Videotape) Glendale, Calif.: The Strecker Group, 1988.

(62)   Douglass, W.C., AIDS: The End of Civilization. Clayton GA: Valet, 1989.

(63)   Staver, Sari, "One in 250 HIV-infected sticks transmits virus -- studies." Am. Med. News. Jan. 13, 1989.

(64)   Jones, Laurie, "CDC: 2 of 1,000 collegians are HIV-positive." Am. Med. News, June 2, 1989.

(65)   Levy, Jay A., "Human immunodeficiency viruses and the pathogenesis of AIDS." J. Am. Med. Assn., May 26, 1989.

(66)   Marx, Jean L., "Drug-resistant strains of AIDS found." Science, March 24, 1989.

(67)   Chase, Marilyn, "Experimental AIDS therapy gets boost." Wall Street Journal, Feb. 9, 1989.

(68)   "FDA OKs human testing of AIDS drug." (United Press International) San Diego Union, April 28, 1989.

(69)   Clark, Cheryl, in San Diego Union, June 6, 1989.

(70)   Steinbrook, Robert, "Salk reports test success of HIV virus treatment." Los Angeles Times, June 9, 1989.

(71)   Dalakas, Marinos et al., "AIDS and the nervous system." J. Am. Med. Assn., April 28, 1989.

(72)   "Studies of AIDS' effect on mind show conflicting results." American Medical News, May 12, 1989.

(73)   Huminer, David, et al., "AIDS in the pre-AIDS era." Rev. Infect. Dis., 9: 1102-1108, 1987.

(74)   Garry, Robert F., et al., letter, "HIV infection in 1968," J. Am. Assn., April 21, 1989.

(75)   The Associated Press, July 28, 1989.

(76)   "AZT is found to delay AIDS development." San Diego, Union, August 4, 1989.

(77)   "U.S. says AZT slows AIDS onset." San Diego Union, Aug. 18, 1989.

(78)   New York Times News Service, Aug. 18, 1989.

(79)   Associated Press. Jan. 16, 1990.

(80)   Farber, Celia, "Sins of omission: the AZT scandal," Spin Magazine, November 1989.

(81)   Adams, Jad, AIDS: The HIV Myth. New York: St. Martin's Press, 1989.

(82)   Altman, L.K., "Unusual microbe, once dismissed, is now taken more seriously." New York Times, Jan. 16, 1990.

(83)   Booth, W., and M. Specter, "Microbe may play role in AIDS, other diseases." Washington Post, Jan. 5, 1990.

(84)   Lo, S-C et al., "Identification of mycoplasma incognitus infection in

patients with AIDS: an immunohistochemcial, in situ hybridization and ultrastructural study." Am. J. Trop. Med. Hyg, Nov. 1989.

(85)   Lo, S-C, et al., "Virus-like infectious agent (VLIA) is a novel pathonegic mycoplasma: Mycoplasma incognitus." Am. J. Trop. Med. Hyg, Nov. 1989.

(86)   Lo, S-C et al., "Association of the virus-like infectious agent originally reported in patients with AIDS with acute fatal disease in previously healthy non-AIDS patients." Am. J. Trop. Med. Hyg, Sept. 1989.

(87)   Lo- S-C, et al., "Fatal infection of silvered leaf monkeys with a virus-like infectious agent (VLIA) derived from a patient with AIDS." Am. J. Trop. Med. Hyg, April 1989.

(88)   Fumento, Michael, The Myth of Heterosexual AIDS. Basic Books, 1990.

(89)   Lublin, Joann S., "Some rodents given high doses of AZT develop cancer, AIDS drug maker says." Wall Street Journal, Dec. 6, 1989.

(90)   Associated Press, March 11, 1990.

(91)   "Compound Q -- the real story." San Francsico, PI Perspective (Project Inform), Nov. 1989.

(92)   Bishop, Jerry E., "U.S. scientists suggest Kaposi's sarcoma is caused by a sexually transmitted agent." Wall Street Journal, Jan. 22, 1990.

Chapter Three

HIV-1,HIV-2, etc.:
THE MAGICAL MYSTERY VIRUSES

From the beginning, the convenient allopathic notion that a single submicroscopic piece of protein surrounding some genetic material ("the AIDS virus") could be the single cause of the devastating, immunity-bashing syndrome AIDS became mired both in concepts and semantics.

The notion was complicated in 1986 by the discovery of yet another "AIDS virus" and even by some research suggestions that there may be more to be discovered.[97,98]

And this complication of course preceded the finding by Dr. Lo that a *non*-virus he had found in AIDS patients not only could be inoculated in test animals, but killed them with AIDS-like diseases [see Chapter Two].

A historical note here: the Koch-Pasteur "germ theory of disease" of the 19th century turned medicine on its ear. It initiated a tidal wave of interest in microscopic organisms that might be causing all the diseases known to man. The terms "microbe" and "bacteria" were bandied about in society talk as well as cancer wards. The idea was that all human pathology might ultimately be explained by "microbes." As late as the second decade of this century, it was believed by many that scurvy was caused by some kind of infectious agent rather than by a deficiency of a nutrient (Vitamin C).

In this century, the discovery of viruses -- visible only with electron microscopes and far tinier than bacteria and other microorganisms -- set off a fresh wave of allopathic endeavor: if bacteria and parasites did not lurk behind many human diseases, then perhaps viruses did. The viral obsession became dominant in orthodox Western medicine by mid-century and is still a major component of medical-biochemical research.

The seemingly sudden advent of AIDS immediately translated into many research minds as a single concept: there must be a new virus out there. And the hunt was on.

49

Skip bacteria, parasites, deficiencies -- look for that virus. From the time the original descriptions of "the AIDS virus" were rendered ("human T-lymphotropic virus-III" by Robert Gallo and the American viral research establishment in general; "AIDS-related virus" by Californian Jay Levy; "lymphadenopathy-associated virus" by France's Luc Montagnier) to the time a dispute over words and patents was resolved in favor of "human immunodeficiency virus" (HIV), scientists sought to link the new discoveries to animal viruses.

As we note elsewhere, there are many animal viruses which produce AIDS-like symptoms in their species and there are viruses which "jump species" from animal to animal. To the point of embarrassment, Western researchers attempted to link the evolution of HIV-1 (in distinction to HIV-2, essentially limited to West Africa but with a few cases now occurring in Europe and America) to viruses in other species.

The development of the theory that African green monkeys, bearing a close relative of HIV-1, somehow must be the source for human AIDS, was dominant until 1987.

There is, after all, simian immunodeficiency virus (SIV) and monkeys are relatives of man. However, by 1987/88 it was becoming clear that the variety of simian immune-depleting viruses that had been studied were molecularly distinct from HIV-1 -- similar to, yet different from -- so the notion that a green monkey must have bit an African at some point in time with a species-jumping virus which later spread throughout humans and went on to demolish entire immune systems in whole groups of people was quietly abandoned.

The fact is that as of this writing the actual origin of HIV-1 or HIV-2 or any other HIV is simply unknown, however similar these microscopic, parasitical structures are to microscopic, parasitical structures in other animals.

The presence of apparently HIV-like infections in otherwise healthy human populations dating back to the 1950s and 1960s skewered both time and geographic frames for the supposed human transmission of one or more animal-derived viruses.

The many problems inherent in attempting to determine the origin of HIV have inevitably led to consideration of the possibility that the virus is man-made, by design or error (see Chapter Eleven), a splice-together of pre-existing animal viruses. This concept is as good as any other, since at least a dozen countries, and probably more, have the technological wherewithal to manufacture viruses.

"HTLV-III" was misnomered from the beginning because of U.S. researcher Robert Gallo's insistence on interconnecting a presumed family of related human viruses. The "HTL" portion of the acronym originally referred to "human T-cell leukemia/lymphoma", and indeed HTLV-I, so striking in geographical and transmission routes to HTLV-III, does seem to be correlated to a very rare form of human leukemia. HTLV-II seems to do little of anything, although it may be related to "hairy cell" leukemia, a rare form of cancer. But "HTL" now refers to "human T-cell-lymphotropic" to indicate "tropism" -- or attraction for -- human T-cells of the immune system.

It is now apparent that HIV is "tropic" for more than simply human immune system cells, even though these cells are still the apparent first and major targets.

HIV is classed both as a retrovirus (that family of viruses which must translate genetic information from RNA to DNA in order to divide, or "replicate") and as a lentivirus, or slowly activating virus, due to its apparently lengthy incubation period, one which now seems to range from a few days to an entire lifetime.

Its presence as a pathogen, or disease-causing organism or structure, is insidious because medicine has never been able to actually cure "viral" let alone "retroviral" diseases.

In their natural history, viruses -- which, as parasites, can only grow, develop and evolve within carriers, or hosts -- adapt to their host organisms and over time are less and less pathogenic. Whether HIV will turn out to be simply another human-carried virus which over time "evolves down" to inconsequential status or "evolves upward" through rapid mutation to far more virulent forms susceptible of multiple routes of transmission are among the unknowns of "the AIDS virus."

If HIV-1 or HIV-2 really do promote the HIV/AIDS infection curve, then they are among the most fickle, let alone mysterious, of disease-causing agents known to man.

For, as of 1990, it could be said of the presumed central role player, HIV-1, that:

51

-- While it may be recovered from most (but by no means all) AIDS patients, and while the blood of most (but by no means all) AIDS patients tests positive for HIV antibodies,[17,18,23,69,78,79] nonetheless:

-- Large proportions of people who test positive for "AIDS virus" antibodies have no AIDS disease and have been "incubating" "the AIDS virus" for considerable periods of time.[1,2,3,4,5,15,25,48,80,81]

-- Despite various estimates of quick death from "fast AIDS" and various estimates as to how long "full-blown" AIDS patients will survive, a growing number of terminal AIDS and advanced ARC-level patients are surviving well beyond normal spans of time, virtually all of them doing so on "unorthodox" programs, or programs of mixed "unorthodox" and "orthodox" therapies.[95,96]

-- Actual HIV virus often cannot be found in HIV antibody positive people, and in some cases the virus itself may be present and later not be present.[101,102]

-- Despite statistical correlations between HIV and male homosexuality in the Western World, HIV infection occurs in the Western World among heterosexuals as well, and anal intercourse may not be a factor in this occurrence.[48,49,50]

-- "AIDS virus" antibodies and AIDS itself are statistically highly correlated to homosexual activity in males in the U.S.A. yet fully half or more of the Africans, Haitians and others in whom HIV is said to flourish are either heterosexuals or women or both.[6,7,8,9,10,76]

-- "AIDS virus" has been isolated from blood, sweat, tears, semen, urine, breast milk, cerebrospinal fluid, lymph nodes, saliva, bone marrow, heart and brain tissue, yet seems relatively difficult to transmit,[17,19,20,21,22,23,24,74,83] leading to the officially adopted position in the U.S.A. that "casual contact does not spread AIDS."

-- There are instances in which "the AIDS virus" is recoverable from the body but the blood remains negative for antibody[12,13,14,15,16] though it is now understood antibodies may not appear for months or even years.

-- The period of incubation may range from as few as six days to several years to a lifetime.[1,27,28,29,30,82] Therefore, it cannot precisely be determined if and when a person is infectious. Orthodoxy considers any "HIV-positive" person to be potentially infectious.

--   In the natural history of HIV and progression to intermediate stages and actual AIDS in groups of AIDS carriers, there are huge time lapses between presumed infection and development of symptoms, due not only to the groups of infectees but to other unknown factors.

--   There is little or no correlation between antibodies to "the AIDS virus" and Kaposi's sarcoma in Africa, at least the "classical" variety thereof (KS being a potentially lethal form of crypto-cancer which frequently[9,11] strikes AIDS victims in the U.S.A., particularly male homosexuals.) And even in the U.S., it was learned in 1990 that KS may not be "AIDS" at all! [see Chapter Two].

--   At present, a positive blood test for HIV antibodies cannot tell a person if he actually has the virus, or is going to develop an AIDS-related disease; conversely, a negative blood test cannot prove the individual is not harboring the virus or will not contract it in the future,[12,13,14,16] leading to speculation as to just how valuable the various serological assays for "the AIDS virus" really are.

--   Patients or others who carry the immunological alterations, particularly an inversion in the T4 ("helper") and T8 ("suppressor") lymphocytes, usually associated with AIDS, may have antibody-negative HIV blood tests.[29,31,32]

--   Patients or others with positive HIV blood tests may have no such T-cell inversion.[3,30]

--   Only some of a group of persons receiving transfusions of blood allegedly contaminated with HIV eventually became seropositive for HIV.[25]

--   None of 22 HIV seropositive recipients of factor VIII (blood product) patients in a U.S. study[70] developed full-blown AIDS even though several developed ARC.

--   Only some of a group of women receiving semen from an HIV infected donor (for artificial insemination) became HIV positive.[33]

--   Only some spouses and some children of HIV infected heterosexual males had positive HIV antibody tests.[49]

--   There are instances, particularly in end-stage AIDS, when neither "the AIDS virus" nor HIV antibody is recoverable from body tissues,[17] although this may be explained by the virus' apparent ability to demolish part of the immune system and remove all traces of the destruction (namely, the T4 cells).

-- So far, inoculations of animals with human HIV have been unable to transmit the actual disease[34] except to chimpanzees, where the illness is mild and not fatal. HIV successfully infected rabbits and mice in 1988.[121,122]

-- The structure of "the AIDS virus" can change as it is passed from one person to another.[35,36]

-- The ability of HIV to constantly mutate and protect itself from immune surveillance mechanisms greatly complicates the development of a vaccine.[37] It reproduces 100 to 1,000 times faster than similar viruses.[77]

-- While semen-to-blood and blood-to-blood (and, by implication, blood-to-semen) seem to be primary routes of transmission for HIV, AIDS has also been associated in some areas with parasites and "insect vectors"[38,39] and may invade the central nervous system directly.[40,41,42,43,44]

-- The "insect vectors" hypothesis is said not to have held up to closer scrutiny so far.[120]

-- HIV infections in health care workers, while extremely rare, may only lead to transient symptoms.[27,45]

-- Antibody to the virus has been known to appear and disappear in healthy people.[46,47,119]

Each new revelation about HIV -- or, more appropriately, a whole family of similar viruses -- has been like peeling off one more layer of an onion only to discover yet another layer.

Some of the above cited mysteries about HIV -- particularly as to when antibodies form, when viral antigens may appear, and what they mean -- were both solved and others created by an important 1989 study by David Imigawa *et al.* The UCLA research[123] which tracked the blood changes of homosexual men still engaging in risky sexual practices found that actual antibodies to HIV may not appear for up to *three years* following infection. This meant that the vaunted "window period" between when an individual allegedly is infected and when antibodies appear is much longer than earlier estimated -- a reality which placed into question the safety of blood donations from many "high risk" people and did nothing to solve the issue of whether such "silent infections" are capable of being transmitted.

Dana-Farber Cancer Institute AIDS researcher William Haseltine noted[124] that the new findings were "both encouraging and disquieting" and that "the observation that in some people the infection is controlled at least for a time, or silent infections are established, suggests that it may be possible to suppress the expression of the virus." And there is the matter of how many T4 cells HIV allegedly infects, and what infection means. While earlier research suggested that the infection rate was 1 in every 10,000 to 100,000 T4 lymphocytes, a 1989 study led by Steven M. Schnittman of the National Institute of Allergy and Infectious Disease found[133] that in a patient with active AIDS, HIV can infect 1 percent (that is, 1 of every 100) of the T4 cells. The higher the "virus load," the more difficult it is to develop a therapy to knock out the virus, according to the current wisdom. (This does not answer the question whether HIV in infected cells is active or dormant.)

More and more ways to "find" HIV -- whole virus, particles (virions, antigens), sophisticated antibody tests -- were developed as scientific industry moved into high gear. Though voices of caution were still questioning single-mode causality, the Western allopathic paradigm, viral subdivision, went charging ahead.

HIV could be found in a tremendous range of human tissues. The fact that levels of HIV-1 were found to be "much higher than previous estimates" in plasma and the cells of peripheral blood,[134] and that these levels seemed to be predictive of clinical disease together with declining "helper" T4 cells[135] led the traditionalist *New England Journal of Medicine* (through AIDS researchers David Baltimore and Mark B. Feinberg) to muse that "although the data should dispel any lingering doubts about whether HIV is the true culprit in AIDS, they are silent about matters crucial to understanding the details of viral transmission."[136] This was, at best, an understatement.

In 1990, the pharmaceutical firm Upjohn brought together a wide array of scientists and investigators for a multidisciplinary symposium. Its results, as parlayed through the establishmentarian *Journal* of the American Medical Assn., could have been titled "We Still Don't Understand."

Despite copious information available on every facet of HIV, said Upjohn Cancer and Infectious Diseases

Research Unit Director Wendell Wierenga: "... we still can't explain the full depletion of CD4 ["helper" cells] in AIDS patients."

And the "transcription complex .. is still an enigma ... we still don't understand what controls processing and how protease [an enzyme said to be involved in the process whereby HIV utilizes reverse transcriptase] acts where it acts..."

More baffling, after outlining various systems proposed and in use for "clinically staging" HIV infection, the research consensus was "we still don't have any useful staging system or markers for disease progression."[137]

By 1990, many mainstream researchers, who had been committed to the HIV-as-the-single-cause-of-AIDS theory, were beginning to backtrack sufficiently to speak of "co-factors" as necessary in explaining HIV's capability to do such damage in some people over a short period of time and leave others seemingly untouched for years. (Our original monograph, *AIDS: TERROR, TRUTH, TRIUMPH,* published in 1986, was among the first papers which called into question the monofactoriality of AIDS causation. But various holistically minded physicians and researchers, well credentialed to do so, also doubted a new virus could be the single culprit.)

From the beginning of the announcement of the HIV connection to AIDS, numerous researchers had been wary about jumping to ipso facto conclusions.

Assessing serological evaluations of 2,000 residents of the United Kingdom, R. Cheingsong-Popov *et al.* in 1984 found that although "these data confirm the close association between HTLV-III and AIDS and PGL [persistent generalized lymphadenopathy] and show that infection with HTLV-III is also prevalent in the populations in whom these syndromes are most likely to develop ... it would be unwise to presume that AIDS will necessarily develop in seropositive subjects."[57]

Dr Jay A. Levy, University of California-San Francisco, commenting[25] on the peculiarities of HIV, stressed that virtually every AIDS-virus isolate is unique because of the virus' "uncanny" ability to generate variants, a point of view now held to be obvious.

Researchers from Litton Bionetics, Walter Reed Army Institute of Research and the National Cancer Institute, who literally tore apart the genetic code of virus strains isolated from AIDS and pre-AIDS patients, found what the *Wall Street Journal* termed[37] a "striking degree of genetic variation" which is the "characteristic and prominent feature of the AIDS viruses."

Their combined report, said the *WSJ*, "raises the troubling question of whether the virus, through its ability to mutate, possesses a Houdini-like immunologic escape" feature allowing it both to avoid the body's immunological defense mechanisms and drugs administered as preventive treatments.

WSJ quoted Flossie Wong-Stahl of NCI who pointed out that the greatest genetic diversity is located in the gene for the virus' outer "protein envelope" or coat, an essential ingredient in the body's ability to recognize and then destroy the virus. She said that HIV is more similar to "lentiviruses" -- slow viruses that affect certain animals, particularly visna virus in sheep [see Chapter Five] -- than any other kind of virus. (There is one allegation [see Chapter Eleven] that visna virus was used in the man-made creation of "the AIDS virus".)

There were diversities, researchers indicated, between the HTLV-III, isolated in the U.S.A., and LAV, isolated in France, and yet another, the ARV, isolated in California. Yet by 1986 these differences were sufficiently resolved in favor of one major virus -- HIV.

Just how HIV was isolated, who really found it first (and who or what should reap benefits from HIV antibody test kits) was a behind-the-scenes dispute of scientific arrogance and greed at its worst, only some of which has bobbed to the surface.

In 1989, British television journalist Jad Adams, in a book which seemed designed to ruffle allopathic feathers, *AIDS: The HIV Myth*,[138] described the whole shoddy affair, and none of the principals come out untarnished. Damningly, he noted that the AIDS researchers were not looking for a cause -- they were looking for a virus. They found one, or maybe two.

But aside from bird-dogging the notion of an "AIDS virus", the gang-up on Africa as a source of the infection (a likelihood ever more remote), the in-fighting between the American cancer establishment and France's Pasteur Institute, Adams came up with perhaps the most important fact:

The French homosexual from whom the Montagnier group originally isolated "LAV" in 1982 (and which virus may have been the real, genuine, first "HIV") had been found to be alive and well in 1988, or 6 years later! While Western orthodoxy trumpeted the certainty of death from "HIV infection," the individual from whom the alleged causative agent was first isolated was alive and well. Of course, with an ever-lengthening "incubation period" for the allegedly tricky, sinister, murdering virus, anything is possible. . .

A constantly-mutating virus with a "Houdini-like" escape mechanism and which can constantly change its "costume", while greatly complicating the search for a vaccine, does not entirely rule out the possibility of one, yet most investigators agree the development of such a "cross-reactive" vaccine is years away.

Research into HIV persistently has come up with *more* mystifying news about this will-o'-the-wisp structure:

It is now known that HIV not only decidedly infects the "helper" T4 cells (the inversion between T4:T8 lymphocytes, the T8s increasing and then declining as T4s continue to decrease to the vanishing point) but that AIDS patients may already have a missing or inactive subset of these cells[53,54].

Whether HIV selectively targets not only T4 cells in general but a special group of them must be considered. (As we comment elsewhere, T4:T8 alterations are also known to be caused by other viruses and other conditions).

By 1986, researchers were able to announce[75] that the specifics of how HIV targets T4 cells had been determined (the viral protein gp110 binds to the T4 protein on T4 cells). (How HIV attacks other cells has been the subject of much advanced research since that time, with key mysteries still outstanding, particularly as to HIV infectability from cell to cell or as extracellular virus.)

By 1987, it was clear that, despite or perhaps because of the onrushing information about HIV, the submicroscopic structure posed more questions than answers.

And open war had erupted between researchers even within the allopathic model: Berkeley molecular biologist Peter Duesberg, an expert in retrovirology, forthrightly denied that HIV could cause AIDS, and other researchers began looking more seriously for co-factors, suspecting that HIV at least alone could not be doing all that it was said to be doing, with the U.S.' Robert Gallo, "co-discoverer" of HIV, blasting the idea that HIV is *not* the cause of AIDS as "crazy."

But by 1988, even Gallo -- who had admitted the year before on a television program that syphilis, endemic to the central African areas where HIV is also thought to be endemic, might be a co-factor -- wrote (with Luc Montagnier, isolator of LAV in France) that:

"Although HIV kills T4 cells directly, it has become clear that the direct killing of these cells is not sufficient to explain the depletion seen in AIDS. Indirect mechanisms must be at work."[84]

Faced with the growing anecdotal evidence that HIV/AIDS acts very differently in people in the matter of whether or not they are infected, the extent to which they are infected, the time of onset of symptoms, the severity of symptoms -- all grist for the multifactorial model of HIV/AIDS causation and management, yet not well grasped by the allopathic thought process -- Gallo and Montagnier also concluded:

"Although it is clear that a large enough dose of the right strain of HIV can cause AIDS on its own, co-factors can clearly influence the progression of the disease. People whose immune systems are weakened before HIV infection may progress toward AIDS more quickly than others ... Interaction with other pathogens may increase the likelihood that AIDS will develop." This was a monumental shift in concept since the earlier AIDS years.

In fact, at the Fifth International AIDS Conference in Montreal in 1989, Gallo stated flatly that other viruses are known to act as co-factors.[125] He cited his earlier announced HTLV-1 virus, another virus (papovavirus JC) linked to progressive multifocal leukoencephalopathy (one of the neurological complications of AIDS) and the newly discovered human herpesvirus-6 (HHV-6). The latter, he said, might infect as much as 70 percent of the U.S. population.

Further complicating the quest for the presumed agents of AIDS were announcements of new human herpesviruses said to be "tropic" for human T lymphocytes[126] and the delineation of subtypes of HIV, with such subtypes said to help determine the prognosis of AIDS and of death from the disease.[127]

By 1989, researchers doubting that HIV alone could cause AIDS included not only Duesberg (and the AIDS-as-syphilis doctors) but also Harvard Nobel laureate Dr. Walter Gilbert, while Dr. Joseph Sonnabend continued to insist on a multifactorial model for AIDS causation. As research writer Clemmer Mayhew III belled the cat:

"(HIV) was quickly embraced during the Reagan administration as the primary causative factor of what is called acquired immune deficiency syndrome. Fueled by a race for millions of dollars in medical research money, grants and prizes, scientific fact has been subject to deregulation and consensus.

"There are certain undisputed facts that the general public keeps forgetting. Many AIDS patients die without ever testing positive for the virus. All chimpanzees inoculated with the AIDS virus during the past two years have not developed AIDS. Inhalation is the primary path of all pneumonia..."[132]

The primacy of HIV as the sole cause of AIDS is primarily vital to two schools of though in the controversy -- the "establishment" position, which is erecting a huge industry around HIV; and the AIDS-as-end-of-civilization doomsayers for whom the unstoppable, allegedly manmade virus represents the true finale of humankind.

We are not belittling here either position -- only pointing out that the argument is *not* closed.

Scientists at the National Cancer Institute and Chester Beatty Laboratories earlier detected neutralizing antibodies against HIV.[36] And cases in which HIV antibody appeared and disappeared while the carriers stayed healthy[46,47] indicated possible immunological defense within healthy people even against a "Houdini" virus and strongly hinted that exposure need not lead either to disease or to a permanent carrier state.

There may be genetic predispositions to explain why some people are infected by HIV, and others are not. Two kinds of white blood cells called "human leukocyte antigen" (HLA) -- HLA DR5 and HLA B35 -- have been associated either with Kaposi's sarcoma or HIV/AIDS progression.[105]

Earlier research indicating that a protein called "group complement" is indicative of higher likelihood of

HIV infection has so far not been confirmed. Anecdotal assessments have led some to believe that Orientals are perhaps less succeptible to HIV infection -- if only, epidemiologically speaking as of 1989, because there is so little HIV infection so far in the Orient.

Of the many mysteries concerning HIV, the lack of actual AIDS disease developing within the conservative estimate of, now, many millions of carriers, and the lengthy periods of incubation which may or may not follow such exposure/infection, are among the more salient.

Retrospective analyses of a black American male who died in 1968 have confirmed that he died of causes related to AIDS, that he was positive for HIV or something very much like it 15 years before "the AIDS virus" was discovered.[85] New York retrospective cases suggest that one or two people still alive today may have been incubating HIV since 1974. Research on stored blood in central Africa has indicated the existence of HIV at least as early as 1959[97] and 1972.[86] The latter case involved school children who were apparently free from disease.

The Venezuelan study reported November 16, 1985,[2] found HIV antibodies in serum samples collected from 224 aboriginal Amazonian Indians, with three of the sera having been collected in 1968. "All individuals tested were apparently healthy at the time of the study," reported Luis Rodriguez *et al.* They noted that HIV or a "closely related cross-reactive virus" may be endemic in the area and stressed its presence in non-negroid Latin America.

The Venezuelan Indians, then, may have been harboring the virus since *at least* 1968, and, when this was reported in 1985, still had no disease -- that is, 17 years *later.*

Some investigators now feel that both the ubiquity of malaria and parasites in parts of central Africa and elsewhere in the tropics might account for some "false positive" HIV tests.

This explanation might undercut the findings of alleged HIV in stored blood from Africa dating back 30 years, and possibly that of the Venezuelan aborigines, but it is difficult to state that HIV was not present in 1968, when -- apparently -- the first American died of AIDS-like conditions, for both the clinical features and the finding of HIV in the blood are parallel.

All of these various laboratory results cry out for clarification: are the tests not really very good (as was the case with some African HTLV-1 and HIV "positives" later determined to be "negatives"?[106,107]) Is HIV positivity so fickle it may simply be a marker for malaria and parasites? Can it really, truly, be the *cause* of HIV/AIDS? Is it a "marker", a "passenger" or simply inconsequential?

At the Fourth International Conference on AIDS in 1988, researchers reported[100] that actual AIDS is unlikely to develop sooner than 12 months after "seroconversion" (the blood turning positive for antibodies), that almost 80 percent of HIV-infected people are free of actual AIDS for up to 60 months following exposure.

This jibes with the updated San Francisco "cohort" study of San Francisco homosexual males followed since the advent of a hepatitis B vaccine study. Some 23 percent of these were reported by 1989 to have survived symptom-free for an estimated 11 years.[128] It also jibes with the aforementioned UCLA study (Imigawa) indicating that it might take as long as 3 years for antibodies to appear. The larger the "cohort" studied, the more long-term symptom-free infected people there are.

In terms of incubation, it became common wisdom in 1988/1989 to speak of an HIV "incubation period" of "at least" 14 years -- the assumption being that persons whose blood (on retrospect) bad HIV antibodies as early as 1977 must have had those antibodies since at least 1974 or 1975 -- and it might take "at least" 10 years for symptoms to appear.

As we noted in Chapter Two, a British estimate was that the larger the "cohort" studied, the fewer the amount of patients showing symptoms, so that in most of such cluster studies, as of 1988, 50 percent or fewer had symptoms. This led to the conclusion that some HIV infectees might remain "symptom-free for the whole of their natural lifespan."[82]

Indeed, HIV co-discoverer/designator Gallo covered his retrospective bets in 1988 by noting[84] that "it was tentatively concluded that HIV has infected human beings for more than 20 years but less than 100."

Some cynics might suggest that such mystifying data suggest a virus in search of a disease, or the development of *reductio ad absurdum* in wondering when AIDS might spring form an HIV infection, real or imagined.

At the outside, then, HIV incubation may be a matter of many years.

On the other hand, as the 1985 Cooper study in Australia, showed[30], in one case an incubation period of *six days* followed presumed exposure to what the researchers called ARV (AIDS-associated retrovirus), one of three names for what the American government researchers, at least, believed to be one and the same virus. In three other subjects in the Sydney AIDS Study Group analysis, "seroconversion" occurred 19, 32, and 56 days after the onset of acute symptoms.

By September 1985, Centers for Disease Control (CDC) investigators admitted to broad ranges of incubation.[1]

They noted that the virus "has been isolated months to years after the onset of symptoms from 85 percent or more of seropositive individuals with AIDS, lymphadenopathy, or other associated conditions",[60,61,62] that in investigations of cases of transfusion-associated AIDS, HIV was isolated from 22 of 23 seropositive blood donors an average of 28 months after the implicated donations,[68] and, intriguingly, that all but one of the high-risk donors were without symptoms at the time of the donations, and 15 of 22 of them remained so when the virus was isolated from 1 to 4 years later.

HIV was also isolated from the blood of eight of 12 homosexual males who had been symptomless while seropositive for from 4 to 69 months.[69] Curran *et al.* then noted that earlier studies estimated the mean incubation period for transfusion-associated AIDS to be 4.5 years and the average interval between seroconversion and diagnosis of AIDS in homosexual men exceeded 3 years.[1]

Once a person is diagnosed with "full-blown" AIDS, the general theory is that he has little time to live, despite the growing numbers of "anecdotal" case histories of long-term survivors. By the end of the decade, life extensions were attributed to earlier drug intervention, particularly against Kaposi's sarcoma and Pneumocystis pneumonia, and the pattern was emerging of a slowly debilitating chronic infection whose endpoint nonetheless is death.

A study of 526 AIDS patients at a New York City hospital, presented at the Fourth International AIDS Conference in 1988,[99] showed that survival depended largely on the kind of "opportunistic infection" under treatment: Kaposi's sarcoma cases had the longest median survivals (14 months), and tuberculosis-associated cases the worst (4 months.) Neither this group of cases nor rapidly developing caseloads elsewhere reflect the life extensions being reported through the use of one or more "unauthorized" drugs, or the survival rates on eclectic/holistic programs (Chapter Thirteen).

With, now, the presumption of massive infection of HIV in Africa with only a limited -- but growing -- number of actual AIDS cases in that area, the link between "the virus" -- if indeed there is only one and if indeed it is the trigger, catalyst or cause -- is only a few levels beyond circumspect.

The earlier Curran report, and others, admitted to no end of puzzlement over African AIDS. Citing an earlier study in 1985, it noted that "..antibody was reported to have been in 75 serum samples collected from healthy children in Uganda as early as 1972 and 1973. Since AIDS has not been reported from Uganda, the interpretation of this finding is unclear."

Particularly unclear, one might add, unless either the virus referred to is not HIV or is a mutant form of it that is not dangerous, or the virus, or viruses, are not particularly damaging in otherwise healthy people,or the viruses simply do not, in and of themselves, cause AIDS. (There is also the question of how much re-use of hypodermic needles in African clinics -- and elsewhere -- may be a factor in viral spread[67,68].)

As we point out at several points, some investigators from the very beginning doubted how HIV acting alone could in and of itself (themselves) cause AIDS. The general opinion among these multifactorialists was that, at least in the cases seen in the U.S.A., an AIDS patient needed to be severely immunocompromised, actually "sick", before the virus could actually "take".

Malcolm Martin, MD, chief, Laboratory of Molecular Microbiology of the National Institute of Allergy and Infectious Diseases, noted[24]that "a lot of us working in this field suspect that the virus isn't highly contagious. We think there are a lot of defective particles. We know from epidemiologic evidence that multiple contacts are needed to make a 'hit'; that is, to induce antibody.

"I suspect that either the virus isn't terribly contagious or that there are multiple defective forms of the virus and it takes a lot of virus to get a fully infectious agent ... It's not like contagious viruses, such as influenza or poliomyelitis, which can spread like wildfire among susceptible populations. It's relatively hard to acquire the disease naturally ... This ... doesn't mean that one couldn't get the disease from a single sexual encounter with someone who had AIDS or by receiving a single unit of blood that has the virus in it...."

And, one should understand, Dr. Martin was discussing the presumed sexual mode of transmission almost exclusively.

HIV's now well known modus operandi is its making of a copy of its genome (genetic structure) and inserting that copy of its viral RNA (ribonucleic acid) in the form of DNA (deoxyribonucleic acid) into the chromosomes of the infected cell--usually the T4 "helper" cells, but also into other kinds of cells. Being a "retrovirus" -- or RNA-containing -- the structure needs the activity of the enzyme reverse transcriptase, hence giving rise to some therapies which seek to suppress the action of that enzyme.

The insertion of HIV genetic material into a T4, or any other cell, is the equivalent of the "hijacking" of that cell. For, over time and due to factors only guessed at by researchers, HIV may lie dormant in an infected cell or start "replicating" until the cell itself becomes a factory producing carbon copies of the invader.

The history of HIV now indicates that the virus may infect other cells including the macrophage/monocyte part of the immune system, where it can in effect "hide out" and escape immune surveillance -- a reason some people may test "false negative" on an antibody test.

Even so, the big questions are why there is such immune devastation when HIV actually infects only a small number of T4 cells, what factors allow HIV to gain entry, what factors determine whether and how long it is dormant, when and how it will start to "replicate." There are also differences of opinion as to how much HIV infection is cell-to-cell or by "free virus."

The central insidious feature of HIV remains its affinity for that very part of the immune system (T4 or "helper" cells) which is designed to inhibit viral invaders. If someone had wished to design a submicroscopic biological warfare weapon he could not have done better than HIV.

The presence of HIV is detected by various antibody tests. Antibodies, produced by the immune system in response to the virus or parts of it (antigen), may not occur for 3 to 12 weeks or up to three years following exposure, and then the tests may be misleading. The common antibody test is ELISA (enzyme-linked immunosorbent assay), and it is usually confirmed by the more specific Western Blot test.

More experimentally, there are the RIPA (based on radioisotopes) and indirect immunofluorescence assays. There are increasingly fewer "false positives" and "false negatives", according to health authorities, but even so a variety of other conditions (particularly other infections) can "throw off" these tests.

A blood test to detect the HIV envelope protein antigen (gp120) has found HIV presence as early as 2 weeks after exposure. Part of the HIV virus (antigen p24) may be "captured" by a monoclonal or polyclonal antibody test. A 10-minute SUDS (single-unit diagnostic system) test is in the offing.

There also are methods of "culturing" whole virus of parts of it out of blood. By 1988 the polymerase chain reaction (PCR) experimental test was said to be able to detect HIV infection even months before antibodies appeared and when P24 viral antigen and other tests were negative.[117] (To these, the experimental French R-HEV and the U.S. HIV-AG assays have recently been added.)

Parallel to tests for HIV antibodies, whole virus or viral particles is the standard immune panel test -- with the absolute numbers of T4 ("helper") cells, and to a lesser degree, the ratio between helpers and T8s ("suppressors") being of prime importance. Consistently falling T4 numbers are suggestive (but not confirmatory) of HIV/AIDS infection.

(The research frustration over predictability values of various immune responses in HIV/AIDS patients has led some clinicians and researchers, as we will see, to disregard T-cell tests almost completely. A University of California-San Francisco study suggested[118] that beta-2 microglobulin (B2) and HIV p24 antigen tests are independent and better predictors of AIDS than are T4 counts and are comparable predictors of progression from ARC to AIDS.)

T4s are the major targets of HIV infection (along with the central nervous system) but there is no clear picture of exactly how HIV, striking in varying and small amounts, can actually obliterate the body's ongoing supply of these immune-system cells.

Laboratory experiments suggest that there are other ways large amounts of T4 cells might be destroyed (the formation of many merged cells, or syncytia, stimulated by a particular action of HIV, being one). Redfield noted [115] that HIV "replication" in infected cells may increase when these cells become activated for various reasons, as when they take part in an immune response either to HIV itself or to other viruses in other cells.

"Thus the very process that should defeat HIV -- an immune response -- has the diabolical effect of increasing the proliferation of the virus," he wrote. He also described a method by which "free viral gp 120" -- parts of HIV -- may circulate in blood and lymph and bind to uninfected T4 cells causing them to provoke an attack on themselves by the immune system.

These various methods of seeming trickery and connivance by HIV are laboratory experiments; it remains to be demonstrated that they actually occur in the body.

In viral infections, the indication the body is producing antibodies is generally a sign the host is mounting a successful challenge to the invader. Yet this is held not to be so in the matter of HIV, at least by the majority of AIDS researchers committed to the single-cause theory.

Dr. B. Frank Polk of Johns Hopkins, commenting [116] on an ongoing 8-year study, said in 1987 that "I suspect that the antibody response early in the course of infection probably is protective." The Boston research indicates that patients with low levels of antibodies to HIV are five times as likely as those with high levels to come down with AIDS within 15 months.

It was brought to our attention several times that "high-risk" people might "test negative" for HIV several times within a year and still suddenly come down with "full-blown AIDS." In one case, a New York patient in ordinarily good health before and "testing negative" twice on ELISA tests during 1987 suddenly entered the hospital in

December of that year with Pneumocystis pneumonia. Only weeks later his blood revealed a low level of antibodies to HIV.

In his case and that of many others, negativity for HIV (either because the virus was "hiding" in macrophages or the tests are not particularly meaningful anyway) was no indication he was not already well into the HIV/AIDS infection curve.

Attacking HIV is, among many other things, made all the more difficult by the fact that the same carrier may harbor multiple forms of the virus, and, in contrast to other retroviruses, this particular one is "very heterogeneous" in genomic structure (Martin) with its various genes being "very unstable."

It has also been found that if any one of the genes unique to HIV is defective, the virus cannot replicate, yet inactive genes in one virus may be replaced by active genes in another virus, a virological process called "complementation."[24]

Even if HIV makes a "hit", it is now obvious that AIDS may not develop.

The first reported case of appearing-and-disappearing HIV antibodies was reported in October 1985.[47] The wife of a hemophiliac patient who apparently contracted AIDS from blood-clotting products (and later died of *Pneumocystis carinii*) underwent a blood test in January 1984 in which she was both positive for HIV antibody and had a slightly depressed T4:T8 ratio. Yet four months later there were no HIV antibodies nor was her immune system depressed.

Dr. William Robinson, a Stanford specialist in infectious diseases and one of the authors of the report, was succinct: "I think this was a perfectly healthy woman with a normally functioning immune system who became infected with the virus and then recovered." The case was followed up in 1987;[87] the woman still had no HIV antibodies.

In 1987, researchers at Johns Hopkins Hospital were studying "at least three people" who had tested negative for HIV after earlier repeated retesting had produced positive results. The Hopkins study individuals had not developed any of the life-threatening infections or cancers associated with AIDS, and Dr. Homaycon Farzadegan said: "The tests were quite accurate. In fact, we've ruled out the possibility of a laboratory mix-up."[119]

Robert C. Gallo, MD, credited with isolating HTLV-III in the U.S.A. as "the AIDS virus",[17] based his work on studies of the earlier defined T-lymphotropic retroviruses HTLV-I and HTLV-II which, as we have noted, have important divergences from HIV. HTLV, which some researchers believe to be a family of related T-cell lymphotropic retroviruses, is the first class of viruses specifically correlated to human cancer (namely, rare forms of leukemia).[17,53] Again, correlation is one thing -- causality another.

Because it is similar to, but far from being, HTLV-III, the prototypical virus HTLV-I was of considerable interest to Gallo and other researchers. The epidemiology of HTLV-I has greatly colored the notion of the now questionable "African genesis" of HIV.

From studies in Africa, it was believed that HTLV-I originally infected one species of monkey but later was transmitted to humans, that it spread to Japan in the 16th century through the black servants of Portuguese traders and to other parts of the world through the slave trade. Because this particular form of potential leukemia may take up to 30 years to develop, if it develops at all, control measures are obviously challenged.

The *Wall Street Journal* reported in late 1985[55] that in the process of tracking down "the AIDS virus" researchers found higher-than-expected numbers of male homosexuals and drug addicts in America who had been exposed to the leukemia virus; that is, HTLV-I is appearing with more frequency in the "risk" populations also targeted by HIV. It was obvious by 1990 that large segments of the human population are "carrying" HIV-I and HTLV-II (especially prostitutes and drug addicts) but most of them are not dying of leukemia, on anything else "caused" by these viruses.

Most importantly, HTLV-I is able -- in *in vitro* tests under certain circumstances -- to transform normal T cells. The widespread African connection in HTLV-I[17,54,55] is the dominant factor in the geographical linkage of the alleged migration of HIV -- a linkage now considerably in question.

For, as Hunsmann *et al.*, have shown,[51] although sub-Saharan Africa is an endemic area for HTLV-I, "the data suggest that HTLV-III was rare in Africa until recently, and still is rare in much of the continent. It would seem that the epidemic of AIDS started at about the same time as, or even later than, epidemics in America and Europe. Our results do not support the hypothesis that HTLV-III virus originated in Africa."

Nonetheless, it is now the standard view that AIDS "suddenly appeared" at about the same time (late 1970s) in the U.S.A., Caribbean and sub-Saharan Africa.

Nor do all researchers leap to the conclusion of the connections between the "three HTLVs." Assessing the other HTLV viruses in the United Kingdom, Tedder *et al.* found that "infection by HTLV-I and HTLV-II retroviruses thus occurs more frequently in ELAS (extended lympha-denopathy) patients and drug addicts than in the U.K. population as a whole, but the low prevalence of these infections in ELAS and AIDS patients indicates that these two strains of lymphotropic retroviruses have no aetiological role in ELAS and AIDS."[58]

And a study of 440 AIDS patients reported by Robert-Guroff *et al.* summarized that "although HTLV-I-specific antibodies are more prevalent in AIDS patients than in healthy U.S. donors, the difference is not sufficient to suggest an association of HTLV-I with the disease. The low rate may indicate an opportunistic infection of AIDS patients by HTLV-I, or a crossreaction with the recently described HTLV variant, HTLV-III..."[59]

At the University of California-Los Angeles, investigators following a group of male homosexuals at high risk for AIDS reported in October 1985 that two patterns of T4 cell activity were seen in the seropositive groups -- in one, low normal values were maintained (paralleled by limited evidence of clinical deterioration) while in the others (persons who advanced to actual AIDS) T4 cell counts fell progressively.

"These observations suggest that another factor(s), besides HTLV-III/LAV infection, is needed for substantial lowering of T4 cell levels and progression to the full-blown AIDS," they wrote.[32]

Archer and Glinsmann pointed out[71] that although attention to immunostimulation to halt destruction of the T4 subset by HIV should be a part of therapy and prevention, the increase in the T8 population "should not be treated lightly or overlooked."

They suggested that, while increases in T8 populations are characteristic of many infections, HIV, in addition
to destroying T4 cells, may be responsible for an expansion
of T8 cells, particularly the T8Leu7 subpopulation, which
"makes the host more permissive for the effects of HTLV-
III."[72]

But in some cases elevated T8s seem to be associated with a symptom-free state, as our Mexican
research group found. *In vitro* research also suggests
this.[102]

San Francisco AIDS researcher Jay Levy has been
pre-eminent not only in earlier defense of the possible multifactoriality of predisposing AIDS factors but also in indicating the possible HIV-blocking effects of the T8 or
"suppressor" cells. He reported[129] in 1989 that "further
work has shown that only HIV-infected individuals have
[suppressor] cells that can suppress virus replication in infected cells. One mechanism for this antiviral effect is the
production by CD8+ cells of a lymphokine whose structure
is not yet defined. ... Most asymptomatic subjects, in contrast to patients with AIDS, require only low numbers of
[suppressor] cells to control HIV replication by cultured
cells . . . The extent of anti-HIV suppression probably
depends on the intrinsic function of a selected subgroup of
the CD8+ cell population."

If there is a self-destruct mechanism inherent in
HIV infection (by some kind of action by the "suppressor" or
T8 cells) this is a bit of virological good news. Levy added
that "the individual who can maintain a resistant state in
which HIV production in the body can be suppressed can
expect a relatively asymptomatic course and even a return
of CD4+ (T4 or 'helper') lymphocytes to near-normal
numbers."

But no one at this writing knew what factors might
be involved in such suppressor activity.

On a gloomier note, researcher Bani Bolognesi at
Duke University at about the same time assessed[130] the
series of HIV-connected immunological events this way:

"As the immune response intensifies, viral activity is
suppressed and remains so throughout the asymptomatic
phase of the infection. However, several unique properties
of HIV, notably its ability to spread by cell-to-cell transmission, its capacity to diversify in the face of an immune

response, and its potential for suppressing immune function, gradually tip the balance in favor of the virus."

All such assessments depend, again, on the assumption of HIV as the single cause of AIDS.

The major challenge to the HIV etiology of AIDS was mounted in 1987 by molecular biologist Peter H. Duesberg of the University of California.

His main arguments have been[88,89,90,91] that HIV as a single cause of HIV/AIDS violates the so-called Koch postulates three different ways. Most importantly, AIDS as free virus, provirus or viral RNA cannot be detected in all cases and cannot be isolated in from 20 to 50 percent of AIDS cases. Even antibodies often do not appear in HIV/AIDS cases.

He argued that HIV is not biochemically active in the syndrome for which it is named, that it cannot affect sufficient T4 cells at any given time to pose a meaningful challenge to immunity, that "it is paradoxical that HIV is said to cause AIDS only after the onset of antiviral immunity ... because most other viruses are not pathogenic before immunity," that "the long and highly variable intervals between the onset of antiviral immunity and AIDS, averaging 8 years, are bizarre for a virus that replicates within 1 to 2 days in tissue culture and induces antiviral immunity within 1 to 2 months after an acute infection."

In essence, Duesberg was saying that the emperor has no clothes, and the American medical establishment was quick to attack him, usually arguing simply that the molecular biologist who has done major research on retroviruses simply does not understand AIDS. The fact is, he articulated the suspicions of many researchers that HIV is not the cause of HIV/AIDS; at the very least, "the AIDS virus" cannot be working alone.

The "establishment" position[93] is that wherever AIDS breaks out it is still apparently preceded by HIV, that HIV antibodies in blood prepared for transfusions are associated with the HIV/AIDS infection curve later, that AIDS cases on retrospect, through a study of stored blood, normally reveal HIV antibodies.

In truth, the anti-HIV theorists do not fare well in demolishing HIV as an absolutely irrelevant feature in the picture, although they may argue that just because HIV antibodies may be found in blood later found to have infected hemophiliacs or persons who needed blood transfusions, any number of other viruses, antibodies and particles may have been transferred as well.

At the present time, virologists are not of a single mind as to the behavior of, and body reactions to, these tiny parasitical structures, and their mutual name-calling does not resolve any issues.

No small part of the argument revolves around how little is, in fact, known about particles so minuscule that they cannot be seen by regular optical microscopes.

Their presence and actions may be seen by the "scanning electron microscope" but only after they have, in effect, been killed. The behavior of a virus in the test tube, or *in vitro*, is not evidence of what is going on in the body itself -- *in vivo* -- and the fact that a given virus may be "cultured" from human blood outside the body through a series of laboratory procedures is not firm evidence of what is going on within the living organism, either.

Even the fact that particles of HIV seem to be active for a considerable time outside the host has almost nothing to do with how virulent or non-virulent HIV as an intact virus may be within the body.

These nuances and distinctions are normally not relayed through the lay media in dealing with "the AIDS virus" or when describing how someone who has been described as "positive" for antibodies to "the AIDS virus" -- *not* for the virus itself -- is now an "AIDS carrier."

What was known about HIV by 1990 was that it is an incredibly complex structure with affinity for both immunological and neurological cells. Nine genes had been discovered in the structure by molecular biologists as of 1988.

David Baltimore, PhD, a Nobel laureate virologist, described the genome of HIV as "a plethora of little genes" and asked rhetorically: "Why does this virus have so many genes, and what tricks are these genes really allowing the virus to play on the people it affects?" [103]

The variability of "the AIDS virus" was the topic of a meeting held in July 1988 at the National Institutes of Health, Bethesda, MD. The University of Alabama's George Shaw noted that "the data imply that there is no such thing as an 'AIDS virus isolate.' You probably have enormous numbers of slightly different viruses in an individual."[104]

The great variability of HIV makes it difficult to come up with a vaccine let alone a specific drug to kill or inhibit the structure. Yet as devilish at it seems to be, HIV is not perfect. It needs the enzyme reverse transcriptase in order to be able to translate RNA genetic material to DNA. National Institute of Environmental Health Sciences (NIEHS) researchers were on hand at the meeting to note that HIV reverse transcriptase "errs" more often than other reverse transcriptases.

Other scientists at the Bethesda meeting pointed out that in a similar infection -- equine infectious anemia virus (EIAV) in horses -- the host mounts a vigorous antibody defense, the viral infection declines and so do the antibodies.

However, in chimpanzees, the only other animal species in which HIV has so far been successfully inoculated (except for rabbits and mice in 1988 studies), neutralizing antibodies against the same strain have been produced continuously up to 4 years. Humans also apparently are generating antibodies to a parent strain indefinitely. Yet humans may become sick and die, and nothing of consequence happens to chimpanzees.

In the Stanford tests on mice, none of the HIV infected mice showed signs of illness, "a fact that some researchers find curious,"[131] though some of the offspring of these animals developed illnesses similar to the AIDS syndrome in humans, and some died -- "the first time that any animal other than a human has died of an HIV-caused syndrome."

Another challenge to the single etiology theory was proposed by both clinicians and researchers, which also cast doubt as to HIV's importance in HIV/AIDS being much more than that of a "marker": that the full span of HIV/AIDS infection is only a modern expression of syphilis, that the signs and symptoms associated with full-blown AIDS are all historically known to be associated with syphilis.

This West German/American research was gathering adherents in 1989-90, and the treatment of AIDS symptoms with aqueous penicillin and other antibiotics was reportedly lengthening lives (see Chapter Twelve).

There remain other etiological theories as to AIDS as well.

One was raised by physician/researcher Alan Cantwell, MD, who first was particularly smitten by the work of Dr. Virginia Livingston-Wheeler and others and later by the Strecker man-made virus theory. Both these theories are well described in his two excellent AIDS-related books. [108,109]

The Livingston-Wheeler research is the modern-day manifestation of earlier theories that there may be a microscopic, form-changing (pleomorphic) structure which may be at the root of all cancer and possibly of all disease -- but only specialized microscopes can detect this ever-changing, minute germ.

As we note in Chapter Fourteen, San Diego inventor Royal Rife claimed in the 1930s to be able to see "the cancer virus" as well as to be able to kill it with a certain device. Eleanor Alexander-Jackson, Irene Diller, Florence Seibert and Georges Mazet are among scientists who have dedicated much of their professional lives to tracking "the cancer microbe."

Dr. Virginia Livingston-Wheeler baptized [110,111] the form-changing structure with the intriguing name *Progenitor cryptocides* ("ancestral hidden killer") to indicate its coexistence in man from earliest times. It may or may not be what Wilhelm Reich defined as "bions" or Gaston Naessens classed as "somatids." Rife and Naessens developed high-resolution microscopes through which they claimed such disease-causing, ever-changing forms could be seen.

Our Bradford Research Institute darkfield/brightfield fiber-optic microscopic system has also seen things most optical microscopes do not, including waves of ill-defined structures that we have simply defined as "bacteria," particularly swimming in the blood of diseased people. The B.R.I. was also pre-eminent in the world in finding "pleomorphic" forms of *Candida albicans*, the fungus/yeast infection prevalent in HIV/AIDS people, in its body-wide state.

Dr. Cantwell found what he considered to be "bacteria" in Kaposi's sarcoma tissues and in AIDS-infected tissue in general.

With some researchers claiming the presence of a cancer-causing virus as endemic to cancer in general, and cancers of various forms occurring in upwards of a quarter of all AIDS patients, for some investigators it became appropriate to think of AIDS as simply a form of cancer. Other investigators, noting the presence of inexplicable microscopic structures in other diseases, might agree with Dr. Livingston-Wheeler that there was indeed an "ancestral hidden killer" underlying all disease. (All of these are allopathic notions looking for single-mode causes rather than emphasizing the prior disposition of the host in which such microbes, germs or pathogens might or might not flourish.)

Among the many grave difficulties with viral diseases -- which HIV/AIDS is held to be -- is that (a) no viral disease, let alone retroviral disease, has itself ever been "cured" in the full sense of that word; and (b) no non-electron microscope with the possible exception of some new laser-beam devices ever actually "sees" "living" viruses.

The various electron microscopes, up to now the only devices in which viruses can be visually detected, really only "see" dead or immobilized material. At least a version of the Naessens microscope is said still to exist, and pictures of "somatids" have been published. The Naessens microscope is described as using ultraviolet and laser-beam technology.[112]

But until these experimental systems are more commonly in place, and not simply hinted at, no existing optical microscope is capable of "seeing" viruses at work, and virtually all that is known about viruses is derived from laboratory "culturing" of such structures and immune responses to their presumed presence.

It is instructive that the new AIDS parameters announced by the Centers for Disease Control (CDC) in 1987[92] include guidelines to diagnose AIDS even in the absence of HIV positivity -- for antibodies or actual virus -- in lab workups.

In the area of logic, it is easy to see the enormous challenge posed to the accepted dogma of HIV-as-single-cause-of-AIDS by the notion that HIV is not the cause (and therefore billions of dollars in research funds examining every scintilla of, and screening mass populations for antibodies to, this virus have largely been wasted and profits on antibody test kits inappropriately made) or that history's most famous masquerading infection -- altogether curable -- or an "ancestral hidden killer" is the genuine culprit.

Or that Dr. Lo's "mycoplasma incognitus" is, after all,
the villain in the piece.

REFERENCES

(1)   Curran, James W., et al., "The epidemiology of AIDS: status and future prospects." Science, vol. 229:1352-1357, Sept. 27, 1985.

(2)   Rodriguez, Luis, et al., "Antibodies to HTLV-III/ LAV among aboriginal Amazonian Indians in Venezuela." Lancet, Nov. 16, 1985.

(3)   Kestens, Luc, et al., letter, "Absence of immunosuppression in healthy subjects from eastern Zaire who are positive for HTLV-III antibody." N. Eng. J. Med.,v vol. 312, no. 23, June 6, 1985.

(4)   Biggar, Robert J., et al., "Seroepidemiology of HTLV-III antibodies in a remote population of eastern Zaire." Br. Med. Jour., vol. 290, March 16, 1985.

(5)   Dr. William A. Haseltine before Special Hearing for Funding for AIDS, Labor, Health and Human Services, Education Subcommittee, U.S. Congress, Sept. 26, 1985.

(6)   Hunter, Pat, "AIDS variations slow doctors searching for vaccine." Honolulu Advertiser, Feb. 20, 1985.

(7)   Clumeck, Nathan, et al., "Seroepidemiological studies of HTLV-III antibody prevalence among selected groups of heterosexual Africans." J. Am. Med. Assn., 254:18, 2599-2602, Nov. 8, 1985.

(8)   Serwadda D., et al., "Slim disease: a new disease in Uganda and its association with HTLV-III infection." Lancet, Oct. 19, 1985.

(9)   Anderson, R.E., and Jay A. Levy, "Prevalence of antibodies to AIDS-associated retrovirus in single men in San Francisco." Lancet, January 26, 1985.

(10)   Goedert, James J., et al., "Determinants of retrovirus (HTLV-III) antibody and immunodeficiency conditions in homosexual men." Lancet, Sept. 29, 1984.

(11)   Kestens, Luc, et al., "Endemic African Kaposi's sarcoma is not associated with immunodeficiency." Int. J. Cancer 36: 49-54, 1985.

(12)   Budiansky, Stephen, "False test results raise doubts." Nature, vol. 312, Dec. 13, 1985.

(13)   Perkins, Herbert A., "The risk of AIDS from blood transfusion." San. Med., April 1984.

(14)   Salahuddin, S.Z. et al., "HTLV-III in symptom-free seronegative persons." Lancet, Dec. 22/29, 1984.

(15)   Giorgi, J.V. and J.L. Fahey, "Acquired immune deficiency syndrome: effects of HTLV-III on T-cell population." Lab. Management, May 1985.

(16)   Carlson, J.R., et al., "AIDS serology testing in low- and high-risk groups." J. Am. Med. Assn., 254:15, Oct. 18. 1985.

(17)   Broder, Samuel, and Robert C. Gallo, "A pathogenic retrovirus (HTLV-III) linked to AIDS." N. Eng. J. Med., Nov. 5, 1984.

(18)   Sarngadharan, M.G., et al., "Antibodies reactive with human T-lymphotropic retroviruses (HTLV-III) in the serum of patients with AIDS." Science, 224:506-8, 1984.

(19)   Ziegler, John B., et al., "Postnatal transmission of AIDS-associated retrovirus from mother to infant." Lancet, April 20, 1985.

(20)   Zagury, D., et al., "HTLV-III in cells cultured from semen of two patients with AIDS." Science 226:449, 1984.

(21)   Ho, D.D., et al., "HTLV-III in the semen and blood of a healthy homosexual man." Science 226:451, 1984.

(22)   Groopman, J.E., et al., "HTLV-III in saliva of people with AIDS-related complex and healthy homosexual men at risk for AIDS." Science 226:447, 1984.

(23)   Fujikawa, L.S., et al., "Isolation of human T-lymphotropic virus type III from the tears of a patient with the acquired immunodeficiency syndrome." Lancet 2:529, 1985.

(24)   Marwick, Charles, "AIDS-associated virus yields data to intensifying scientific study." J. Am. Med. Assn., 254:20, 2865-2870, 1985.

(25)   Silberner, J., "On the AIDS trail: work continues on test, cure, vaccine." Science News, vol. 27, 1985.

(26)   Fauci, A., "Acquired immunodeficiency syndrome (AIDS) -- an update." Am. Gastroent. Assn. meeting, New York, May 13, 1985.

(27)   Weiss, Stanley H., et al., "HTLV-III infection among health care workers." J. Am. Med. Assn., 245:15, 2089-2093, Oct. 18, 1985.

(28)   Rogers, Martha F., "AIDS in children: a review of the clinical, epidemiologic and public health aspects." Pediatric Infec. Dis., 4:3, 230-236, 1985.

(29)   Ranki, Annamari, et al., "Immunosuppression in homosexual men seronegative for HTLV-III." Ca. Res. (Suppl.) 45, 4616s-4618s, 1985.

(30)   Cooper, David A., et al., "Acute AIDS retrovirus infection." Lancet, March 9, 1985.

(31)   Krohn, Kai, et al., "Immune functions in HTLV-III antibody positive homosexual men without clinical AIDS." Lancet, Sept. 29, 1984.

(32)   Schwartz, Kendra, et al., "Immunological changes in lymphadenopathy virus positive and negative symptomless male homosexuals: two years of observation." Lancet, Oct. 12, 1985.

(33)   Stewart, G.J., "Transmission of human T-cell lymphotropic virus type III (HTLV-III) by artificial insemination by donor." Lancet, Sept. 14, 1985.

(34)   Francis, Donald P., "Human retrovirus in acquired immunodeficiency syndrome (AIDS)," in Proc. Intl. Conf. on RNA Tumor Viruses in Human Cancer, Denver, Colo., June 10-14, 1984. Boston: Nijhoff, 1985.

(35)   "AIDS virus final name may spell money," Medical World News, Oct. 14,

1985.

(36)   "Two more groups have detected neutralizing antibody to HTLV-3," On-
         cology Times, VII:9, Sept., 1985.

(37)   Chase, Marilyn,   "AIDS study finds virus varies greatly in genetic
         makeup." Wall Street Journal, Aug. 16, 1985.

(38)   Pearce, Richard B., "HTLV, missionaries and parasites." Lancet, Oct. 20,
         1984.

(39)   Biggar, Robert J., et al., "ELISA HTLV retrovirus antibody reactivity
         associated with malaria and immune complexes in healthy Africans."
         Lancet, Sept. 7, 1985.

(40)   Smith, Fran, "AIDS ravages victims' brains, studies find." San Jose (Ca.)
         Mercury, April 23, 1985.

(41)   Levy, Jay A., et al., "Isolation of AIDS-associated retroviruses from
         cerebrospinal fluid and brain of patients with neurological symptoms."
         Lancet, Sept. 14, 1985.

(42)   Radding, Wilson, "Is AIDS caused by a neurotropic virus?" J. Am. Med.
         Assn., 253:19, May 17, 1985.

(43)   Thomas, Christopher S., et al., "HTLV-III and psychiatric disturbance."
         Lancet, Aug. 17, 1985.

(44)   Shaw, G.M., et al., "HTLV-III infection in brains of children and adults
         with AIDS encephalopathy." Science 227:177-82, 1985.

(45)   "AIDS virus infects two workers." AP & UPI in San Francisco Chronicle,
         Sept. 27, 1985.

(46)   Valle, Sirkka-Liisa, et al., "Diversity of clinical spectrum of HTLV-III
         infection." Lancet, Feb. 9, 1985.

(47)   Perlman, David, "Case reported of vanishing AIDS virus. "San Francisco
         Chronicle, Oct. 16, 1985.

(48)   Papaevangelou, G., et al., "LAV/HTLV-III infection in female
         prostitutes." Lancet, Nov. 2, 1985.

(49)   Redfield, Robert R., et al., "Frequent transmission of HTLV-III among
         spouses of patients with AIDS-related complex and AIDS." J. Am. Med.
         Assn., 253:11, 1571-1573, March 15, 1985.

(50)   Redfield, Robert R., et al., "Heterosexually acquired HTLV-III/LAV dis-
         ease (AIDS-related complex and AIDS)." J. Am. Med. Assn., 254:15, 96,
         1985.

(51)   Hunsmann, G., et al., "HTLV positivity in Africans." Lancet, Oct. 26,
         1985.

(52)   Shilts, Randy,   "AIDS loses out to African politics." San Francisco
         Chronicle, Nov. 25, 1985.

(53)   "Critical defect is identified in immune systems of AIDS patients." New
         York Times News Service, San Jose (Ca.) Mercury, July 11, 1985.

(54)   Lane, H. Clifford, in New Eng. J. Med., July 11, 1985.

(55)   Bishop, Jerry E., "Scientists fear that cancer virus may spread in same

way as AIDS." Wall Street Journal, Nov. 4, 1985.

(56)   Montagnier, L., et al., "Isolation of a new retrovirus from a patient at risk of AIDS." AIDS Opportunistic Infection in Hemophiliacs. Stuttgart: Schattauer Verlag, 1984.

(57)   Cheingsong-Popov, R., et al., "Prevalence of antibody to human T-lymphotropic virus type III in AIDS and AIDS-risk patients in Britain." Lancet, Sept. 1, 1984.

(58)   Tedder, R.S., et al., "Low prevalence in the UK of HTLV-I and HTLV-II infection in subjects with AIDS, with extended lymphadenopathy, and at risk of AIDS." Lancet, July 21, 1984.

(59)   Robert-Guroff, Marjorie, et al., "HTLV-I specific antibody in AIDS patients and others at risk." Lancet, July 21, 1984.

(60)   Barrei, F., et al., Science, 220:868, 1983.

(61)   Gallo, R.C., et al., Science, 224:500, 1984.

(62)   Levy, J.A., et al., Science, 225:840, 1984.

(63)   Feorino, P.M., et al., N. Eng. J. Med., 312:1293, 1985.

(64)   Jaffe, H.W., et al., Ann. Intern. Med., 102:627, 1985.

(65)   Saxinger, W.C., et al., Science, 227:1036, 1985.

(66)   Barin, F., et al., "Serological evidence for virus related to simian T-lymphotropic retrovirus III in residents of West Africa." Lancet, Dec. 21/28, 1985.

(67)   Wykoff, Randolph F., "Female-to-male transmission of AIDS agent." Lancet, Nov. 2, 1985.

(68)   Pape, J. et al., paper presented to International Conference on the Acquired Immunodeficiency Syndrome (AIDS), Atlanta, Ga., April 17, 1985.

(69)   Redfield, R.R., and Donald S. Burke, "HIV infection: the clinical picture." Scientific American, October 1988.

(70)   Evatt, B.L., et al., in N. Eng. J. Med. 312, 484-486, 1985.

(71)   Archer, Douglas L., and Walter H. Glinsmann, "Enteric infections and other cofactors in AIDS." Immun. Today, 6:10, 292, 1985.

(72)   Lewis D.F., et al., in J. Infect. Dis., 151:555-558, 1985.

(73)   Weber, J.N., and Robin A. Weiss, "HIV infection: the cellular picture," Scientific American, October 1988.

(74)   Saviteer, Susan M., et al., "HTLV-III exposure during cardiopulmonary resuscitation." N. Eng. J. Med., Dec. 19, 1985.

(75)   "Scientists find how AIDS attacks body." Associated Press, in San Francisco Chronicle, Jan. 17, 1986.

(76)   National Sunday Mail, Harare, Zimbabwe, Feb. 9, 1986.

(77)   Perlman, David, "Drug users started AIDS epidemic, doctor says." San Francisco Chronicle, Oct. 18, 1985.

(78)   Duesberg, Peter H., "Retroviruses as carcinogens and pathogens: expectations and reality." Cancer Research, 47, March 1, 1987.

(79)   Duesberg, Peter H., "HIV is not the cause of AIDS." Science, 241, July 20,

1988.

(80)   "AIDS virus could wait 8 years to strike." (Associated Press) San Diego Union, Aug. 20, 1987.

(81)   "Battling AIDS: a report from the front lines." San Francisco Examiner, May 31, 1987.

(82)   Steel, Michael, "Fourth international AIDS conference." Lancet, July 2, 1988.

(83)   "Transmission of HIV by human bite." Lancet, Aug. 29, 1987.

(84)   Gallo, R. C., and Luc Montagnier, "AIDS in 1988." Scientific American, October 1988.

(85)   Garry, R.F., et al., "Documentation of an AIDS virus infection in the United States in 1968," J. Am. Med. Assn., 250: 14, Oct. 14, 1988.

(86)   Stein. Rob, "A medical mystery: researchers hunt for the longest-surviving AIDS patients." Los Angeles Times, March 28, 1988.

(87)   Chaitow, Leon, and Simon Martin, A World Without Aids. Great Britain: Thorsons Publishing Group, 1988.

(88)   Duesberg, Peter H., Cancer Research, loc. cit., 1987.

(89)   Booth, William, "A rebel without a cause of AIDS." Science, 239, March 20, 1988.

(90)   Miller, Jeff, "AIDS heresy." Discover, June 1988.

(91)   Lauritsen, John, "Kangaroo court etiology." New York Native, May 9, 1988.

(92)   Centers for Disease Control (CDC), Atlanta GA, August 1987.

(93)   Blattner, W., et al., "HIV is the cause of AIDS." Science, 241, July 20, 1988.

(94)   Mann, J.M., et al., "The international epidemiology of AIDS." Scientific American, October 1988.

(95)   Grady, Denise, "AIDS survivors." American Health, September 1988.

(96)   Gavzer, Bernard, "Why do some people survive AIDS?" Parade, Sept. 18, 1988.

(97)   Collin, J., "Regarding Strecker's view of AIDS." Townsend Letter for Doctors, April 1988.

(98)   Whelan, Elizabeth, "AIDS: everything you must know." U.S.A. Today, October 1987.

(99)   "Coverage, Fourth International Conference on AIDS." American Medical News, July 22, 1988.

(100)   Ibid.

(101)   Michaelis, B.S., et al., "Recovery of human immunodeficiency virus from serum." J. Am. Med. Assn., 257:10, March 13, 1987.

(102)   Walker, C.M., et al., "CD8+ lymphocytes can control IV infection in vitro by suppressing virus replication." Science, Dec. 19, 1986.

(103)   Marx, J.L., "The AIDS virus can take on many guises." Science, 241, August 26, 1988.

(104)   Goldsmith, M.F., "Small scientific steps important in 'gigantic' AIDS control mission." J. Am. Med. Assn., 260:7, Aug. 19, 1988.

(105)   Jennings, C., Understanding and Preventing AIDS. Cambridge MA: Health Alert Press, 1988.

(106)   Karpas, A., et al., "Lack of antibodies to adult T cell leukemia virus and to AIDS virus in Israeli Falashas." 319:794, 1986.

(107)   Weiss, R.A., et al., "Lack of HTLV-I antibodies in Africans." Nature 319: 794, 1986.

(108)   Cantwell, Alan, Jr., AIDS: The Mystery and the Solution. Los Angeles CA: Aries Rising Press, 1984.

(109)   Cantwell, Alan, Jr., AIDS and the Doctors of Death. Los Angeles CA: Rising Press, 1988.

(110)   Livingston, Virginia, Cancer: a New Breakthrough. Los Angeles CA: Nash Publishing Corp., 1972.

(111)   Wuerthele-Caspe Livingston, V., and A.M. Livingston, "Demonstration of Progenitor cryptocides in the blood of patients with collagen and neoplastic disease." N.Y. Acad. Sci. 34 (5) 1972.

(112)   Brown, Raymond K., AIDS, Cancer and the Medical Establishment. New York: Speller, 1986.

(113)   "Coverage, Fourth International Conference on AIDS." American Medical News, July 22, 1988.

114)   "AIDS in childbirth." San Diego Union, March 3, 1988.

(115)   Redfield, Robert R., and Donald S. Burke, loc. cit.

(116)   "Research isolates factors that help AIDS prediction." Los Angeles Times, Jan. 8, 1987.

(117)   "PCR test now available." AIDS Treatment News (San Francisco), July 15, 1988.

(118)   "Coverage," loc. cit.

(119)   "Tests hint some victims rid selves of AIDS virus." (Associated Press) San Diego Tribune, Nov. 12, 1987.

(120)   Castro, K.G., et al., "Transmission of HIV in Belle Glade, Fla.: lessons for communities in the United States." Science, 239: 193:197, 1988.

(121)   "Poison offers possible AIDS treatment." (Associated Press) Escondido CA Times Advocate, Sept. 22, 1988.

(122)   CBS News, Dec. 27, 1988.

(123)   Imigawa, David, et. al., "Human immunodeficiency virus type 1 infection in homosexual men who remain seronegative for prolonged periods." New Eng. J. Med., June 1, 1989.

(124)   Haseltine, William A., "Silent HIV infections." New Eng. J. Med., June 1, 1989.

(125)   Clark, Cheryl, "AIDS conference ends on optimistic note about less potent strains of virus." San Diego, Union, June 10, 1989.

(126)   Becker, W.B., et. al., "New T-lymphotropic human herpesviruses." Lan-

cet, Jan. 7, 1989.

(127)   Tersmette, M., et. al., "Association between biological properties of human immunodeficiency virus variants and risk for AIDS and AIDS mortality." Lancet, May 6, 1989.

(128)   Clark, Cheryl, in "Infant AIDS rate alarms N.Y. health official," San Diego Union, June 6, 1989.

(129)   Levy, Jay A., "Human immunodeficiency viruses and the pathogenesis of AIDS." J. Am. Assn., May 26, 1989.

(130)   Bolognesi, Bani, "Prospects for prevention of and early intervention against HIV." J.Am. Med. Assn., May 26, 1989.

(131)   Raymond, Chris, "Once again, mice come to research's rescue, this time as infection models in AIDS studies." J. Am. Med. Assn., Feb. 3, 1989.

(132)   Mayhew, Clemmer, "AIDS virus theory grows ever emptier." Palm Beach Post, April 19, 1989.

(133)   "AIDS virus infects more cells than scientists once believed." The Associated Press in Escondido, Calif., Times-Advocate, July 21, 1989.

(134)   Ho, David H., et al., "Quantitation of human, immunodeficiency virus type 1 in the blood of infected persons." N. Eng. J. Med., Dec. 14, 1989

(135)   Coombs, Robert W., et al., "Plasma viremia in human immunodeficiency virus infection." N. Eng. J. Med., Dec. 14, 1989.

(136)   Baltimore, David, and Mark, B. Feinberg, "HIV revealed." N. Eng. J. Med., Dec. 14, 1989.

(137)   Goldsmith, MArsha F., "Midwest symposium seeks therapeutic answers to global AIDS problem." J. A. Med. Assn., Jan. 19, 1990.

(138)   Adams, Jad, AIDS: The HIV Myth. New York: St. Martin's press, 1989.

83

Chapter Four

OF BLOOD AND SEMEN:
IS AIDS A 'GAY DISEASE'?

In November 1985 the Harvard Medical School assessed the totality of information pouring in about AIDS both from the American and international aspects.

The medical school's newsletter summarized[1]: "The fact that AIDS was first identified in certain seemingly well-defined groups -- intravenous drug abusers, homosexually active men, hemophiliacs, and Haitian immigrants -- has probably led to a false sense of security in people who do not belong to these groups."

The Harvard researchers, fully committed to the "one-mode" etiological agent causation theory of AIDS, somberly added:

"As information about HTLV-III and AIDS has accumulated, another explanation [other than that certain 'high risk' groups are more vulnerable] has emerged that is more plausible. Unfortunately, its implications are grave.

"According to this hypothesis, the people in the original high-risk groups simply had the bad luck to be in the way of a newly emerging infectious agent as it first began to spread. In each case, there were also factors in their lifestyle or medical history that increased the efficiency with which the virus was transmitted to them."

At least, this is the case in the United States and the Western world -- for, as continuing research shows, the vast majority of HIV-infected and/or AIDS/ARC cases in Africa are neither homosexuals nor drug users.

The homosexuality component in the overall HIV/AIDS picture in the U.S.A. (which as of early 1990 still accounted for more than half the full-blown AIDS cases in the world, despite the estimates of millions of infected Africans) continues to fall.

In 1981, when the first few U.S. cases of AIDS-related diseases were reported, the correlation between homo-sexuality and AIDS was 100 percent (but, as we shall see, it was equally correct to say that the correlation between drug abuse and AIDS was also 100 percent in 1981.)

In 1988, it was reported[35] that 63 percent of the victims of AIDS had been homosexual or bisexual men without a history of intravenous (IV) drug abuse, 19 percent were men and women who were IV abusers, 7 percent were homosexual or bisexual men who also were IV drug users, 4 percent were men and women with a history of sexual relations with HIV-infected people, 3 percent were blood transfusion cases, 1 percent were hemophiliacs, 3 percent were "undetermined" (though some retrospective analyses could claim that all these fell into known categories after all), and there was a rapidly growing rate of pediatric AIDS cases.

By 1990, the most rapidly growing aspects of the U.S. caseload were male and female drug users and infant cases. Heterosexual women seem to be infected at a higher rate than heterosexual men.[36]

In southern Europe, "IV drug users" are often the top category of HIV/AIDS sufferers,[37,38] as is now the case where reported AIDS seems belatedly to be taking hold, as in Thailand and the Philippines.[39] The port of entry of HIV/AIDS into the Philippines seems to have been almost entirely female prostitutes who picked up the infection(s) while "servicing" U.S. military bases there.[40]

The enormous contrasts between the HIV/AIDS profile in central Africa, with its alleged millions of cases (yet comparatively few actually reported full-blown cases), where sexual persuasion itself seems to be of no importance, and the United States, where male homosexuality is still the major "reservoir", though continually declining, still baffle observers.

But social bias may account for the early instantaneous labelling of AIDS as 'a gay disease. Because the very first Centers for Disease Control report[41] on the first cases of reported AIDS referred to the "active homosexuality" of the few victims in the first paragraph, one had to proceed through many lines of type to find that all of them were also drug abusers.

What was the whim of CDC reporting to emphasize the homosexuality rather than the drug-abuse nature of these first few victims? We may never know.

But once out of the bag, the description stuck, and for a long while it lulled all but promiscuous male homosexuals into a false sense of security that somehow this strange malady was self-limited not only to one sex but to a subpopulation of one sex.

The early cases of reported AIDS in the United States dealt almost exclusively with young men who were, indeed, homosexuals. But they almost always were users of some form of drugs as well. As we show in Chapter Six, it is a misleading statistic of the Centers for Disease Control (CDC) to segregate "intravenous drug users" from simply "drug users," inasmuch as all forms of drug use are rampant in many communities -- drugs may be intravenous, smoked, sniffed, snorted, or orally ingested.

When *all forms* of drug use are considered within the U.S. database, we find that probably 79% of AIDS patients (rather than just 25% in the "IV drug user" category) have been drug abusers. This strongly suggests that, at least statistically (Austrian research is even more eloquent on the subject, as noted in Chapter Six) AIDS could as easily be seen as a "drug-users' disease" as it is a "gay plague." (If "legal" drugs in the form of overuse of antibiotics and steroids are included, the correlation approaches 100%!)

In the U.S.A. and the Western world, it is not homosexuals *per se* who are at risk, but rather that subgroup of homosexuals in whom the statistically correlated factors of passive anal intercourse, multiple sex partners, prior venereal infections, and concurrent multiviral infections are also present.

This book also strongly points to other factors in immune depression, including "malnutrition of the affluent" through food processing, vitamin/ mineral deficiency, overuse of antibiotics and other medications, and even fluoridated water.

This does not lessen the burden on the high-risk subgroup of homosexuals in whom these factors are present -- it simply means that homosexuality *per se* is not the "cause" of AIDS, yet one important factor in homosexual practices -- unprotected passive anal intercourse -- is without a doubt a major sexual way in which AIDS is spread.

There is nothing biologically unique to homosexuals in this practice, however, and heterosexual men and women engage in this sexual expression as well. Indeed, as the information from non-homosexual cases grows, it is evident that AIDS correlates more with multiple partners -- extreme promiscuity -- than specific sex acts themselves.[2,3,4,46,47]

It was never really correct to call AIDS a "homosexual" disease in the Western world -- but it was largely proper, at least at the beginning, to call it an "anal intercourse disease." The assumption that all male homosexuals practice this sex act, or that homosexuals define themselves by this single act, is an erroneous social myth, not a demonstrated fact.

In 1987 and 1988 statistical and mathematical studies[48,49,50] made the clear connection between transmission and the overwhelming predominance of anal sexual intercourse, and Trichopoulos et al. in Greece noted:[51]

"This finding [that by far the most important risk factor for HIV seroconversion in male homosexuals is receptive anal intercourse] points to the potential importance of role separation (active vs. passive) among male homosexuals as a population variable in models of the AIDS epidemic. If all male homosexuals were either active or passive, but never both, the proportion of male homosexuals would not be critical to understanding the past or predicting the future spread of AIDS. Those practicing insertive anal intercourse would not be at increased risk because of the inherently low risk of their practice; those practicing receptive anal intercourse would not be at very high risk, because of the low prevalence of HIV among their sexual partners, and they would not transmit the infection further."

There clearly is, and this has been evident from the first caseloads of AIDS, transmissibility in semen and blood. The promiscuous sex/intravenous drug use/hemophiliac correlation to AIDS established such a link, and it has only tended to grow with the years.

In terms of semen, the relationships to AIDS are the possible immunosuppressive effects of semen itself (almost certainly the lesser of factors) and the contact between semen and blood at the very area where there might be sufficient lacerations and tears from traumatic sexual acts or venereal lesions to accomplish the contact: almost overwhelmingly, the anal-rectal area in both sexes and, possibly of real but lesser importance, the vaginal-cervical area in women.

Subsequent research has suggested there is probably more anal intercourse practiced among heterosexuals than earlier thought, and that transmission of AIDS agents through normal vaginal intercourse is probably easier than at first thought, leading to greater dangers for women from being infected by men than vice-versa.

As epidemiological studies have continued, there are now scattered reports of possible infection by oral intercourse alone and female-to-female transmission, but these cases are so far beyond the evolving norm as to be statistically insignificant.

In 1984, Shearer and Levy noted[5] the "possible contributions of semen, HLA alloantigens, and lack of natural resistance" in a multifactorial model of AIDS causation. They were among researchers suggesting "antigen overload"[9] aspects in AIDS and questioned early in AIDS research whether a single agent could possibly be the cause.

"It is remarkable that a putative infectious agent with such devastating immunological consequences has been limited to the groups that it infects and has not spread to the general population..." Shearer and Levy wrote, just as the presence of AIDS in heterosexuals was beginning to be noted.

Immune suppression can be induced by sperm and semen -- at least in mice,[6] and "if sperm and semen can reach the lymphatics and vascular system of passive partners of anogenital sex, immune suppression could occur, rendering these individuals susceptible to AIDS," according to scientists.[7,8]

Sperm has indeed been found to be highly immunogenic[31] and homosexual males have been reported to have higher serum levels of Igm antisperm antibody than do heterosexual men.[32] Also, in a study of 20 homosexual pairs, sperm-induced allogenic immunization was found to correlate with immune dysregulation.

There is no doubt, anatomically, that it is simply easier for insertive damage to occur in the anorectal area than in the vagina, due to the structure of these separate tissues, with one doctor noting[11] that "the passage of semen into the circulation is likely because the unprotected, nonstratified cuboidal epithelium of the rectum bears the brunt of traumatic intercourse [in homosexual males]. In contrast, the stratified epithelium of the vagina prevents such an occurrence in heterosexuals." To which it should be added, "most of the time."

Investigators pondering the immune suppressing effects of sperm note the Witkin study[12] in which lymphocyte proliferation by sera from rectally inseminated male rabbits was inhibited. Morgan discussed[55] the possible cause of AIDS from a "virus-like interaction between sperm cells and the immune system", emphasizing the "strong functional resemblance that exists between viruses and sperm cells: both inject genetic material into a cell, which is then transformed by the injected material."

"Antigen overload" from many different seminal depositions was looked at early in the AIDS controversy, and as it was examined it became more and more obvious that numbers of partners correlated with cases of AIDS.[13,14] This later became apparent in caseloads from Africa, in which promiscuity (rather than heterosexuality vs. homosexuality) seemed to be key.

The Goedert et al. study of determinants of retrovirus antibody and immunodeficiency conditions in homosexual men[14] pointed out that "the lifestyle risk factors for HTLV-III seropositivity were large numbers of homosexual partners and receptive anal intercourse, with an apparent synergistic interaction between these two activities."

It is significant that the Goedert study correlated seropositivity with sex practices and nitrite inhalant (poppers) use, though poppers and five of the sex practices were statistically unrelated.

The three factors correlating to higher HIV seropositivity were: number of partners, receptive anal intercourse, and a particular practice known as "fisting." The links between multiple partners and receptive anal intercourse and AIDS in U.S. male homosexuals can be considered without a doubt firmly established.[15,16,17,18,19,20,21,35]

Early in such research, however, not only was multiple anal intercourse implicated, but aberrant practices even within that more noted practice were traced, with "fisting" -- the actual insertion of whole hands, fists and parts of the arm into the anorectal area -- occurring. (Eleven of 62 in the Goedert study practiced fisting and higher percentages have been reported in other groups).[25]

It can hardly be said that "fisting" represents a common practice among the world's homosexuals, even though anal intercourse plays a relatively high role.

It was largely the Mavligit study in 1984 which mired the anal-intercourse connection in controversy, since the authors concluded[8] that "chronic, repeated exposure to sperm during anal intercourse results in a high frequency of allogeneic immunization and may play an important role in the development of [AIDS] in homosexual males."

But if this were even a primary cause of immune depression, then why, as Drs. Owen and Campbell asked,[22] had AIDS not occurred before? After all, they wrote, "anal-receptive homosexual (and heterosexual) intercourse has been practiced at least since the beginning of recorded human history."

Part of the defense posed by Mavligit[23] was that "the epidemic of AIDS first detected in the summer of 1981 is in our opinion the result of a major behavioral change among homosexuals.

"This statement is based on information from a ten-year study by Masters and Johnson (1968-77) ... It is ... quite conceivable that the vast increase in the practice of anal intercourse, which took place some time around 1978-1979, coupled with an extensive degree of promiscuity, may have catapulted the evolution and epidemic spread of the putative infective agent causing AIDS."

A substantial number of homosexuals would strongly doubt that there has been a "vast increase in the practice of anal intercourse" over the span of this century or any other. They might agree, however, that in certain subgroups within subgroups within the self-identified homosexual community there might have been increases in experimental sex, including such highly dangerous and laceration-causing traumatic practices as "fisting."

In fact, all that can be said of unprotected anal intercourse itself is that it probably makes it easier for infective viruses to enter the bloodstream than does vaginal intercourse. All that can be said of multiple partners involved in anal intercourse is that such elevated numbers increase the risk. Promiscuity and anal sex, while frequent among some homosexuals, can hardly be said to define the homosexual lifestyle in its entirety. (And particularly if, as the Kinsey studies of three decades ago indicated, at least 10 percent of the American population may be homosexual.)

That is, in excess of 23 million Americans, men and

women, may be homosexual, and if half of these are male it would indicate that a subgroup within this group -- that which is extremely promiscuous, is involved in receptive anal sex, is weakened by prior infections, and is involved in drug abuse -- is at extremely high risk for AIDS, but not that homosexuals *per se* are at such risk.

Indeed, in the "gay mecca" of San Francisco, where sexual promiscuity, experimental sex, and the presence of a visible, organized and substantial homosexual community are apparent, estimations as to just how many male homosexuals are probably infected by "the AIDS virus" -- by percentage -- have tended to decline rather than advance.

In January 1985, Anderson and Levy reported[24] that "our data suggest that AIDS-associated virus exposure in San Francisco is common (37% among single men with homosexual contacts) but less prevalent than previously reported." (Namely, 65% of men attending a venereal disease clinic.)

The well organized homosexual community response to HIV/AIDS had, by 1988, led to falling numbers of new cases and a veritable revolution in the "gay lifestyle" in which rampant promiscuity was largely replaced with monogamous relationships or even celibacy.[42] As the 1970s had marked an era of sweeping "gay revolution" and the assertion of a homosexual lifestyle, then the 1980s, almost singly because of AIDS, put a brake on the movement. The cases now being reported are more often than not infections acquired at least several years prior.

In sociological terms, the lack of a change in lifestyle among IV drug users, and the disproportionate rates of new HIV/AIDS cases in minorities, particularly blacks and Hispanics, pose major challenges as a new decade begins.

In sexual-transmission studies, such elements as genital ulcers from various diseases and even uncircumcised foreskins are achieving more importance in determining the relative ease or difficulty of "AIDS virus" transfer.

Concerning oral intercourse, a practice widespread in heterosexuals as well as homosexuals, the Harvard Medical School Health Letter pointed out[1] that "oral exposure to semen may or may not be an effective route of transferring HTLV-III" despite the possibility of viral transfer from saliva to a raw exposed mouth surface. But up to now there have been too few correlations between oral sex and AIDS to implicate this practice as much of a danger, though it still must be considered "high risk."

In June 1988 Rozenbaum *et al.* reported[53] five cases of HIV infection in persons who had denied either anal sex or other risk factors other than oral copulation for three months or more before "seroconversion" -- that is, testing positive for antibodies. This led to their conclusion of an increased risk in oral sex.

These findings were later assailed by others[54] on the basis of the ever-expanding presumed period of incubation of "the AIDS virus" and the fact that isolation of the virus antigen or its DNA component have occurred as early as 42 months ($3^{1}/_{2}$ years) before "seroconversion" -- so, they reasoned, an absence of any other factors than oral-genital sex for at least three months before production of antibodies does not mean much of anything.

Rozenbaum *et al.* responded that the polymerase chain reaction (PCR) test for HIV viral DNA well in advance of the presence of antibodies remains to be fully established, and that no antigen could be found in three of the five patients prior to their "seropositive" antibody tests.

These mixed findings can be read several ways: either oral sex is a minimum but real risk factor in HIV transmission, or -- once again -- the obsession with attempting to find HIV antibodies, viral particles, antigens and DNA borders on the irrelevant since they do not "cause" at all or may only be co-factors or "markers" for something else connected with AIDS.

In a large cluster of homosexuals (400 consecutive patients screened for AIDS and pre-AIDS in south Florida between January-November 1983), Drs. Whiteside and MacLeod found[26] that "only receivers or passive partners in anal intercourse had symptoms of AIDS or AIDS-related complexes."

So the primary elements in homosexuality which correlate to AIDS are greater numbers of partners and passive anal intercourse. There is nothing in these two elements that are the exclusive domain of homosexuals, and it is now clear that non-anal intercourse between heterosexuals (as well as anal intercourse between heterosexuals) provides transmission of AIDS.

One study in 1985[27] found "frequent transmission of HTLV-III among spouses of patients with ARC and AIDS" and demonstrated that "HTLV-III can be transmitted by repeated heterosexual contact." Earlier, these same researchers found in examining AIDS patients at Walter Reed Army Medical Center in Washington that 37% (15 of 41) had acquired the infection from a partner or partners of the opposite sex.[28]

They summarized: "The method of sexual activity did not appear to be related to disease acquisition; however, this study clearly demonstrated that receptive anal intercourse was not a requirement."

In Africa, "homosexuality, intravenous drug abuse, and blood transfusion did not appear to be risk factors" in patients in Zaire;[2] of a prospective study in Rwanda of AIDS patients "most of the men were promiscuous heterosexuals and 43% of the females were prostitutes [and] no patient had a history of homosexuality, intravenous drug abuse or transmission in the previous five years."[3]

An Italian study[30] found both female-to-male transmission in cases of AIDS and ARC, including five children born to seropositive parents. In Greece,[29] 12 out of 200 registered prostitutes were positive for HIV yet had no symptoms of AIDS or ARC.

We point out in Chapter Six that even the connection between seropositivity for HIV and female prostitution seems to be strongly associated with intravenous (and by implication, other) drug use and may have little or nothing to do with the actual form of sexual expression engaged in by prostitutes or their notable promiscuity.

In one of these studies, that in Pordenone, Italy,[33] it was also demonstrated that the presence of HIV antibodies in 95 male intravenous drug users was 52% vs. 15% for 30 male homosexuals.

Since the great majority of individuals thought to be carrying "the AIDS virus" are indeed Africans and since homosexuality (let alone drug abuse and blood transfusion) do not strongly correlate to HIV/AIDS in Africa, then the syndrome would at first blush seem to be a disease for all seasons, with an implied threat to the population as a whole -- particularly to those elements who are already somehow immune compromised because of any of many other factors.

Yet, as of 1990, the great majority of known sexual partners of HIV-infected patients were either not positive for HIV, or, if they were, most were not sick. HIV/AIDS was growing among heterosexuals -- but far more readily through drug addiction and mother-to-infant transmission.

The Harvard assessment in 1985[1] is instructive:

"Until more data are available, the safest assumption is that exposure of mucous membranes to blood, semen, or saliva involves some risk of acquiring AIDS. Unprotected anal intercourse is most certainly the higher-risk behavior but vaginal intercourse clearly carries some level of risk to the woman.

"Over time, even 'less risky' behaviors could become important routes of transfer. If, for example, receptive anal intercourse with someone infected by HTLV-III had one chance in 50 of transmitting the disease, whereas an episode of intense kissing with that person had only one chance in 5,000, the risk of transmission from 100 episodes of deep kissing would be equivalent to that from a single occasion of receptive anal intercourse. This calculation is purely hypothetical -- nobody knows the actual rates of transmission -- but it illustrates a real and disturbing possibility: that intimate behaviors which are relatively common have a theoretical potential to transmit AIDS, merely because they are common."

And also, one might add, if AIDS is more than anything a viral disease.

In the area of HIV seropositivity and saliva, David Ho and colleagues at Massachusetts General Hospital found[34] that only one of 83 saliva samples from 71 homosexual men seropositive for HIV was positive for the virus, vs. isolation of the virus from 28 of 50 blood cultures of these men, who had been under observation for a year.

Their conclusion: "Therefore, we conclude that HTLV-III is present infrequently in the saliva of infected persons. When it was detected in the saliva of one patient with intraoral disease, the amount of virus present was small. These findings are consistent with epidemiologic data indicating that casual transmission of HTLV-III does not occur."

In 1988, one study[52] showed that something in saliva apparently inhibits HIV.

Whatever the route of transmission, by 1990 it could be said that HIV/AIDS remained far more difficult to "catch" than venereal diseases and hepatitis.

REFERENCES

(1)   "AIDS: update (part 1)." The Harvard Medical School Health Letter, XI:1, November 1985.

(2)   Piot, Peter, et al., "Acquired immunodeficiency syndrome in a heterosexual population in Zaire." Lancet, July 14, 1984.

(3)   Van de Perre, Philippe, et al., "Acquired immunodeficiency syndrome in Rwanda." Lancet, July 14, 1984.

(4)   Van de Perre, Philippe, "Female prostitutes: a risk group for infection with human T-cell lymphotropic virus type III." Lancet, Sept. 7, 1985.

(5)   Shearer, Gene M., and Robert B. Levy, "Noninfectious cofactors in susceptibility to AIDS: possible contribution of semen, HLA alloantigens, and lack of natural resistance." Ann. N.Y. Acad. Sci., v. 437, 1984.

(6)   Hurtenbach, U., and G.M. Shearer, "Germ-cell induced immune suppression in mice. Effect of inoculation of syngeneic spermatozoa on cell-mediated immune responses." J. Exp. Med. 155:1719-1729, 1982.

(7)   Sonnabend, J.S., et al., "Acquired immune deficiency syndrome, opportunistic infections, and malignancies in male homosexuals," J. Am. Med. Assn. 249: 2370-2374, 1983.

(8)   Mavligit, G.M., et al., "Chronic immune stimulation by sperm alloantigens: support for the hypothesis that spermatozoa induce immune dysregulation in homosexual males." J. Am. Med. Assn., 251:237, 1983.

(9)   Levy, J.A., and J.L. Ziegler. "Acquired immunodeficiency syndrome is an opportunistic infection and Kaposi's sarcoma results from secondary immune stimulation." Lancet, i:78-81, 1983.

(10)   Langone, John, "AIDS special report." Discover, December, 1985.

(11)   Kondlapoodi, P., "Anorectal cancer and homosexuality." J. Am. Med. Assn., 248:17, 2114-2115, Nov. 5, 1982.

(12)   Witkin, Steven S., "Inhibiton of lymphocyte proliferation by sera from rectally inseminated male rabbits." Ann. N.Y. Acad. Sci., vol. 437, 1984.

(13)   Levine, A.S. "The epidemic of acquired immune dysfunction in homosexual men and its sequelae -- opportunistic infections, Kaposi's sarcoma, and other malignancies. An update and interpretation." Cancer Treat. Rep. 66:1391-1395, 1982.

(14)   Goedert, James J., et al., "Determinants of retrovirus (HTLV-III) antibody and immunodeficiency conditions in homosexual men." Lancet, Sept. 29, 1984.

(15)   Goedert, J.J., et al., "Determinants of lesser AIDS." Proc. Am. Soc. Clin. Onco. 3:14, 1984.

(16)   Goedert, J.J., et al., "Decreased helper T lymphocytes in homosexual men:1. sexual contact with high-incidence areas for the acquired im-

munodeficiency syndrome." Am. J. Epidem., 1984.

(17) Goedert, J.J., et al., "Decreased helpter T lymphocytes in homosexual men: II. sexual practices." Am. J. Epidemiol., 1984.

(18) Curran, J.W., "AIDS--two years later." N. Eng. J. Med. 309: 609-11, 1983.

(19) Marmor, M., et al., "Risk factors for Kaposi's sarcoma in homosexual men." Lancet, i:1083-1087, 1982.

(20) Marmor, et al., "Kaposi's sarcoma in homosexual men: a seroepidemiologic case-control study." Ann. Int. Med., 100: 809-815, 1984.

(21) Jaffe, H.W., et al., "National case-control study of Kaposi's sarcoma and Pneumocystis carinii pneumonia in homosexual men. Part I: epidemiologic results." Ann. Intern. Med. 99: 145-151, 1983.

(22) Owen, William F., and James M. Campbell, "Spermatozoa and immune dysregulations in homosexual men." J. Am., Med. Assn., 252: 9, 1130, Sept. 7, 1984.

(23) Mavligit, Giora, reply, J. Am., Med., Assn., 252:9, 1130, Sept. 7, 1984.

(24) Anderson, Robert E., and Jay A. Levy, "Prevalence of antibodies to AIDS-associated retrovirus in single men in San Francisco." Lancet, Jan. 26, 1985.

(25) "A cluster of Kaposi's sarcoma and Pneumocystis carinii pneumonia among homosexual male residents in Los Angeles and Orange Counties, California." MMWR, 31: 305-307, June 18, 1982.

(26) Stockwell, Serena, "Dengue arbovirus could be marker for AIDS; possible link to mosquitos being studied." Oncology Times, VII:10, October 1985.

(27) Redfield, Robert R., et al., "Frequent transmission of HTLV-III among spouses of patients with AIDS-related complex and AIDS." J. Am. Med. Assn., 253:11, 1571-1573, March 15, 1985.

(28) Redfield, Robert R., et al., "Heterosexually acquired HTLV-III/LAV disease (AIDS-related complex and AIDS)." J. Am. Med. Assn., 254: 15, 2094-2096, Oct. 18, 1985.

(29) Papaevangelou, G., "LAV/HTLV-III infection in female prostitutes." Lancet, Nov. 2, 1985.

(30) Luzi, G., et al., "Transmission of HTLV-III infection by heterosexual contact." Lancet, Nov. 2, 1985.

(31) Alexander, N.J., "Immunological aspects of vasectomy." In Boettcher, B., ed., Immunological Influence on Human Fertility. New York: New York Academic Press, 1977.

(32) Witkin, S.S., and J. Sonnabend, "Immune responses to spermatozoa in homosexual men." Fertil, Steril. 39: 337-342, 1983.

(33) Tirelli, Umberto, et al., in "HTLV-III antibody in prostitutes." Lancet, Dec. 21/28, 1985.

(34) Ho, David D., et al., "Infrequency of isolation of HTLV-III virus from saliva in AIDS." N. Eng. J. Med., Dec. 19, 1985.

(35) Heyward, W.L., and J.W. Curran, "The epidemiology of AIDS in the U.S."

Scientific American, October, 1988.

(36)   Clark, S., "Women warned on risk of AIDS virus." San Diego Union, Sept. 20, 1987.

(37)   Casabona, J., et al., "The impact of the revised case definition of AIDS." J. Am. Med. Assn., 260: 15, 2213, Oct. 21, 1988.

(38)   Mann, J.M., et al., "The international epidemiology of AIDS." Scientific American, October, 1988.

(39)   Ibid.

(40)   Bulletin Today, Manila, Jan. 28, 1986.

(41)   Morbidity and Mortality Weekly Report, Centers for Disease Control, Atlanta GA, June 5, 1981.

(42)   "San Francisco successful in cutting HIV infection rate." American Medical News., Nov. 27, 1987.

(43)   Stamm, W.E., et al., "The association between genital ulcer disease and acquisition of HIV infection in homosexual men." J. Am. Med. Assn., 260: 10, 1429-1433, Sept. 9, 1988.

(44)   Simonsen, J.N., et al., "Human immunodeficiency virus infection among men with sexually transmitted disease." New Engl. J. Med., 319: 3, 274-278, Aug. 4, 1988.

(45)   Heyward, et al., loc. cit.

(46)   Padian, N., et al., "Male-to-female transmission of human immunodeficiency virus." J. Am. Med. Assn., 258: 6, 788-790, Aug. 14, 1988.

(47)   Monzon, O.T. and J.M.B. Capellan, "Female-to-male transmission of HIV." Lancet, July 4, 1987.

(48)   Kingsley, L.A., et al., "Risk factors for seroconversion in human immunodeficiency virus among male homosexuals." Lancet, i: 345-49, 1987.

(49)   Johnson, A.M., "Social and behavioural aspects of the HIV epidemic: a review." J.R. Statist. Soc. A., part 1, 1988.

(50)   Isham, V., "Mathematical modeling of the transmission of HIV and AIDS: a review." J.R. Statist. Soc. A., part 1, 1988.

(51)   Trichopoulos, D., et al., "Homosexual role separation and spread of AIDS." Lancet, Oct. 22, 1988.

(52)   "Saliva somehow inhibits AIDS virus, study finds." Associated Press (San Diego Union), May 6, 1988.

(53)   Rozenbaum, W., et al., "HIV transmission by oral sex." Lancet, June 18, 1988.

(54)   Dassey, David; R. Detels, B. Visscher; W. Rozenbaum et al., "HIV and orogenital transmission." Lancet, Oct. 29, 1988.

(55)   Morgan, James, "Concerning the genesis of AIDS." Med. Hypotheses, 13: 357-358, 1984.

Chapter Five

THE MULTI-VIRAL CONNECTION

The onrush of scientific research which continues to pour in from all sides, particularly from the "orthodox" or allopathic medical community, makes it increasingly obvious that "the AIDS virus" -- or viruses -- cannot possibly be the cause of the syndrome by themselves.

This point of view does not indicate an "establishment" embrace of the multifactorial models proposed by holistic and eclectic physicians and researchers (Chapter Thirteen) but it does point to the blind alley of single-mode etiology posed by the continually unravelling mysteries of HIV.

As noted earlier, the Fifth International AIDS Conference in Montreal in 1989 -- like its predecessors a forum overwhelmingly tipped toward allopathic procedures, concepts and doctrines -- revealed more statistical links for viral "co-factors" even to HIV. These included the first of the Gallo "lymphotropic" viruses to be discovered -- HTLV-I, as well as the more recently described human herpesvirus 6 and papavovirus JC, said to cause the "opportunistic" viral infection progressive multifocal leukoencephalopathy, one of the lethal late-stage consequences of neurological involvement in AIDS.

Indeed, if so much attention had not been turned toward HIV-I (formerly HTLV-III) because of the AIDS pandemic, HTLV-I, showing up in the same target populations as HIV, would probably have received the research funds and adverse publicity.

And HHV-6, now said to be rampant in the human population (See Chapter Three), is an isolate of a particular immune-depressing if apparently not lethal complex of maladies variously called "Lake Tahoe" or "Incline Village" syndrome.

It became legitimate in the 1980s to wonder just where HTLV-I, HTLV-II (possibly linked to the rare human cancer called hairy cell leukemia), HTLV-III (now HIV-1), HHV-6 and other viruses have been all this time. Are they just now being "discovered" because of new technology, having been there all along?

Were some of them, as conspiracy theorists contend (Chapter Eleven), man-made, as at least highly suggested by existing literature and the technological realities of at least a dozen countries?

Or are these irrelevant "passenger" viruses, cohabiting in humans with dozens of others and, in themselves, of little importance?

However one might review or rewrite human virological history, it is almost certain that at least some of the virally-connected (or induced) conditions involving what some referred to by 1989 as "chronic fatigue/immune dysregulation syndrome" (CFIDS) and including such spin-offs or variants as"Lake Tahoe Syndrome" on the one hand, and AIDS on another, are *new*. This would suggest that their organizing agents (if not inducers) are themselves *new*.

While numerous physicians in the Western world had been grappling with aspects of this overall syndrome (CFIDS, with elevated Epstein-Barr Virus titers, outbreaks of yeast infection, chronic fatigue, unexplained muscle weakness, fevers, sleep and neurological disturbances all involved), for years, the U.S. medical monopoly waited for more years -- until the period 1987-1989 -- even to admit the syndrome existed.

At a San Francisco conference in May 1989 on CFIDS, called by some "yuppie flu," and now officially tagged CFS (Chronic Fatigue Syndrome) by the Centers for Disease Control (CDC), internist R. Dennis Collins was specific: "It's clear to me that we have a real syndrome although we don't quite understand it." And AIDS researcher and virologist Jay Levy said of the presumptive cause of CFS: "I think this is a new agent, it's not necessarily a virus, although it may be . . . it is not easily recoverable, or we would have found it."[60]

The "yuppie flu" of CFS or CFIDS does not specifically target homosexuals or intravenous drug users in America, nor, characteristically, are its carriers positive for HIV. However AIDS-like (particularly at the ARC level) it may be, it escapes the classification of AIDS simply because of the concept that HIV is the *sine qua non* of AIDS.

There can be no doubt, now, that for AIDS actually to occur, or for HIV to "take", there must surely be an adequate substrate of other immunologically compromising factors. Much of this book deals with a variety of these factors including some which have been obviously overlooked or ignored, for whatever reason.

From the beginning of AIDS, it was clear to many researchers that the syndrome, if there was a viral "trigger" to it at all, must surely involve the work of other viruses -- if, indeed, AIDS were to be defined as a viral disease at all.

The several announcements, in late 1983, that a putative AIDS "cause" had been found -- be it identified as human T-lymphotropic virus III (HTLV-III), lymphadeno-pathy-associated virus (LAV), or, perhaps more correctly, AIDS-related virus (ARV), or some constantly mutating form of all of these -- hardly put the interviral argument to rest, even when the term Human Immunodeficiency Virus (HIV) was coined.

At the time, the front runners as alleged viral co-factors with HIV -- and there are those who still believe HIV or a close associate is actually the co-factor to any one of these other viruses or viral products -- were cytomegalovirus (CMV), Epstein-Barr (EBV), herpes simplex 1,2, the "new" HHV-6, and hepatitis B.

Both herpes simplex and hepatitis B may play stronger roles than at first thought, and both are strongly associated with sexual transmission.

And also, at least in the U.S.A, a philosophical/ sociological terrain was set by the "sexual liberation" which broke out in the 1960s and spread through the 1970s, replete with the encouragement of multiple sexual partners for heterosexual men and women quite aside from the already prevalent rampant promiscuity of a certain percentage of homosexual men.

Hepatitis B or a strain of it still has its champions as the primary trigger. Kelly has suggested[1] that "AIDS could be caused by a mutant hepatitis B virus or even a prion-like agent..." Indeed, Japanese research[2] pointed to a combination of the hepatitis and HIV viruses as inducing the syndrome. Herpes simplex and herpes zoster (shingles), frequently related to AIDS cases,[3,4] must be assumed to play a role.

The fact is, all or most of these suspect viruses may exist together and may all be available at the time of AIDS diagnosis, or on autopsy. CMV, EBV, herpes, HHV-6, varicella zoster (VZV) and similar viruses are all members of the herpes family and, noted Britton et al.,[5] may affect any level of the nervous system by either direct viral invasion or immunological mechanisms, as HIV apparently does. Inasmuch as alterations in the ratios of T4:T8 cells of the immune system, and other immunological markers, are classic signs of AIDS, it is vitally important to understand that the herpesvirus family has effects on the immune system and that there are alterations in the helper-suppressor (T4:T8) ratio brought about by factors *other* than HIV. We examine some nutritional factors involved in immune system compromise elsewhere (Chapter Nine).

But in terms of virus, as Anthony S. Fauci of the National Institutes of Health, pointed out[6], quite aside from HIV's own recognized attack on the helper T4 cells, "patients with AIDS are generally infected with cytomegalovirus and Epstein-Barr virus, both of which are B-cell activators. HTLV-III, which infects the T-4 cell, may induce the T cell to secrete activating factors ... and may infect the cell directly. Cytomegalovirus or Epstein-Barr virus may transform the B cell and make it more susceptive to infection with HTLV-III."

Because CMV, EBV and other factors can influence the T4:T8 ratio[7,8,14,15] the "T-cell test" for immune deficiency, while pointing to either an acute or chronic immune depression, is not confirmatory for AIDS even though a persistent or increasing reversal of the T4:T8 ratio, and consistently declining T4 cells, must at all times be regarded as suspicious.

Typical of the multiviral assays in AIDS patients -- both homosexual and essentially non-homosexual - are studies from Great Britain and Zambia.

In 1984 analyses of 16 Zambian patients with Kaposi's sarcoma (the Zambian population not regarded as "at risk" because of homosexuality or drug abuse), all 16 had antibodies to CMV, 15 had antibodies to EBV, 13 to HTLV-1 (human T-cell leukemia virus -- not HTLV-III), and five had evidence of previous infection with hepatitis B virus.[36]

In a 1985 study of British homosexual men with HIV antibodies, seropositive men had a significantly higher prevalence of infection with hepatitis B virus than did the seronegatives,[37] now regarded as a fairly common finding in the West.

In 1988, a University of California-San Francisco study[59] indicated that hepatitis B infection might accelerate the development of AIDS in HIV-infected people. The study found that a hepatitis B viral protein triggered proliferation of HIV in an experiment in which hepatitis viral fragments were placed into human cell cultures containing cloned HIV. One suggestion of the study was that persons at "high risk" for, but not currently infected with, HIV might benefit from vaccination against hepatitis B.

In view of the observations elsewhere in this book that the hepatitis B vaccine itself might have triggered AIDS or have somehow catalyzed AIDS in New York City in 1978, and also in view of the riskiness of any vaccination for presumably HIV-infected people (whether currently antibody positive or not) the suggestion is of questionable merit.

The consideration of CMV as the essential factor in AIDS dominated much research at least until the advent of HIV and still remains important in consideration of viral co-factors. To begin with, the pathology of cytomegalovirus fits into everybody's overview of what AIDS is.

Herpes-like virus particles were identified in tissue culture lines derived from the biopsies of American Kaposi's sarcoma patients, and serum antibodies to CMV were detected a few years later in elderly European and U.S. KS patients[9,10,11,12]. CMV was known to have a particular relationship to KS even before the latter's appearance as part of the AIDS epidemic in the West[13].

Later, and more astonishingly, CMV antibodies were found in the sera of more than 90% of homosexual men tested (94% in one sample), while such antibodies occurred in only 3.8% of serum specimens randomly collected from volunteer male blood donors.[14,15,16]

Noted Drew and Mintz[14]: "Data on the prevalence of CMV Igm antibody further suggest that homosexual men experience repeated episodes of CMV infection ... [antibodies] tended to appear, disappear and then reappear again over the course of time." In one study[15], CMV virus was found in the urine or semen of 11 of 30 healthy homosexual men, who as a group had lower T4:T8 ratios (0.8 to 0.4) than did heterosexual controls (1.8 to 1.4).

However, KS in Africa is not necessarily connected either with AIDS itself, or with immunodepression,[16,17] nor is AIDS in Africa associated with homosexuality, intravenous drug use or even hemophilia[18]. Hence, the association between CMV and HIV in the U.S.A. may not be "homosexual-specific" even though sexual promiscuity and increased numbers of partners (common to, but by no means limited to, homosexuality) are clearly AIDS factors. In 1989, a British study of 108 HIV-infected hemophiliacs established that CMV infection is associated with a more rapid progession to HIV disease.[61]

Epstein-Barr virus (EBV) presents a number of intriguing mysteries and relationships to AIDS. It is problematic in that it is virtually ubiquitous in the human population and not thought of generally as a pathological problem, at least in the West, until it advances to infectious mononucleosis (IM), sometimes called the "kissing disease," and more often than not its reactivation is linked to promiscuous sex and/or an affluent lifestyle.

Primary infection usually occurs in childhood without any clinical evidence of disease and leads to a lifelong presence and development of certain immunological responses, particularly in the B lymphocytes. Only humans and certain primates apparently harbor the virus.

In the Third World, some 99% of children are infected by the age of three,[19] and in Western countries with higher physical standards of living 80% of the population usually becomes infected.

When infection takes place in adolescent or adult life, as Epstein himself has demonstrated,[20] there is a 50% chance that it will be accompanied by the symptoms of infectious mononucleosis, similar to the ARC or "pre-AIDS" or actual AIDS conditions themselves.

"Everything known about the biology of EB virus and the immunological changes in AIDS makes it obvious that the agent will be active in flourishing AIDS patients and likely to give rise to EB virus carrying B-lymphoid tumors in such people," he says. EBV is in fact associated with Burkitt's lymphoma and other non-Kaposi cancers connected with the AIDS syndrome.[21]

EBV is an important element in CFS/CFIDS, a rapidly advancing condition going into the 1990s which also was usually accompanied by systemic infection with *Candida albicans*, itself a virtual "marker" for HIV/AIDS. In fact, many cases of what this writer came to call "AIDS without AIDS" were seen in which a wasting syndrome, swollen glands, chronic fatigue, mood swings, memory disturbances, etc., were all present -- without positivity for HIV.

Sonnabend[22] and others believe that episodes of reactivation of EBV are part of the multifactorial causation of AIDS.

Roulette William Smith adduced[23] the concept that EBV products are the primary culprits in AIDS, and that they set the stage for the syndrome when other factors (such as possible malnutrition and drug abuse) are present. He believes that viruses and virus-like phenomena may *not* underly "slow, progressive disease",but that "context-specific ribonucleoprotein complexes that are progressively released in multiple quantities, thereby mimicking viral transmission and replication," may actually be causes.

"In general, my results indicate that many SPD [slow, progressive diseases] may be consequences of abnormal RNA processing -- possibly secondary to some viral infection. In regard to AIDS in humans, available evidence now implicates Epstein-Barr viruses (EBV) as the principal contributors underlying immune modification with subsequent autoprogressive phenomena mimicking secondary viral infections," he wrote.

In a follow-up letter to interested researchers,[24] he summarized that "even at this date (in mid-1985) my evidence suggests that the Epstein-Barr virus (EBV) may be the cause of the initial immune modification in AIDS, with LAV/HTLV-III being obligate opportunistic cofactors." In fact, he said some research indicated that EBV is the major contributor to the diversity of genes now recognized in the alleged AIDS retrovirus.

He based part of his work on that of Sigurdsson, who described[25] the development of four AIDS-like diseases in sheep in Iceland as early as 1933, coinciding with the importation from Germany of 20 Karakul sheep.

One of the viruses involved was visna/maedi, which, like HIV and human T-lymphotropic viruses, and together with such animal viruses as caprine arthritis-encephalitis virus and avian leukosis virus, are retroviruses, "are nearly always associated with herpes viruses and are likely to be obligate opportunistic cofactors in AIDS."

The EBV, EBV-product interviral immunological cross-reactivity may explain why AIDS patients are open to only certain specific opportunistic infections, diseases which in and of themselves are usually rare, Smith noted. He also stressed the need for a continual assessment of AIDS epidemiology:

"What remains ... would be to determine if particularly virulent strains of EBV are the causative agents or if social, cultural, or environmental factors have created a dose-dependent (or titer-dependent) cause for AIDS ...

"Evidence favoring particularly virulent strains of EBV should be sought from an analysis of travel patterns (e.g., Belgians traveling to Zaire, Haitians traveling to Zaire, Cubans traveling to Angola, Angolans traveling to Cuba, Cubans traveling to Haiti, Haitians traveling to Cuba, male homosexuals traveling to Haiti, male prostitutes in Haiti, Cubans entering the United States in large numbers in 1980 (of which substantial numbers were male homosexuals), Haitians traveling to the United States, and from malarial statistics.

"These particular travel patterns are cited because of increased traffic in all these categories during the past five years ... and the proximity of Angola to Zaire. The correlation between outbreaks of malaria and infections by EBV (and especially Burkitt's lymphoma) may be especially important ... The correlation between malaria and EBV infectivity ... may have a substantive basis that was overlooked in the past because possible virulence of secondary products of EBV was never suspected."

The gradual build-up of infectivity -- dose and titer dependency -- becomes an "equally attractive candidate for explaining the magnitude and profoundness of the AIDS problem," wrote Smith, with initial support for the thesis coming from findings that "most unconventional slow viruses are dependent on titer and dilution."

In the meantime, multiple herpesviruses and other probable co-factor viruses continue to appear in AIDS and ARC patients, raising a number of cause-and-consequence questions, none of which is resolved by the assumption that HIV, acting alone, is the single "cause" of AIDS.

Holmberg *et al.* investigated herpesviruses (including CMV, EBV, and HSV-1 and HSV-2) in separate studies[38,39] which indicated the complexity of attempting to find how co-factors might operate even in concomitant multiviral infections. Their conclusions were that the herpesviruses themselves were not co-factors in AIDS although

HSV-2 (herpes simplex virus 2) might be a "risk factor for subsequent or concurrent HIV infection."

Other researchers had made HIV-herpesvirus connections[40,41] even though the precise way in which one or more of these structures might enhance, catalyze or work synergistically with HIV was not fully expostulated.

By 1988, San Francisco researchers continued to note a relationship between CMV and Kaposi's sarcoma, as also suggested by other scientists. And a French study[43] found concomitant infection by the "new" herpesvirus, HHV-6, HTLV-1 (the leukemia-associated virus originally thought to be connected in some way with HIV) and the "new" AIDS virus, HIV-2.

Just what HHV-6 and HTLV-1 may have to do with the "AIDS viruses" (HIV-1, HIV-2), remains very much open to question, the former being the new viral kid on the block, as a renamed version of HBLV (human B-cell leukemia virus).

As we have seen, HHV-6 is suspected in the "Lake Tahoe Syndrome" as perhaps a causative agent of unknown origin and transmissibility. (One B.R.I-Mexico patient with this syndrome was seropositive only for HHV-6 as well as bearing very modest elevations in "titers" of EBV, with no immune distortions.) One 1988 study[44] on HHV-6 in male homosexuals both positive and negative for HIV antibodies failed to make any firm conclusions as to how HHV-6 might "potentiate" HIV.

But this new member of the herpes family does show up in the multiviral screens of HIV/AIDS patients, along with HTLV-1, Dr. Gallo's first HTLV "family" member now associated with adult T-cell leukemia and said to have a very long incubation period. HTLV-1 seems to be highly correlated with drug addicts, so much so that by 1988 a whopping 21% of California's drug addicts (particularly IV users, apparently) tested positive for this structure, described as "related to the AIDS virus."[45]

Another 1988 study[46] indicated that persons infected by HIV-1 might be more likely to develop actual AIDS if they are also infected by HTLV-1. An experiment carried out by molecular virologists at UCLA showed that HTLV-1 apparently activates HIV by stimulating HIV-infected white blood cells to divide. Study leader S.Y. Chen noted: "The chances of any individual being infected by both viruses are very slim, but among selected populations, such as intravenous drug abusers, the chances are quite high."

Such studies open the door to HTLV-1 as a viral catalyst for HIV-1 particularly in the rapidly expanding population of AIDS patients identified by drug abuse as a "high-risk" group.

Yet another possible co-factor is another distinguished member of the herpes family, herpes zoster, which causes shingles. A rapid, painful attack of this condition is increasingly being seen as a sign of immune depression and an early warning signal that the HIV/AIDS infection curve is under way.[47]

Separate studies[48,49] have linked HTLV-1 to multiple sclerosis, an autoimmune disorder which is frequently suspected both of contagiosity and viral connections,and one found more "cross-reactivity" between HTLV-1 and HIV-2, the "second AIDS virus."

The insistence in some circles that HIV itself "jumped species" from other animals to man, and the similarity between certain human and animal viruses and the manner in which they are spread -- for example, by coughing, biting and ingesting, quite aside from blood-to-blood contact through sexual relations -- makes the animal virus connection to human ills more than idle speculation.

It also theoretically calls into question about how complacent we can be that "the AIDS virus" (or viruses) are transmitted only by blood and semen -- when so many closely related animal viruses which produce AIDS-like conditions are transmitted so many other ways.

Drs. Mark Whiteside and Carole MacLeod maintained for some time that the unusually large concentration of AIDS cases in one poor town in subtropical Florida, Belle Glade, strongly indicated not only "insect vectors" (typically, mosquitoes) in AIDS transmission but suggested other insect-related viruses as co-factors.[50,51] The Whiteside/ MacLeod assertions as to a high percentage of "no identifiable risk" factor "AIDS carriers" in Belle Glade upset the standard AIDS research concepts in the U.S.A.

The research establishment did not take long in attempting to refute the theory that mosquitoes, let alone other insects, might be transmitting AIDS, particularly since some U.S. groups helped spread the notion that in-

107

sects might be "flying hypodermic needles" waiting to be injected into the blood.

Castro *et al.* set about reinvestigating AIDS transmission in Belle Glade and reached the conclusion that even the allegedly "no indentifiable risk" victims in this poor, largely minority (Haitian, British West Indian, Hispanic) community really did fall into "high-risk" groups whether they originally seemed to or not -- IV drug use and homosexual and heterosexual relations allegedly accounting for the high-risk activity, at least within the parameters of U.S.-dominated Western medicine.[52,53]

French research[54,55] had also reported that DNA sequences matching the DNA of HIV -- suggestive of, but not confirming, the presence of HIV in insects -- had been found in mosquitoes, ant lions, tsetse flies, cockroaches, ticks and bedbugs from central Africa, yet not in insects from Paris. There was allegedly no evidence of either free virus or viral "replication" within insects in which these viral particles were found.

A further possibility of the "insect vector" had been suggested by one laboratory study[56] in which HIV was cultured from bedbugs up to four hours after they had gorged on blood containing high concentrations of HIV, concentrations far higher than those cultured from the blood of HIV-infected humans. Even at such concentrations, the insects were said not to be able to transmit HIV from infected to uninfected blood during uninterrupted feeding.

The Whiteside studies had the virtue of duplicating in a U.S. setting conditions obtaining in poor tropical areas of the world, including Haiti and central Africa, in terms of poor hygiene and heterosexuality, with the addition of IV drug use. However, despite U.S. medical orthodoxy's fascination with the single-virus etiology of HIV/AIDS, Whiteside and other investigators are probably onto something by insinuating a multiviral etiology which might involve viruses from other species.

In November 1985, AIDS, while represented by only 10 of 395 oral and other presentations at the 34th Annual Meeting of the American Society of Tropical Medicine and Hygiene in Miami,[26] dominated the conference to some extent and seemed to place veterinarians against classical medical allopaths in arguing over AIDS viral transmission.

Dr. G.K. Ogilvie, College of Veterinary Medicine,

University of Illinois, discussed animal retroviruses as a model of human infection,[27] noting in particular how the animal viruses are a major source of information as to how retroviruses -- and the HTLV viruses are considered to be retroviruses -- are transmitted and how they cause disease. Indeed, the primary modes of transmission are "mechanical transmission" by insects and respiratory aerosols, he noted.

Ogilvie discussed the visna virus (the structure Smith noted as causing the early AIDS-like disease in Icelandic sheep in the 1930s) and which is most closely related to the putative AIDS virus in humans. Visna, which causes death from progressive lung and brain disease, so strikingly similar to the human AIDS picture, is transmitted by respiratory aerosols when sheep cough on each other under crowded conditions.

Ogilvie developed the vaccine against feline leukemia virus, which causes an immune deficiency syndrome similar to human AIDS. In fact, it was work on the feline leukemia virus which may ultimately have led to the isolation and naming of HTLV-I, a retrovirus associated with human leukemia[28,29] and indicating the first correlation between viruses and human cancer.

He discussed several animal retroviruses, including bovine leukemia virus, equine infectious anemia virus, visna and the above-mentioned feline leukemia virus. These viruses are spread in blood by biting insects, by saliva and through respiratory aerosols, with the feline virus in particular spread by all three routes. He pointed out that bovine leukemia virus and equine infectious anemia virus (a *lentivirus* or "slow virus", as is the putative AIDS agent) are transmitted by biting insects such as horseflies.

At the meeting, Drs. Whiteside and MacLeod pointed out that half of all their "no identifiable risk" AIDS patients from Belle Glade had antibodies to one or more of the insect-transmitted viruses, known as arboviruses (or arthropod-borne viruses). These viruses combine with each other to produce infections and stimulate retroviruses.

As Dr. Grauerholz paraphrased the Whiteside-MacLeod thesis:[26] "So, not only is it possible that the AIDS virus [*sic*] itself could be transmitted by insects, but other insect-transmitted viruses could act as co-factors in the development of immune depression."

(In terms of the HTLV-I, or so-called adult T-cell

leukemia virus, a slowly moving retrovirus par excellence in that it takes as long as 30 years to incubate, the fact that it had been found in higher-than-expected numbers in homosexuals and drug addicts led early on to some fears that HIV may spread the same way HTLV-I does and may take an extraordinarily long time to reveal itself).[30]

Dr. Whiteside pointed to Type 1 of the dengue virus as being "an epidemiological marker for the introduction of AIDS into the Western hemisphere."[35] He noted that dengue first appeared in the U.S.A. in 1977, a year before the first cluster of AIDS was reported in this country and in Haiti, where, he has stated, most Haitians have had multiple exposures to at least one type of dengue fever.

The variable incubation period, prodromal signs and symptoms, and pathologic changes caused by AIDS are strikingly similar to those of repeated infection by dengue virus and possibly other arboviruses, assessed Dr. Whiteside. Repeated bouts of dengue and other flu-like diseases associated with insect-transmitted arboviruses can cause increasing degrees of immunosuppression and eventual activation of dormant retroviruses -- including HIV -- he has pointed out.

He told *Oncology Times:*[31] "Most people think that HTLV-III is the cause of AIDS, but we think it is more likely to be a marker for immunosuppression or a cofactor." He added that it has been known for some time that arboviruses can activate retroviruses in animals.

Drs. Whiteside and MacLeod,reviewing the records of 400 consecutive homosexual patients screened for AIDS in South Florida between January-November 1983, found that since 1977 "a large majority... of these men had either traveled to the Caribbean... or had sexual contact with Puerto Ricans, Dominicans, Haitians, Jamaicans, or Cubans... Only receivers or passive partners in anal intercourse had symptoms of AIDS or AIDS-related complexes."

They told a tropical medicine conference that the data suggest that "a new agent was introduced into the Western hemisphere" possibly in 1978 or before. They found widespread presence of antibody to various arboviruses.[32,33]

They found substantial numbers of patients with antibodies to *maguari*, a Bunyamwera serogroup virus, with one panel excluding Haitians and denoting travel patterns suggesting that only two had travelled outside the U.S.A. "Presence of antibody to (maguari) in NIR patients who have not traveled strongly suggests that this virus has been introduced into South Florida, and that it plays an important role in the pathogenesis of AIDS," they said.[34]

Further, Dr. Whiteside noted the close relationship between AIDS and tuberculosis, concluding that "milder degrees of infection and immunosuppression by arboviruses are known to cause TB. Most people recognize that TB is environmental. We are seeing similar patterns of AIDS and TB in long-term residents of the same poor neighborhoods of Southern Florida. We believe that AIDS is a tropically based, environmental disease."

The possible effects of animal viruses in man are not limited to speculations on arboviruses. The conspiracy theorists of the synthetic origins of HIV (Chapter Eleven) believe the structure is a splice-together of two animal viruses whose adaptation to human existence evolves with each new human carrier.

That there might be a connection between AIDS and viruses in animals other than insects and green monkeys drew interest from the beginning. One of the AIDS-like animal diseases is African swine fever, whose outbreaks in 1978 in Zaire, the Dominican Republic, Brazil and Haiti are, as in the case of the hepatitis vaccine experiment in New York, chronologically convenient for the belated arrival of AIDS in all of these places.

A primary apostle of the AIDS-swine fever connection has been Charles Ortlieb, publisher of *The New York Native*[57] who, citing *The Boston Globe*, wrote that the American CIA brought swine fever into Cuba in the early 1970s and as a result some 800,000 pigs in Cuba had to be slaughtered.

Swine fever produces an immune deficiency in pigs similar to that allegedly produced by HIV in man. The extrapolation of these considerations is that somehow mutated swine fever virus may have been introduced into humans, possibly as a result of a political maneuver, or through some unusual kind of exposure.

The U.S. government argument that the swine fever virus does not infect people founders on the realities of viruses and retroviruses: they mutate and adapt, and swine-fever virus affects other animals.[58]

111

It is *not* clear that repeated everyday exposure to such parasitical structures as the swine-fever viruses (such as walking around on a farm, for example) is without risk.

It was striking to this writer from the early days of AIDS research that consideration of animal virology, well-known to veterinarians, seemed to be pooh-poohed by the AIDS research establishment, at least in the U.S.

While one wonders why, at least some alarming possibilities present themselves.

A considerable number of animal viruses which cause immune depression are spread by methods *other than* blood and semen. These viruses also mutate from species to species. If the AIDS establishment is forever wedded to the HIV etiology of the syndrome, then why is it relatively silent on the possibility HIV might mutate to spread in ways common to animal retroviruses?

In asserting, for a time, the African-green-monkey-bites-man theory of HIV origins in the Dark Continent, the U.S. AIDS research network was adrift in controversy: on the one hand it was insisting that "casual contact" (by implication, with saliva, if not outright biting) could not spread AIDS, yet it was suggesting that a non-sexual mode of transfer (biting) must have occurred at some point allowing the "species jump" from primate to man!

With MacLeod/Whiteside not yielding on their warnings concerning insect vectors[62] and with those interested in human virology noting that human viruses do indeed mutate, it is entirely too early to argue that it is chiseled in stone that there is no other route of HIV infection other than by blood and semen.

It is also, of course, too early to discount multiviral connections with both humans and other animals -- and, happily, we believe, too late to defend much further the idea that HIV alone causes the syndrome.

REFERENCES

(1)   Kelly, Thomas A., "Acquired immune deficiency syndrome (AIDS)." Medical Hypotheses 14: 347-351, 1984.

(2)   From Science, cited in Aleshire, Peter, "AIDS appears more likely to strike if immune system is already frail." Oakland (CA) Tribune, Aug.

112

14, 1985.

(3)   "AIDS poses complex research puzzle, say N.Y.investigators." Amer. Med. News, Aug. 5, 1983.

(4)   De Mauberge, J. et al., "Syndrome d'immunodefience acquise (AIDS) revele par un herpes genital severe." Dermatologica 168: 105-111, 1984.

(5)   Britton, Carolyn B., et al., "A new complication of AIDS: thoracic myelitis caused by herpes simplex virus." Neurology 35: 1071-1074, 1985.

(6)   Goldsmith, M.F., "Not there yet, but, 'on our way' in AIDS research, scientists say." J. Amer. Med. Assn., 253: 23, 3369-3384, 1985.

(7)   Seligmann, Maxime, et al., "AIDS -- an immunologic reevaluation." N. Eng. J. Med, 311: 20, 1286-1292, 1984.

(8)   Hirsch, Martin S., and Donna Felsenstein, "Cytomegalovirus-induced immunosuppression." Ann. N.Y. Acad. Sci. 437, 1984.

(9)   Ioachim, Harry L., "Acquired immune deficiency disease after three years: the unsolved riddle." Laboratory Investigation, 51: 1, 1-4, 1984.

(10)   Giraldo, G., et al., "Herpes-type virus particles in tissue culture of Kaposi's sarcoma from different geographic regions." J. Natl. Cancer Inst., 49: 1509, 1972.

(11)   Giraldo, G., et al., "Antibody patterns to herpes virus in Kaposi's sarcoma. II.Serological association of American Kaposi's sarcoma with cytomegalovirus." Int. J. Cancer 22: 126, 1978.

(12)   Giraldo, G., et al., "Antibody patterns to herpes virus in Kaposi's sarcoma: serological association of European Kaposi's sarcoma with cytomegalovirus." Int. J. Cancer 15: 839, 1975.

(13)   Drew, W.L., et al., "Cytomegalovirus and Kaposi's sarcoma in young homosexual men." Lancet: 1: 125, 1982.

(14)   Drew, W.L., and Lawrence Mintz, "What is the role of cytomegalovirus in AIDS?" Ann. N.Y. Acad. Sci., 437, 1984.

(15)   Lange, Michael, et al., "Cytomegalovirus isolation from healthy homosexual men." J. Am. Med. Assn., 242: 14, 1908-1910, Oct. 12, 1984.

(16)   Kestens, Luc, et al., "Endemic African Kaposi's sarcoma is not associated with immunodeficiency." Int. J. Cancer 36: 49-54, 1985.

(17)   "The acquired immune deficiency syndrome (AIDS) -- a multidisciplinary enigma." West. J. Med. 140: 66-81, Jan.1984.

(18)   "AIDS: where do we go from here?" WHO Chronicle 39: 3, 98-103, 1985.

(19)   Henle, W., and G. Henle, in The Epstein-Barr Virus. Berlin: Springer Verlag, 1979.

(20)   Epstein, M. A., "Immunological control of Epstein-Barr virus infection: possible lessons for AIDS." Ann. N.Y. Acad. Sci., 427, 1984.

(21)   Klein, G., "The Epstein-Barr virus and neoplasia." N. Eng. J. Med., 293: 1353, 1975.

(22)   Sonnabend, J.A., "The etiology of AIDS." AIDS Research, I:1, 1-12, 1983.

(23)   Smith, Roulette Wm., "AIDS and slow viruses." Ann. N.Y. Acad. Sci., 437,

1984.

(24)   Smith, Roulette Wm., letter to researchers, privately published, summer
         1985.

(25)   Sigurdsson, Bjorn, Br. Vet. J., 110: 255-270, 307-322, 341-354, 1954.

(26)   Grauerholz, John, "AIDS invades conference in tropical medicine." New
         Solidarity (weekly), p. 4, Nov. 22, 1985.

(27)   Ogilvie, G.K., "Animal retroviruses as a model of human infection," ad-
         dress, 34th Annual Meeting, American Society of Tropical Medicine and
         Hygiene, Miami, Fla., Nov. 3-7, 1985.

(28)   Esajian, Jeanie, "Feline leukemia studies led to UCD test for AIDS,"
         Sacramento Union, Dec. 9, 1984.

(29)   Hunter, Pat, "AIDS variations slow doctors searching for vaccine."
         Honolulu Advertiser, Feb. 20, 1985.

(30)   Bishop, Jerry E., "Scientists fear that cancer virus may spread in same
         ways as AIDS." Wall Street Journal, Nov. 4, 1985.

(31)   Stockwell, Serena, "Dengue arbovirus could be marker for AIDS; possible
         link to mosquitoes being studied." Oncology Times III:10, October, 1985.

(32)   MacLeod, Caroline E., et al., "Dengue, an old disease in new guise
         (AIDS)?" (Abstract of paper) Tropical Medicine Program, University of
         Miami, 1985.

(33)   Whiteside, Mark E., et al., "Antibodies to arboviruses in patients with the
         acquired immunodeficiency syndrome (AIDS)." Abstact of paper
         presented to American Society of Tropical Medicine and Hygiene/Royal
         Society of Tropical Medicine and Hygiene, Baltimore, Md., Dec. 3 - 6,
         1984.

(34)   MacLeod, C.L. et al., "Antibody to maguari in patients with the acquired
         immunodeficiency syndrome (AIDS)." Abstract of paper presented to the
         American Society of Tropical Medicine and Hygiene, Miami, Nov. 4 - 7,
         1985.

(35)   MacLeod, C.L., et al., "Dengue immunologic enhancement studies in
         Haitian patients with the acquired immunodeficiency syndrome (AIDS)."
         Abstract of paper presented to the American Society of Tropical Medicine
         and Hygiene/Royal Society of Tropical Medicine and Hygiene, Baltimore,
         Md., Dec. 3 - 6, 1984.

(36)   Downing, R.G., et al., "African Kaposi's sarcoma and AIDS." Lancet,
         March 3, 1984.

(37)   Carne, C.A., et al., "Rising prevalence of human T-lymphotropic virus
         type III (HTLV-III) infection in homosexual men in London." Lancet,
         June 1, 1985.

(38)   Holmberg, S.D., et al., "Prior herpes simplex virus type 2 infection as a
         risk factor for HIV infection." J.Am. Assn. 259: 7, Feb. 14, 1988.

(39)   Holmberg, S.D., et al., "Herpesviruses as co-factors in AIDS." Lancet,
         Sept. 24, 1988.

(40) "Herpes-AIDS link probed." Am. Med. News, Oct. 23 - 30, 1987.

(41) Quinnan, G.V., et al., "Herpesvirus infection in the acquired immune deficiency syndrome." J. Am. Med. Assn., 252:72-77, 1984.

(42) Drews, W.L., et al., "Declining prevalence of Kaposi's sarcoma in homosexual AIDS patients paralleled by fall in cytomegalovirus transmission." Lancet, Jan. 2/9, 1988.

(43) Agut, H., "Concomitant infection by human herpesvirus 6, HTLV-1 and HIV-2." Lancet, March 26, 1988.

(44) Fox, J., et al., "Antibody to human herpesvirus 6 in HIV-1 positive and negative homosexual men." Lancet, Aug. 14, 1988.

(45) Peterson, S., "21% of state's addicts tests positive for leukemia virus." The (Orange County) Register, Feb. 6, 1988.

(46) "Leukemia virus might trigger AIDS." (The Associated Press) The (Orange County) Register, May 20, 1988.

(47) Melbye, M., et al., "Risk of AIDS after herpes zoster." Lancet, March 28, 1987.

(48) Kaprowski, Hilary, et al., "Diagnosis of multiple sclerosis by detection of human T-cell lymphotropic virus IV or antibodies thereto, and vaccine for multiple sclerosis." Immunochemistry, 107:553, 1987.

(49) Ohta, M., et al., "Sera from patients with multiple sclerosis react with human T-cell lymphotropic virus-I GAG protein but not with ENV proteins -- Western blotting analysis." Chem. Absts. 106: 478, 1987.

(50) Whiteside, M.E., et al., "Outbreak of no identifiable risk acquired immunodeficiency syndrome (AIDS) in Belle Glade, Fla.," First Intl. Conf. on AIDS, Atlanta GA., April 17, 1985.

(51) Interview with Dr. John Grauerholz in AIDS is More Deadly Than Nuclear War, Natl. Democratic Policy Committee, 1985.

(52) Castro, K.G., et al., "Transmission of HIV in Belle Glade, Fla.: lessons for communities in the United States." Science, 239: 193-197, 1988.

(53) "Acquired immunodeficiency syndrome (AIDS) in Western Palm Beach County, Fla." Morbidity and Mortality Weekly Report, 35: 609-612, 1986.

(54) Becker, J.L., et al., "Infection of cultured insect cells with HIV, the causative agent of AIDS, and demonstration of infection in African insects with this virus." C R Acad. Sci. III: 303: 303-306, 1986.

(55) Chermann, J.C., et al., "HIV related sequences in insects from central Africa." Third Intl. Conf. on AIDS, Washington D.C., June 1, 1987.

(56) Lyons, S.F., et al., "Survival of HIV in the common bedbug." Lancet, 2:45, 1986.

(57) Cited in Null, Gary, "The AIDS cover-up," Penthouse, December 1985.

(58) Teas, Jane, "Considerations in searching for the cause of AIDS." Ann. N.Y. Acad. Sci., V:437, 1984.

(59) "Hepatitis B seems to worsen AIDS infection." Washington Post, Nov. 1, 1988.

115

(60)   Staver, Sari, "Meeting sheds light on chronic fatigue." American Medical News, May 26, 1989.

(61)   Webster, A., et al., "Cytomegalovirus infection and progression towards AIDS in hemophiliacs with human immunodeficiency virus infection." Lancet, July 8, 1989.

(62)   Douglass, William C., AIDS: The End of Civilization. Clayton GA: Valet Publishers, 1989.

Chapter Six

THE DRUG CONNECTION

Since the beginning of the AIDS epidemic, a connection between drug use and the syndrome was apparent -- and to some observers it was just as easy to see AIDS as a "junkies' disease" as it was to view it as the "gay plague."

It is also obvious that some of the mononucleosis-like and wasting symptoms frequently seen among drug users may actually have been cases of AIDS, yet not reported as such, in the 1970s.

The drug connection in the onset of AIDS has largely been obscured by the reporting techniques of the Centers for Disease Control (CDC), which segregate "intravenous drug users" from homosexuals as "at-risk" populations, thereby failing to take into account the substantial use of *non*-intravenous substances by several classes of people, aside from the variable of persons presenting themselves as "drug users" rather than as "gays" and vice-versa.

The first connection between drugs and AIDS was noted in regards to nitrite inhalant substances, better known as "poppers." From the earliest reports of *Pneumocystis carinii* in homosexual males on both coasts, researchers noted a prevalence of "recreational drug" use as reported by the patients themselves.[1] Indeed, all the first five men diagnosed with AIDS as reported to the CDC had used poppers. One also was an IV drug user and only two fit CDC guidelines for unusual promiscuity.

Cesar A. Caceres, MD, and Terry Krieger emphasized[2] the reality for those not aware of the fast-lane lifestyle of some gays let alone of many other kinds of people, using the CDC database: adding the (1985 numbers) 1,163 of 10,003 homosexual and bisexual AIDS patients who were also IV drug users to the 2,342 IV drug users said to be exclusively heterosexual, "we find at least 25% of AIDS patients have been intravenous drug users", they wrote.

But since CDC does not itemize drug use in general, Caceres-Krieger, relying on another figure (from Dr. Harry W. Haverkos, then of the CDC), namely, that 97% of 87 homosexual and bisexual AIDS patients involved in three

CDC studies had used "street drugs" at least once, and 75% used them at least once a week for several years without being IV drug users, and assessing the statistics of other CDC studies, concluded that at least 54% of AIDS patients in general have been abusers of oral drugs. Adding that 54 percent to the 25% who are IV drug users, we are looking at a figure of 79% drug abuse across the board in AIDS patients.

This general assessment holds with the interviewing conducted by the Bradford Research Institute over a 6-year period beginning in 1983 of prospective HIV/AIDS experimental therapy patients, some of whom later entered the program at the B.R.I. Mexico division. All but 6 of 300 interviewees were admittedly homosexual males; all but a dozen admitted some form of drug abuse, only a dozen or so of these others admitting to actual IV drug use.

It is also safe to say that about the same percentage also fit the profile for promiscuity and repeated anal-passive sex.

The variety and amounts of "recreational" and "street" drugs vary considerably. In that subpopulation of the openly gay community which tends to be disco- and bath house-oriented, poppers are drugs of choice, said to enhance the feeling of sexual arousal during sex acts themselves and/or to stimulate non-stop disco dancing. Several AIDS-diagnosed patients known to our group admitted to an actual habituation or possible addiction to poppers themselves.

Not only some homosexuals, but many other people, usually young and usually urban, are committed to drug use of a non-intravenous nature, and reflect far different profiles from the needle-marked, anemic heroin junkie waiting at the bus station for a contact and a fix.

Amphetamines ("uppers" in street parlance), barbiturates ("downers"), LSD and PCP hallucinogens, all of which are taken orally, join cocaine, currently a drug of choice for the "upwardly mobile," poppers and ethyl chloride, all of which are sniffed. Cocaine may also be injected and is thus a bridge into classical IV drug use. Over and above these substances is the naggingly persistent use of marijuana.

It may be said now, including the use of marijuana, that "recreational" and "street" drugs are, among other things, generally immunosuppressive. They may be immunosuppressive in and of themselves, with research in this area ambivalent, but as co-factors to frequent malnutrition or actual starvation are decidedly so.

We have to agree with Caceres-Krieger up to a point when they state: "AIDS patients seem to have been people who already were sick in the sense of having a damaged immune system. Apparently most were sick because they abused drugs."

In 1984, James J. Goedert of the Environmental Epidemiology Branch, National Cancer Institute, reported to the New York Academy of Sciences[3] that various studies of the effects of nitrite inhalants correlated with lowered helper-suppressor T-cell ratios, the classical immune system "marker" for pre-AIDS. The popper factor was the only variable in some cases; in others, sexual promiscuity and other variables played statistical roles.

Marmor et al., noted[4] a 12-fold relative risk for Kaposi's sarcoma among homosexual men with exposure to amyl, but not butyl, nitrite. Jaffe et al. showed in a national CDC study[5] that the use of multiple recreational drugs was related to the risk of developing AIDS, even though no single drug was implicated.

In contrasting studies done by his group with later reports from the CDC, Goedert found that daily inhalation of amyl nitrite vapor by mice resulted in immunological impairment, though animals exposed to isobutyl nitrite had no such damage. *In vitro* studies have indicated significant immunotoxic effects from both amyl and isobutyl nitrite.[6,7]

The Marmor study also implicated cocaine as a possible epidemiological factor in AIDS, as did that part of the Goedert work based on the habits of Danish male homosexuals. Cocaine may be teratogenic in mice.[8]

Assessed Goedert: "Intravenous drug abusers have many immunologic similarities to promiscuous homosexual men, including consistently elevated immunoglobulin M levels, positive results on hepatitis B and syphilis serologic tests, atypical lymphocytosis recognized 15 years ago, and several reports of autoimmune thrombocytopenic purpura."

In 1985, Gangadharam et al., at the National Jewish Hospital and Research Center, Denver, reported[9] that one isobutyl nitrite -- that is, popper -- product, "Rush," tested in mice reduced the animals' ability to fight off *Mycobac-*

119

terium intracellulare, a tuberculosis-producing bacterium which frequently strikes AIDS patients. "We believe our findings establish that inhaling isobutyl nitrite should be considered dangerous to homosexuals and others at high risk," Dr. Gangadharam said.[10]

The same year, Haverkos reported[11] on the increased frequency of use of nitrite inhalants by male homosexuals suffering from Kaposi's sarcoma as contrasted with gays with other manifestations of AIDS or with asymptomatic HIV infection. This led the CDC to conclude[12] that the use of such inhalants as well as the persistent problem of cytomegalovirus infection needed further attention as possible AIDS co-factors.

In a study of 42 homosexual or bisexual men with persistent generalized lymphadenopathy not attributable to an identifiable cause, eight patients advanced to clinical AIDS, an outcome, researchers said, that was "associated with previous heavy nitrite inhalant use."

Among the group of 42 the use of amphetamines, marijuana and cocaine was "common." The authors concluded that "although amyl nitrite is unlikely to be primary in the syndrome of PGL [persistent generalized lymphadenopathy] or AIDS, our findings ... demonstrating an association between heavy nitrite inhalant use and Kaposi's sarcoma (after adjustment for sexual contacts) suggest that these exposures may influence ultimate disease expression. This notion is strengthened by the disproportionate numbers of cases of Kaposi's sarcoma in homosexual males compared with other AIDS risk groups."[18]

The most damning abstract of the popper-AIDs connection, accompanied by an attack on the HIV-as-single-cause theory, was prepared by Lauritsen and Wilson in 1985/86.[24] In 1989, Kaslow *et al.,* reporting on thousands of AIDS cases in a "multicenter AIDS cohort study,"[25] claimed that neither alcohol nor "psychoactive substances" enhanced "the progression of human immunodeficiency virus infection" although such factors were not looked at within a whole spectrum of possible immune-depressing activities.

It is intriguing that as popper use has declined in gay communities in response to the AIDS crisis, so have the levels of KS.

In the meantime, some research continues to implicate marijuana as a possible factor, as well. A 1983 San Francisco Public Health Department study found that both pot and poppers were "popular" in the S.F. gay community. Researchers Edward Morales and Michael Graves found that 75 percent of S.F. gays used marijuana and 58 percent inhaled poppers.[13]

At the University of South Florida, D.K. Blanchard *et al.* noted the suppressive effects in certain immune functions in mice by delta-9-tetrahydrocannabinol (THC), the major psychogenic component in marijuana.[14] Another study pointed to the immunosuppressive effects of barbiturates.[15]

In November 1985 in *The Lancet*, Austrian researcher D. Fuchs *et al.* questioned: "Are homosexuals less at risk of AIDS than intravenous drug abusers and hemophiliacs?"[16] Using June 1985 CDC statistics, and utilizing levels of urinary neopterin, which already had been found to be elevated in 100 percent of AIDS and ARC patients,[17] they analyzed that in terms of actual risk "it is only the large size of the homosexual population that makes them contribute [statistically] the largest number of AIDS cases; the individual risk of contracting AIDS is higher for the other two risk groups."

Fuchs has also correlated increased neopterin levels with receptive anal intercourse. Again, he was only looking at "IV" drug users in studying CDC statistics, but his conclusion points as much, if not moreso, to the "druggishness" of the disease as to the "gayishness" of it.

The drug connection in AIDS is by no means limited to male homosexuals.

At the end of 1985, *The Lancet* reported[19] on findings from England, France and Italy on correlations between drug use, AIDS and heterosexual prostitutes, which conflicted with earlier information from Rwanda,[20] Athens[21] and Seattle, U.S.A.,[22] which tended to make female prostitution a "reservoir" for HIV infection.

In London, S.E. Barton *et al.* reported that 50 English prostitutes, all engaging in vaginal intercourse, 41 in oral sexual intercourse and nine in regular anal intercourse, and only three of whom had used intravenous drugs, were *all* negative for HIV antibodies. Nineteen of the 50 had always insisted on condom use. The sampling of London prostitutes indicated a far more insignificant use of at least IV drugs among prostitutes there than is usually the case in the U.S.A.

In Paris, Brenky-Faudeux and Fribourg-Blanc, analyzing the activities and sera of 56 prostitutes, found that all 56 were HIV-negative. "These women aged 18-60 have sexual intercourse 15-25 times daily and do not routinely use protection," they said, adding that "furthermore, none of the Paris prostitutes was a drug addict."

In Italy, Tirelli *et al.* did a prospective study on 24 female prostitutes, 14 of whom were intravenous abusers, in the town of Pordenone. Controls were 15 women who were not IV drug abusers but were sexual partners of men who were taking part in a study of the heterosexual transmission of HIV. (Prevalence of HIV antibody in 95 male IV drug users and of 30 homosexual men in Pordenone was 52% and 15% respectively.)

Among the intravenous drug-using prostitutes, 71% had antibodies to HIV vs. nine for the non-IV drug users and one of the controls. Also, 75% of the drug users had altered T4:T8 ratios vs. only one of the non-IV drug using prostitutes and 17% of the controls. None had developed actual AIDS. Neither group of prostitutes had had intercourse with IV drug addicts or with bisexual men. Condoms were rarely used by the customers of the drug addict prostitutes but they were always used by customers of the non-addict prostitutes.

The eight stable long-term sexual partners of non-addict prostitutes were men without known AIDS risk factors, whereas the five stable long-term partners of the addict prostitutes were themselves drug abusers.

Concluded Tirelli and his colleagues: "Our data show that, in Pordenone, prostitutes who are not intravenous drug abusers are not at increased risk for AIDS, while those who are should be considered as being at risk of HTLV-III infection."

The data from these three sets of cases also suggest that promiscuity *per se* is not a major factor, nor is anal intercourse, nor necessarily is protection from condoms. The data were silent as to non-IV drugs, but they strongly implicated at least intravenous drugs with HIV positivity in female prostitutes.

An excellent review of research on the many ways

drugs lead to immune depression was published in 1985 --
as the terms "immunotoxicology" and
"immunopharmacology" came into vogue.[23]

Allowing for such variables as the debilitating effects
of actual malnutrition, the absence of the "drug factor" may
account to some extent for the paucity of AIDS cases in
much of the Third World -- for in many places, particularly
Southeast Asia, where homosexual activity is notoriously
rampant, it cannot be said that sexual promiscuity is substantially less than it is in the U.S.A. However, economic
hardship prevails in that part of the world, and the
homosexual community, if indeed it can be so styled, does
not have the funds to engage in the purchase and use of
poppers, marijuana, cocaine and most other drugs.

For American investigators, there will remain the
considerable problem of interviewee honesty and sincere
recall when discussing drug use. I am reminded of one of
our earliest AIDS cases (KS, gay bowel syndrome, opportunistic infections.) Only grudgingly did this individual, a
scholar, admit to prolonged and heavy use of poppers,
marijuana and "uppers" -- not because he was lying but because the practice was so natural to him that he did not
regard the significant use of these substances as a problem
to be noted.

Interviewers also meet with the rejection syndrome
one finds in dealing with alcoholics -- denial that the
problem exists. It is almost a certainty that drug use and
abuse, however much it is now being noted, has still gone
under-reported in the AIDS controversy.

Nor should the "socially sanctioned" drugs -- alcohol,
nicotine, caffeine -- be overlooked in their possible immunosuppressive roles in helping set the stage for
retroviral replication. The extent to which habituation to
these common drugs may interact with the more lethal substances or be immunosuppressive in and of themselves has
not been adequately studied.

The proliferation of the use of antibiotics and
steroids ("legal drugs") -- see Chapter Seven -- is a con-
tributory factor to depressed host resistance and immune
depletion. In fact, if the "high-risk" HIV/AIDS groups
reporting abuse of illegal drugs are added to those who have
used inordinate amounts of antibiotics and steroids, the
drug connection to HIV/AIDS may approach 100 percent.

The continual abuse of drugs, be they legal, illegal, socially sanctioned or not, when complexed with poor diet, bad hygiene, ongoing multiple infections, a promiscuous lifestyle, unnatural water and other elements of the modern world, can make a witch's brew to which HIV, added as a catalyst, may stimulate the HIV/AIDS infection curve.

REFERENCES

(1)   Centers for Disease Control, Pneumocystis pneumonia -- Los Angeles. Morbid. Mortal. Weekly Rep. 30: 250-252, 1981.

(2)   Krieger, Terry, and Caceres, Cesar A., "The unnoticed link in AIDS cases." The Wall Street Journal, Oct 24, 1984.

(3)   Goedert, James J., "Recreational drugs: relationship to AIDS." Ann. N.Y. Acad. Sci., v.437, 1984.

(4)   Marmor, M., et al., "Risk factors for Kaposi's sarcoma in homosexual men." Lancet, i: 1083-1087, 1982.

(5)   Jaffe, H.W. et al., "National case-control study of Kaposi's sarcoma and Pneumocystis carinii pneumonia in homosexual men, Part I." Ann. Intern. Med. 99: 145-151, 1983.

(6)   Marmer, D.J., R.F. Jacobs, R.W. Steele, "In vitro immunotoxicity of amyl nitrite." Clin. Res. 30: 894A, 1982.

(7)   Hersh, E.M., et al., "Effect of the recreational agent isobutyl nitrite on human peripheral blood leukocytes and on in vitro interferon production." Cancer Res. 43: 1365-1371, 1983.

(8)   Mahalik, M.P., R.F. Gautieri, D.E.Mann, "Teratogenic potential of cocaine hydrochloride in CF-1 mice." J. Pharmaceut. Sci. 69: 703-706, 1980.

(9)   Gangadharam, P.R.J., et al., "Immunosuppressive action of isobutyl nitrite." Immunopharmacol. v.7 (3), 1985.

(10)   United Press International, Sept. 12, 1985.

(11)   Haverkos, H.W., et al., paper presented at the First International Conference on AIDS, Atlanta, GA, April 1985. (In Curran, q.v.)

(12)   Curran, James W., et al., "The epidemiology of AIDS: current status and future prospects." Science, vol. 229: 1352-1357, Sept. 27, 1985.

(13)   Harris, Richard F., "Pot and 'poppers' could bring risk of AIDS." San Francisco Examiner, Sept. 12, 1985.

(14)   Blanchard, D. K., et al., "Suppressive effect of delta-9-tetrahydrocannabinol on interferon production by murine splenocyte culture." Int. J. Immunopharmacol. v.7 (3), 1985.

(15)   Spiers, E.M., et al., "Certain barbiturate drugs suppress mitogen-stimulated lymphocyte growth in vitro." Int. J. Immunopharmacol., v.7 (3), 1985.

(16)   Fuchs, D., et al., "Are homosexuals less at risk of AIDS than intravenous drug abusers and hemophiliacs?" Lancet, 1130. Nov. 16, 1985.

(17)   Fuchs, D., et al., "Urinary neopterin in the diagnosis of acquired immune deficiency syndrome." Eur. J. Clin. Microbiol. 3: 70-71, 1984.

(18)   Mathur-Wagh, Usha, et al., "Longitudinal study of persistent generalized lymphadenopathy in homosexual men: relation to acquired immunodeficiency syndrome." Lancet, May 12, 1984.

(19)   Barton, S.E., et al., Brenky-Faudeux, Dominique, and Andre Fribourg-Blanc; Tirelli, Umberto, et al., "HTLV-III antibody in prostitutes." Lancet, Dec. 21/28, 1985.

(20)   Van de Perre, P., et al., "Acquired immunodeficiency syndrome in Rwanda." Lancet, ii: 62-65, 1984.

(21)   Papaevangelou, G., et al., "LAV/HTLV-III infection in female prostitutes." Lancet, ii: 1018, 1985.

(22)   "Heterosexual transmission of human T-lymphotropic virus type III/lymphadenopathy-associated virus." MMWR 34: 561-63, 1985.

(23)   Dean, J.H. et al., eds., Immunotoxicology and Immunopharmacology. New York: Raven Press, 1985.

(24)   Lauritsen, John, and Hank Wilson, Death Rush: Poppers and AIDS. New York: Pagan Press, 1986.

(25)   Kaslow, R.A., et al., "No evidence for a role of alcohol or other psychoactive drugs in accelerating immunodeficiency in HIV-positive individuals." J. Am. Med. Assn., June 16, 1989.

Chapter Seven

THE IATROGENIC CONNECTION

In recent times, it has become obvious that the very medicines produced by the modern pharmaceutical giants allegedly to cure diseases and conditions actually cause new diseases. Indeed, so great has the danger of "doctor-caused" illness become, either through prescription of dangerous substances, over-dependence on them, or improper or dangerous new medical techniques, that the phrase "iatrogenic disease" has now entered the national lexicon.

Iatrogenic disease is implicated in a wide array of chronic, systemic degenerative disease conditions, either as co-factors or actual causes. [See, for example, Illich[1] and Culbert[2]]. It may be no mystery that the explosion of synthetic drugs in the Western World, particularly since World War II, has been accompanied by an exponential increase in the rise and proliferation of all kinds of new conditions and pathological challenges, most of them totally unknown in the last century.

In the late 1970s and early 1980s, a new class of patients began appearing not only at the Bradford Research Institute's affiliated hospital in Mexico (American Biologics-Mexico S.A. Medical Center) but at doctor's offices around the U.S.A. -- and, probably at about the same time, in other offices in other Western European and English-speaking countries.

These patients complained of a Pandora's box of symptomata -- general fatigue, depression, pains in the joints, muscle cramps, sleep disturbances, multiple allergies and sensitivities ranging from mild to severe, skin problems, occasionally swollen glands, unexplained weight loss. At the laboratory level it was noted that they had one or more new or reactivated viral infections, usually of the ubiquitous Epstein-Barr, but increasingly of cytomegalovirus (CMV) and/or other herpesviruses. The presence of visible "yeast infection" on mucous surfaces (*Candida albicans*) became a virtual marker for this constellation of symptoms.

For a time, the general classification Theron Randolph created -- "universal reactor syndrome" -- was as easy a term to apply as any. But despite the names and symptoms, there was little allopathic physicians could do.

As the years went by, many patients progressively got worse, starting to react to practically everything in a burst of autoimmune activity as the body seemed frantically to be turning against itself. As often as not in the U.S.A., patients at the earlier stages of this no-name disease were dismissed as hypochondriacs or psychoneurotics -- and yet the disease conditions were very real.

The B.R.I.-Mexico team began dealing with an ever-growing group of these patients, usually refugees from American medicine who had been told either it was all in their heads or nothing could be done for them, the way cancer patients had been dealt with for some time: through individualized, integrated metabolic protocols involving detoxification, immune balancing, and dietary change. Positive results were seen, but not "cures."

Into the 1980s, many of these symptoms could be explained away by hypoglycemia -- a condition U.S. medical officialdom had taken a long time to admit actually existed -- and later, in women, by elements of PMS (menstrual syndrome). They sometimes could be explained in part by mercury intoxication from too many dental fillings or occasionally by fibromyalgia.

This syndrome of many conditions paralleled the outbreak of HIV/AIDS and, in many instances, mimicked early ARC-level or LAS-level cases. Yet patients characteristically were negative for HIV antibodies and were not regarded as HIV/AIDS patients -- yet surely they were suffering from "AIDS without AIDS."

Characteristically, at the minimum, they had systemic *Candida albicans* infection (a condition also for a long time not recognized by U.S. medical orthodoxy) and elevated titers of Epstein-Barr antibodies. Sometimes they presented as EBV cases, other times as yeast infection patients.

Eventually, it became clear that such patients (once PMS, mercury toxicity, hypoglycemia, endocrine problems or even psychosis had been eliminated as factors) had had long-term treatment with antibiotics, corticosteroids and various synthetic hormones. At times, patients had had literally *years* of such chemicals for everything from acne and sore throats to far more serious conditions.

By 1987 upwards of 20 percent of all patients seen at AB-Mexico Hospital were sufferers of this no-name syndrome. The typical person in this category was a 37-year-old female with 10 prior years of antibiotic or steroid therapy, including years of being on the contraceptive pill.

In short, these people -- and by implication millions more in their late 20s, 30s and occasionally 40s turning up at doctors' offices across the "civilized Western world" -- had been *poisoned.*

The advent of the no-name disease, which American medical orthodoxy finally agreed to call "chronic fatigue syndrome" in 1987/88, also paralleled the rapidly developing interest by some researchers, very much including the Bradford Research Institute, in "oxidology" -- the study of reactive oxygen metabolites in the system and their relationship to health and disease.

Breakdown products of toxic oxygen ("ROTS" -- or reactive oxygen toxic species, of which "free radicals" are the best known) were seen to be involved in the new syndrome -- CFS -- and probably all other degenerative disease conditions and metabolic challenges. The manipulation of ROTS became a B.R.I. pioneered adjunct to total metabolic therapy.

The new syndrome continued to excite plenty of "orthodox" interest, as did outbreaks of seemingly new and dangerous viruses above and beyond the attention accorded HIV/AIDS. The "Lake Tahoe syndrome" seemed to indicate a new viral infection (and human herpesvirus 6 may be a causative agent). Indeed, new viruses seemed to be lining up waiting either to fall into the metabolic miasma of civilized man or to be reactivated or to help reactivate other long-dormant viruses.

The role of Candida yeast infection became paramount in tracking CFS, and led inescapably to the conclusion that the mass population had been poisoned by excessive antibiotics and steroids.

Such substances, we now know, greatly alter the intestinal flora of the gastrointestinal tract, primarily the colon. The disturbance of normal bacteria there, in an area where the digestive and immune systems literally find common ground, helps eradicate benign, necessary bacteria and leads to the proliferation of parasitical organisms normally held in check.

The most notorious of these, *Candida albicans*, proliferates wildly through the system, leading to such visible signs as white specks or splotches in the mouth or nasopharyngeal area ("thrush" -- virtually a marker for both CFS and AIDS), vaginal and rectal distress, and cheesy growths under fingernails and toenails.

Along the way, yeast infection poisons the body with "mycotoxins," and profoundly affects immunity, depressed immunity leads to a reactivation of dormant pathogenic organisms or viruses, and/or helps position the body for an attack by manmade environmental chemicals (no longer blocked because the protective mixed-function oxidase-- MFO--enzyme system has been compromised) and by bacteria, fungi and viruses the body's crippled defense system can no longer overcome.

The body's last-ditch effort to compensate for the loss of its internal defenses is to carom from immune depression to autoimmune excitation, in which the body, losing its ability to distinguish "self" from "non-self," starts behaving as if its own tissues and organs are "non-self," manufactures defenses against them, and begins the precipitous march toward acute autoimmune disease -- the body turning on itself.

No wonder that an explosive growth in autoimmune-related disorders, including lupus, multiple sclerosis, and rheumatoid arthritis, have been part of the rapidly expanding CFS/AIDS picture.

The advent of immune/ autoimmune diseases, matched by multiviral reactivation, historically followed on the heels of the development of the synthetic antibiotics and corticosteroids, a history going back to chloramphenicol, first of the synthetic antibiotics and, in its time, overprescribed and overused. It has caused fatalities and suppressed bone marrow formation.

The drugs commonly developed for use in venereal infections, yeast overgrowth and localized inflammation common in venereal diseases -- ranging from terramycin, vaginal sulfa drugs, cephalosporin, ampicillin, amphotericin and clotrimazole to cortisone creams, doxycycline and metronizadole (Flagyl) -- are all, to various extents, immune depressants.

In their review of the health histories of San Francisco Bay Area homosexual men, Joan McKenna and associates found[3] patterns of persistent use of antibiotics and corticosteroids over many years, with antibiotics being used, often indiscriminately, to treat breakout after breakout of gonorrhea, chlamydia and other sexually-transmitted diseases.

The wholesale dosing of the gay population by tetracycline (sometimes suggested as useful before and after a specific sex act) and many other antibiotics led to a state of immune system alteration waiting to be compromised by something else, just as the continual overuse of antibiotics and corticosteroids by the "straight" population helped set the stage for Chronic Fatigue Syndrome.

Yet a frank admission of the delayed toxic effects of antibiotics and corticosteroids -- "wonder drugs" of an earlier era which have in fact wiped out serious bacterial infections -- would be tantamount to an admission of guilt on the part of the allopathic establishment: that its treatments and nostrums in no small part helped pave the way for serious, perhaps fatal, metabolic disturbances years later.

California homeopathic researcher Dana Ullman described[4] how adverse reactions to (benzathine) penicillin (decreases in white blood cells, skin rashes, persistent chills and fever, prostration, weakness, neuropathy) just happen to be, as well, major symptoms of AIDS.

He analyzed: "Modern medicine is presently doing its best to combat AIDS, but it may also be doing all too much to spread it. It is widely recognized that various recreational drugs have immunosuppressive effects that may allow simple infection of the HTLV-III virus to develop into AIDS. And it is widely ignored how conventional therapeutic drugs have suppressive effects on immune and defense processes which can lead to AIDS when there is concurrent infection with the HTLV-III virus."

It is known that people in the AIDS "risk groups" -- male homosexuals, intravenous drug users, hemophiliacs, recipients of blood transfusions -- are known to be users, and often heavy users, of (benzathine) penicillin and other antibiotics.

Antibiotics alone are far from the only possible guilty partners as co-factors in setting the stage for AIDS, however.

Some 20 cases had been reported as of 1981 of Kaposi's sarcoma -- the uncommon crypto-cancer that commonly strikes AIDS patients -- arising in patients who had undergone various forms of immunosuppressive therapy. Included was the first reported case of KS appearing following steroid therapy for *Pemphigus foliaceus*, a lethal skin disease. The researchers pointed out[5] that "most of the patients with pemphigus ... treated with corticosteroids succumb to the main effects of this therapy..."

In 1984, R. de Long, Department of Biology, Del Mar College, Corpus Christi, set forth mass immunization with live viral vaccines as a possible "cause" of AIDS. He reported[6] that the surge of new diseases appearing in the world might best be explained by mass immunizations, which increase "the probability of genetic recombination between live vaccine viruses and between live vaccine viruses and other viruses."

He included AIDS with Reyes Syndrome, Kawasaki disease, Lassa fever, Marburg disease, non-A, non-B hepatitis and Ebola hemorrhagic fever as immunization-caused illnesses.

He noted that "since 1961 we have been immunizing the human population with attenuated viral vaccines *en masse*. Such unparalleled use of live viral vaccines may be the reason for the appearance of new diseases." This is particularly true, he adds, if cells have become infected with more than one type of virus.

As if echoing his thoughts, a 1985 report in the *Nutrition Health Review*, New York, reported[7] that "ironically, a rather interesting coincidental relationship exists between the rapid outbreak of AIDS and another program of the past decade. In 1978, a group of physicians tested a vaccine for the hepatitis-B virus in Greenwich Village, New York, on a group of homosexual volunteers. The most perplexing result of this study was the death of two subjects who had taken the serum, not of hepatitis, but from an 'unidentified virus.' Could this have been the beginning of AIDS?"

The publication recalled that the first recorded case of AIDS among New York homosexuals occurred in 1979, or one year after the administration of the hepatitis vaccine. (We explore this more deeply in Chapter Eleven).

We discuss elsewhere the possible roles of the smallpox and polio vaccines as wittingly or unwittingly helping spread AIDS in various areas of the world. Whether hepatitis, smallpox and polio vaccines were knowingly contaminated with experimental new viruses (the conspiracy theory) or simply helped trigger pre-existing dormant viruses into a lethal new incarnation remains to be seen.

Suffice it to say that vaccinations -- together with antibiotics and steroids -- have been hallmarks of modern allopathic medicine. But voices of dissent have warned about them from the beginning, including the stilled one of the late Robert Mendelsohn, MD, who believed that allopathic proponents placed too much faith in vaccines and attributed victories to them that were not justified, that as diseases began to die out on their own vaccines were introduced against them so that the vaccination theorists and developers could then take the credit.

Harold E. Buttram, MD, suggested[8] that the increase in immunological disorders during the past decades may be causatively related to large-scale immunization programs involving live virus vaccines.

He also cited the vivid description in a homeopathic journal[9] of how latent viruses become permanently incorporated within genetic material "but it is still recognized by the host as a foreign element. This antigenic response is of necessity autoimmune because the destruction of the 'self' cells, containing the latent virus, is the only way that the foreign element can be removed. As circulating antibodies cannot cross the cell membrane, however, a stalemate may develop while the latent infection persists. Under certain circumstances, a breakdown of this balance might occur, triggering a full-blown autoimmune reaction leading to tissue destruction."

In the earlier days of AIDS research, Haitians, particularly those who had immigrated to the U.S.A., were regarded in and of themselves as a risk group. The Centers for Disease Control (CDC) has more or less quietly dropped Haitians from its "risk" populations, hardly ameliorating the great stigma inflicted upon Haitians in general by their prior association with an alleged risk for AIDS.

Dr. Roulette W. Smith, of the Institute of Postgraduate Interdisciplinary Studies, Palo Alto, California, noted a considerable iatrogenic factor in the earlier presumed "Haitian connection" which deserved further follow-up. In a major paper submitted to the *Annals* of the New York Academy of Sciences in 1984[10], he wrote:

"One curious finding ... is that many Haitians entering the United States in and after 1979 received large doses of diiodohydroxyquin (i.e., iodoquinol), a drug used in treating amebiasis and certain hepatic disorders. This finding .. would not be especially troublesome because the drug has been available for many years .. What is curious .. is that a review of the 1979 edition of the *Physician's Desk Reference* reveals relatively little marketing of the drug in the United States. This was confirmed by its principal pharmaceutical supplier ... Subsequently, the major recipients of the drug have been the Haitian boat people with vastly expanded marketing. Outside of the United States, the drug is frequently administered in Angola and Zaire, two countries also associated with AIDS.

"Thus, the finding that a drug is frequently and almost exclusively used in subpopulations now thought to be at significant risk for AIDS deserves further scrutiny to rule out iatrogenic factors, possibly confounded by additional nutritional factors."

Smith also noted that iodoquinol and a related compound, clioquinol, have been implicated in subacute myeloopticoneuropathy (SMON) in Japan[11], a disease once thought to be caused by "slow" viruses.

This finding took on new dimensions in 1984 and 1985 with the publication of several cases of rapid involvement of the central nervous systems in AIDS.

As Smith analyzed, "because of the substantial possibility that the nervous system and the immune system may share selected functions and molecular mechanisms, investigators must not overlook possibilities that neurological and/or immunological side effects may be associated with one or both of these drugs..."

These considerations are of utmost importance, particularly in light of the widely disseminated view that AIDS somehow originated in central Africa, either as some kind of mutation from a similar virus in the African green monkey (a theory later dropped) or due to some other transcendental event.

One view is that the alleged "AIDS virus" may have spread in human populations because health workers did not use sterile needles when they injected drugs -- mainly penicillin.

It is also known that major pharmaceutical com-

133

panies routinely "dump" huge supplies of antibiotics, (some of them not having passed muster with, for example, the U.S. Food and Drug Administration [FDA] in terms of safety) in Third World countries. This writer has been eyewitness to the over-the-counter (and even on-the-rug) sales of antibiotics, amphetamines and barbiturates in Third World countries where there is little or no medical surveillance for their use.

The poisoning of the human species by wonder drugs, legal drugs, and illegal drugs does not stop with antibiotics, steroids and "recreational" substances.

The 1970s and 1980s turned in an avalanche of warnings and information concerning the toxic reactions in humans of thousands of industrial chemicals used in everything from fertilizers and pesticides to food ingredients. Also, and quite sluggishly, information came to light of the delayed side effects of chemicals used in the recently concluded Southeast Asia War, including manifestations of dementia and immune depression.

Activists such as David Bergh[12] have brought to light the wider-than-expected use of Agent Orange and of its major contaminant TCDD (dioxin) not only in Korea and Vietnam but in wide sectors of North America. In all these places the dioxin family of synthetic chemicals has been used as herbicides. Yet they have subsequently been found to help cause cancer and to lead to immune depression, birth defects and other problems.[13, 14,15]

It is now clear from both animal and human research that dioxin is associated both with Kaposi's sarcoma and non-Hodgkin's lymphoma (NHL), two cancers common to HIV/AIDS patients, as well as the most common immunologic features of the HIV/AIDS infection curve: depressed T4 numbers and inverted T4:T8 ratios.[16,17]

Investigator Paolo Vineis[16] concluded: "The similar immunosuppressive effects of HIV and TCDD dioxin and similar excesses of NHL suggest that the possible association between KS and TCDD is biologically plausible and should be investigated further."

While authorities have dismissed some proponents' arguments that Agent Orange, dioxins and similar compounds are actually *causes* of HIV/AIDS, the role of such chemicals in helping create the groundwork for a new virus can hardly be doubted.

In fact, in the late 1970s the term "immunotoxicology" was coined to describe the harmful effects of environmental agents on various components of the immune system, and led, in 1981, to the delineation of a "unifying model for immunotoxicology," a chain of chemical/immune interreactions just beginning to be discussed at the advent of the AIDS crisis, and -- strangely, it would seem -- less discussed today.[18]

There are political and economic considerations in the development of adequate information concerning the real threat of industrial chemicals in everything from hair dyes to agricultural pesticides, but the knowledge now available suggests that it is only the tip of a very large iceberg.

REFERENCES

(1)   Illich, Ivan, Medical Nemesis. New York: Random House, 1976.

(2)   Culbert, Michael L., What the Medical Establishment Won't Tell You that Could Save Your Life. Norfolk, Virginia: Donning, 1983.

(3)   McKenna, J.J., et al., "Unmasking AIDS: chemical immunosuppression and seronegative syphilis." Med. Hypotheses 21: 421-30, 1986.

(4)   Ullman, Dana, "Penicillin and antibiotics: co-factors in the onset of AIDS," The Sentinel (San Francisco), Page 9, Dec. 5, 1985.

(5)   Ilie, B., et al., "Kaposi's sarcoma after steroid therapy for Pemphigus foliaceus." Dermatologica 163: 455-459, 1981.

(6)   de Long, R., "A possible cause of acquired immune deficiency syndrome (AIDS) and other new diseases." Medical Hypotheses 13: 395-397, 1984.

(7)   "Contradictions of the AIDS epidemic." Nutrition Health Review, page 22, Fall 1985.

(8)   Buttram, Harold E., "Immunizations revisited." Australasian Health and Healing, 5:2, 23-26, Dec. 1985 - Feb. 1986.

(9)   "Immunizations: do they protect our children?" Am. Homeopathy, 1:2, September 1984.

(10)   Smith, Roulette W., "AIDS and 'slow viruses.'" Acquired Immune Deficiency Syndrome, Vol. 437, Annals of the New York Academy of Sciences, 1984.

(11)   SMON Research Commission. Japan J. Med. Sci. Bio. 28 (supplement): 1-293, 1975.

(12)   Bergh, Dave, "AIDS may be tied to chemicals." St. Cloud (Minn.) Daily Times, Sept. 30, 1983.

(13)   Tucker, A.N., et al., "Suppression of B cell differentiation by 2,3,7,8-tetrachlorodibenzo-p-dioxin." Publication of The Am. Soc. Pharmacol. and Exp. Ther., Jan. 15, 1988.

(14)   MacIvar, B., "Agent Orange." Fact Sheet, National Cancer Institute, 1980.

(15)   Letter, David P. Rall, Public Health Service, Dept. of Health and Human Services, to Senator Alan Cranston, April 3, 1987.

(16)   Vineis, P., "Immunosuppressive effects of dioxin in the development of Kaposi's sarcoma and non-Hodgkin's lymphoma." The Lancet, Jan. 29, 1988.

(17)   Hoffman, R.E., et al., "Health effects of long-term exposure to 2,3,7,8-tetrachlorodibenzo-p-dioxin," J. Am. Med. Assn. 255: 2031-38, 1986.

(18)   Dean J.H., and Padarathsingh, eds., Biological Relevance of Immune Suppression as Induced by Genetic, Therapeutic and Environmental Factors. New York: Van Nostrand Reinhold, 1981.

Chapter Eight

THE PARASITE CONNECTION

From the early reporting of HIV/AIDS cases in the U.S.A., it became clear that the syndrome, among many other things, has allowed all manner of parasites, from opportunistic viruses to protozoa, bacteria and fungi, to flourish. Certain parasite-linked conditions known only to specific subpopulations in certain parts of the world and to the immunologically depressed were being seen with frequency and virulence primarily in "high-risk groups."

The connection between parasites and suppression of the immune function -- with parasites either as causal factors or results of existing immune depression -- went overlooked, and is still frequently overlooked, in the overall AIDS clinical picture.

And yet it has tremendous relevance in terms of both partial cause and treatment and is, in turn, at least partially associated with problems of nutritional deficiency and malnutrition, which we explore elsewhere.

In 1977, Sohn and Robilotti, reviewing their experience in dealing with the colorectal problems of 260 gay males in New York City, coined the somewhat misnomered term "gay bowel syndrome" to refer to this collective pathology, or several years in advance of the definition of AIDS.[1] The name is slightly misleading since some of the pathogens involved lead to system-wide dysfunctions.

We discuss in another chapter the "opportunism" of such viruses as Epstein-Barr, cytomegalovirus, hepatitis and herpes viruses, the first two being seen with near-ubiquity in HIV/AIDS patients and homosexual men, and of the fungal parasite *Pneumocystis carinii*, which became the most notorious presenting disease in AIDS as PC pneumonia (PCP).

Selma Dritz, of the San Francisco Department of Health, reported in 1980[24] that "with the expansion of the homosexual community in San Francisco, the number of sexually transmitted enteric diseases ... increased by orders of magnitude; by 1979, amebiasis had risen from 10 cases a year to 250, giardiasis had risen from 1 or 2 a year to 85."

And a New York epidemiologist pointed out that as of 1981 amebiasis was just becoming a serious health problem in the U.S.A., and that it could be traced primarily to male homosexuals and Caribbean immigrants. He suggested that virulence in amebic infection was on the increase.[25]

Another researcher thought that "it may be that the severity of their (homosexuals') illness is determined to a large measure by repeated reinfection associated with frequent oral-anal sexual contacts with individuals who constitute an amebiasis endemic group."[26]

Among the opportunistic infections now associated with HIV/AIDS, and frequently involving intestinal infestation, there are, among the fungi, Candida, Cryptococcus, Aspergillus, Coccidiodes, Histoplasma, and Blastomyces; of bacteria, mycobacterium tuberculosis (*Mycobacterium avium-intracellulare* -- MAI -- now recognized as a common and serious complication of the syndrome),[3] other atypical microbacteria, Legionella, Salmonella, Listeria, and Brucella; and, among protozoa, Toxoplasma and Cryptosporidium. Strongyloides, worms, have also been reported.[2]

Early complications of the overgrowth of these various organisms were diarrhea, fever, weight loss, general wasting away and a huge variety of related conditions and diseases, whether clinically resolved or not. Frequent among AIDS patients are esophageal Candida infection, herpes simplex proctitis, enterocolitis caused by cytomegalovirus (CMV), disseminated mycobacteriosis and such previously rare conditions as cryptospiridiosis.[4,5]

Disseminated histoplasmosis, a rare opportunistic infection occurring in a setting of prior immunological compromise, is now showing up in AIDS,[6,7] though not strictly in homosexual patients.

Giardia lamblia is another offending organism showing up with frequency in AIDS patients.[8] As are *Entamoeba histolytica, Campylobacter jejuni, Clostridium difficile* and *Chlamydia.*[9] Since the "sexual revolution" of the 1960s, moreover, there has tended to be a general proliferation of herpesviruses, hepatitis B, and Chlamydia simply from widespread sexual contact. And the presence of Candida infection in the majority of the population is of increasing concern.

Sidhu and El-Sadr comment[10] that "the overall empirical evidence worldwide seems to suggest that an immunodeficient state secondary to malnutrition or to the interplay of enteric infections and malabsorption is a possible precursor to the second, perhaps irreversible, stage of AIDS initiated by the establishment of HTLV-III/LAV infection in the body" -- evidence, again, that one must already be "sick", in an immune-compromised way, to "get" HIV/AIDS.

Too, they add, "sexual promiscuity, whether in heterosexuals or male homosexuals, appears to be a common central theme in AIDS." Even though it is only a factor, albeit an important one, and may not be of importance in those cases in which the monogamous sexual partners of AIDS-infected individuals also acquire the disease.

There apparently is a vicious cycle involved with intestinal (and other) parasites: they may be festering *because* of immune depression; they then may help to further immune depression; and further immune depression leads to the flourishing of other viruses and parasites.

D.L. Archer and W.H. Glinsman, arguing that repeated enteric infection with multiple pathogenic microorganisms, subsequent colonization in the intestine, and repeated insult to both the large and small bowel leads to malabsorption of essential nutrients and further nutrient loss, and that the presence of microbial products and the loss of essential nutrients lead to compromised immune function and further predisposition to infection, added: "arguing which comes first, the virus or the enteric pathogen-induced malabsorption/malnutrition-derived immunodeficiency ... seems pointless, as both factors are likely involved in the syndrome."[9]

Indeed, Archer and Glinsman divided the U.S. AIDS epidemic into three historical periods,[27] with the first period being an "enteric epidemic" among U.S. homosexual males breaking out in about 1968 and setting the stage for the entry, by 1977, of HIV, with the second stage being HIV introduction, and the third the current "AIDS epidemic."

They recapitulated the earlier clinical evidence that epidemics of amebiasis, giardiasis, shigellosis, and combined infections with these enteric pathogens preceded the development of full-blown AIDS in essentially the same populations.

They wrote: "The clinical evidence suggests a role

for intestinal pathogens and bowel dysfunction in predisposition to AIDS (first historical period) as a possible trigger mechanism or cofactor for HIV infections (second historical period) and in the pathogenic process of AIDS itself (third historical period)."

The routes of entry of parasites are expanded by various kinds of sex acts, by no means limited to homosexuals: fellatio, anal intercourse, rectal manipulation, anilingus, an overlap of functions between the genitourinary and gastrointestinal systems, by no means new in the world.

Dr. Richard B. Pearce, San Francisco, was one of the earlier exponents of the causal links between parasitism and the immune system and detailed various mechanisms whereby parasites depress host immune function.[11,12] He and other researchers studied the continual infection and re-infection patterns of victims of parasitism, with immunodeficiency and antigenic stimulation (continual development of new antibodies) being major elements.

E. histolytica, with an incidence of anywhere from 10 to 40 percent of gay men in a New York study,[13] almost certainly has immunosuppressive capabilities. Giardiasis has been associated with defects in the immune system in mice[14] and men.[15] Some research indicates that anti-parasite antibodies might cross-react with the host's T-lymphocytes, spermatozoa or other elements,[16] leading to effects on the immune system.

Indeed, "antigen overload" -- literally, the production by the body of more immune reactions to invaders than it knows what to do with -- is implicated in AIDS.[17] Pearce quoted Michael Lange, assistant chief, Division of Infectious Diseases and Epidemiology, St. Luke's-Roosevelt Hospital: "Any foreign material can stimulate the immune system -- and other viruses, a common cold, parasites, which produce a lot of foreign antigens and are a problem especially among Haitians. Semen, too. It's these kinds of things that produce what may be a critical load of the AIDS virus."[18]

But despite the prevalence of parasites and immune depression in gay males, they are far from being the only victims of parasitism, however unique their presenting pathological conditions may be. Intravenous drug users are at high risk for parasitic infections, and lactating mothers may spread Giardia to their infants.[11]

140

From the time interest focused on Africa and AIDS, it became clear that populations identified as AIDS reservoirs (other than homosexuals and drug users) are at high risk for repeated, multiple protozoan infections and live in, or are natives of, areas where parasites are endemic.

There is a correlation between seropositivity for HIV and geographical areas where parasitism -- especially malaria -- is endemic.[18] Parasites have been pointed to more than once as possible predisposing factors for Kaposi's sarcoma.[19] Robert J. Biggar et al. demonstrated[20] an ssociation between prevalence of antibodies to HTLV-I, HTLV-II and HIV and malaria in healthy Africans.

Burt et al. reported[21] on a severe AIDS case in a patient with no known risk factors -- a 47-year old Scottish heterosexual who had previously worked in equatorial Africa and had had several episodes of malaria but had never taken treatment for it. Cerebral lymphoma, generalized CMV infection, and cerebral toxoplasmosis were among pathological findings.

Jane Teas traced a possible connection between AIDS and African swine fever virus[22] and noted that this virus has been able to "jump" from one animal species to another, where it produces AIDS-like symptoms. (See also Chapter Five).

In the midst of the U.S. assessment that AIDS primarily affects male homosexuals and, further down the line, intravenous drug users, hemophiliacs and recipients of contaminated donated blood, the case of Belle Glade, Fla., for a time stood out:

As of 1985, some 46 confirmed cases of AIDS had developed in this poverty-stricken, tropical town in Florida, a city of about 20,000 population. The cases made it, by percentage, the "AIDS capital" of America. Yet, intriguingly, half the victims were not thought to be in "high risk" groups.

Dr. Mark Whiteside, co-director of the Institute of Tropical Medicine in Miami, pointed to the "insect vector", mosquitoes in particular, as a mode of transmission of a parasitical agent, and general unhygienic conditions as factors which must be considered in the Belle Glade AIDS epidemic. He strongly doubted the notion that "a single strain of one viral agent, HTLV-III," could be solely responsible for AIDS, and that "this virus can only go by blood or through secretions..."[23]

As we have seen, his considerations marked a point of departure from theories of AIDS etiology and epidemiology in the U.S.A. as well as pointing to considerable new dangers: the possibility of airborne transmission and the co-factors of poor environmental conditions.

While U.S.-led medical orthodoxy wasted little time in refuting the claims concerning "insect vectors"[28,29] in Belle Glade, the fact is that there are co-factors to HIV and that they must occur in U.S. replicas of tropical poverty (Belle Glade being symbolic, aside from IV drug use, of conditions in the economically depressed Caribbean and even central Africa). And such co-factors may indeed include exposure to tropical insects.

Dr. Whiteside argued that in AIDS -- at least in Belle Glade -- what might be involved was repeated exposure to some of the regular insect-transmitted viruses (arboviruses), specially the Bunyamwera group, one of a cluster of the more than 500 insect-transmitted viruses known to science.

His preliminary evidence was that virtually 100 percent of the allegedly non-risk AIDS cases he had tested in south Florida as of September 1985 had antibodies to one of these viruses. He thought such arboviruses might also be "aberrantly transmitted" through blood mechanisms in other risk areas (sexual practices, IV drug use, blood transfusions) and said that "our own particular viewpoint is that retroviruses may not be the prime mover. We're looking at a model in which initial insult may be regular arboviruses which are known to be immunosuppressive."

He also suggested that recombination-mutation between various arboviruses might be bringing about the potential for increased virulence, and what he calls "immunological enhancement" of infection, whereby antibodies to one virus, paradoxically, may stimulate or increase the growth of a related organism, as particularly exemplified by the dengue fever virus.

There is, then, a rich and complicated world of parasites and fellow-travellers infecting humans in different kinds and numbers in different locales, many if not all helping set the stage for immune depression and the conversion of the weakened host into a target for a "new" virus or other disease-causing agent.

142

REFERENCES

(1)   Sohn, N., and J.G. Robilotti, "The gay bowel syndrome." Am. J. Gastroen-
        terol. 67: 478:484, 1977.

(2)   Weller, I.V.D., "AIDS and the gut." Scand. J. Gastroenterol. v.20 (suppl.),
        1985.

(3)   Nyberg, David A., et al., "Abdominal CT findings of disseminated
        Mycobacterium avium-intracellulare in AIDS." AJR (American Roentgen
        Ray Society), 145: 297-299, August 1985.

(4)   Cunningham, A.L., "Aetiology of AIDS: gastrointestinal opportunistic
        infections." Aust. NZ J. Med. v. 15 (suppl.), Feb. 1985.

(5)   Cohen, Jerome D., et al., "Cryptosporidium in acquired im-
        munodeficiency syndrome." Dig. Dis. and Sci., vol.29, no. 8, 773-777,
        August 1984.

(6)   Small, C.B., et al., "Community-acquired opportunistic infections and
        defective cellular immunity in heterosexual drug abusers and homosexual
        men." Ann. Intern. Med. 99: 208-220, August 1983.

(7)   Haggerty, Colin M., et al., "Gastrointestinal histoplasmosis in suspected
        acquired immunodeficiency syndrome." W.J. Med. 143: 244-246, Aug.
        1985.

(8)   Quinn, T.G., et al., "The polymicrobial origin of intestinal infections in
        men." N. Eng. J. Med. 309: 576-582, 1983.

(9)   Archer, D.L., and W.H. Glinsmann, "Intestinal infection and malnutrition
        initiate acquired immune deficiency syndrome (AIDS)." Nutrition
        Research, vol. 5, 8-9, 1985.

(10)   Sidhu, Gurdip S., and Wafaa El-Sadr, "Some thoughts on the acquired
        immunodeficiency syndrome." Nutrition Research, vol. 5, 3-7, 1985.

(11)   Pearce, Richard B., "Parasitism as a possible cause of immune suppres-
        sion in gay men and others." Privately published. San Francisco, 1982.

(12)   Pearce, Richard B., "Do parasites cause AIDS?" Privately published, San
        Francisco, 1983. (See also Pearce letters in Lancet July 2, 1983; June 23,
        1984; Oct. 20, 1984).

(13)   Kean, B.H., "Clinical amebiasis in New York City; symptoms, signs, and
        treatment." Bull. N.Y. Acad. Med. 57: 207, 1981.

(14)   Anders, R.F., et al., "Giardiasis in mice: analysis of humoral and cellular
        immune responses to Giardia muris." Parasite Immunol. 4:47-57, 1982.

(15)   Ament, N.E., and C.E. Rubin, "Relation of giardiasis to abnormal intes-
        tinal structure and function in gastrointestinal immunodeficiency
        syndrome." Gastroenterol 62: 216, 1972.

(16)   Davies, A.J.S., et al., "The biological significance of the immune response
        with special reference to parasites and cancer." J. Parasitol. 66(5):705-
        721, 1980.

(17)   Levy, J.A., and J.L. Ziegler, "Acquired immunodeficiency syndrome is an opportunistic infection and Kaposi's sarcoma results from secondary immune stimulation." Lancet i: 78-81, 1983.

(18)   Pearce, letter, Lancet: p. 927, Oct. 20, 1984.

(19)   Williams, E.H., and P.H. Williams, "A note on an apparent similarity in distribution of onchocerciasis, femoral hernia, and Kaposi's sarcoma in the West Nile District of Uganda." E. Afr. Med. J. 42: 208-09, 1966.

(20)   Biggar, Robert J., et al., "ELISA HTLV retrovirus antibody reactivity associated with malaria and immune complexes in healthy Africans." Lancet, p. 520, Sept. 7, 1985.

(21)   Burt, A.D., et al., "Acquired immunodeficiency syndrome in a patient with no known risk factors: a pathological study." J. Clin. Pathol. 37: 471-474, 1984.

(22)   Teas, Jane, "Could AIDS agent be a new variant of African swine fever virus?" Lancet i: 923, 1983.

(23)   Interview with Dr. John Grauerholz, Sept. 17, 1985, in "AIDS is more deadly than nuclear war." Report of National Democratic Policy Committee, Oct. 1985.

(24)   Dritz, Selma, in N. Eng. J. Med. 302 (8):, p. 463, 1980.

(25)   Fodor, Tibor, "Unanswered questions about the transmission of amebiasis." Bull. N.Y. Acad. Med. 57 (3): 224-226, 1981.

(26)   Imperato, P.J., in Bull. N.Y. Acad. Med. 57 (3): 240-241, 1981.

(27)   Archer, Douglas L., and Walter H. Glinsman, "Enteric infections and other co-factors in AIDS." Immun. Today, 6:10, 292, 1985.

(28)   Castro, K.G., et al., "Transmission of HIV in Belle Glade, Florida: lessons for other communities in the United States." Science, 239: 193-197, 1988.

(29)   Lifson, A.R., "Do alternate modes for transmission of human immunodeficiency virus exist?" J Am. Med. Assn. 259: 9, 1353-1355, 1988.

Chapter Nine

THE POOR NUTRITION CONNECTION

Since the beginning of sudden interest in the major medical conundrum that AIDS represents, some investigators -- particularly those who do not agree with the single-mode concept of AIDS etiology -- have been looking at many possible co-factors.

One of these is the nebulous area of nutrition -- or rather, as they seem to relate to AIDS, undernutrition or malnutrition.

It is axiomatic that in a medical/research setting dominated by the allopathic concepts of disease causation, co-factors would be given far less attention than the endless hunt for the "single etiological agent."

And in American medicine, relationships between nutrition and disease, let alone between nutrition and immune depression, have rarely received adequate attention from the dominant allopathic community.

Among researchers listening to the beat of different drummers was J.A. Sonnabend, who early offered a "multifactorial" model of AIDS etiology.[1] Among the areas he pointed to were poverty and malnutrition.

But many other scientists also were puzzled by seeming disparities: The poverty-malnutrition-disease triad was understandable in Haiti, the Caribbean and tropical Africa, yet would, on the surface, seem less so than in the U.S.A.

Why AIDS in an affluent, seemingly healthy population where sterile measures and cleanliness are the norm?

There also existed the puzzle that only *parts* of the Third World have AIDS cases or prevalence of the putative AIDS-connected retroviruses. Surely, poverty alone (so rampant in Southeast Asia, which has reported negligible cases of AIDS), with accompanying poor sanitation, could not be the only factors.

But what if, as in some parts of the underdeveloped world, despite poverty and despite poor sanitation, nutritional features were *not* negative: that is, people were somehow "eating right," however poverty-stricken they happened to be? This might explain, for example, some notable examples of longevity and general good health among certain groups of non-urban Filipinos, representing a society generally considered as among the most impoverished. These peoples are essentially free of most of the chronic, systemic diseases of "civilization" and certainly are (up to now) reporting very little AIDS and many other "modern" conditions.[2] (In January 1986, 20 cases of HIV seropositivity were detected in prostitutes "servicing" the Subic Bay U.S. Naval base in the Philippines, the first such cluster reported in that country.[27] The number had doubled by 1988 and deaths had occurred by 1989.)

Jain and Chandra have argued that nutritional deficiency predisposes to AIDS and have cited these examples: large numbers of African AIDS patients come from parts of Africa where malnutrition is rampant and where plasma and leukocyte zinc levels are diminished.

They connected protein-energy malnutrition (PEM) with a "profound depression of cellular immunity," part of a possible AIDS substrate. Indeed, PEM itself may lead to an inversion of the T4:T8 ratio, the characteristic immunological sign of AIDS.[3]

They also noted that *Pneumocystis carinii* infections -- the most common presenting disease in U.S. AIDS patients -- are common in malnourished children and that PEM is a "host determinant" for *P. carinii* infection.[4] This kind of pneumonia has been seen both in African children with malnutrition and European children during the Second World War[4,5,6].

Jain and Chandra further noted that subclinical zinc deficiency is "quite common in apparently healthy people" and that deficiencies in other trace elements may be expected in some "high risk" populations, particularly intravenous drug abusers or poor people from parts of Africa and Haiti.

They added that "once the patient develops the major manifestations of AIDS, there may be mutually detrimental interactions between nutrition, immunity and infection.

"Malnutrition will cause suboptimal immunity which will permit infection by the AIDS agent, which in turn will cause severe impairment of immunity. This would lead to secondary infections by opportunistic agents and further deterioration both in immunocompetence and in the nutritional status, thus setting up a vicious cycle which ends only on the death of the patient."

Sidhu and El-Sadr, cited in another chapter, puzzled over parallels between AIDS and nutritional factors, with some of the more *affluent* sections of the population being affected by Kaposi's sarcoma (which, in Africa, may turn out ultimately not to have any direct correlation with AIDS at all), but added: "...The overall empirical evidence worldwide seems to suggest that an immunodeficient state secondary to malnutrition or to the interplay of enteric infections and malabsorption is a precursor to the second, perhaps irreversible, stage of AIDS..."[7]

Archer and Glinsmann, arguing[8] that intestinal parasitical infection and malnutrition (See Chapter Eight) initiate AIDS, pointed out that "malnutrition need not be severe, but may be due to failure to transport one or several nutrients essential for immune functions."

In this model, malnutrition may be secondary to malabsorption caused by enteric infections. The co-factors here could well range from simple unsanitary conditions (proliferation of parasites) to ritualistic religious practices (voodoo, etc.) to repeated high-risk sexual practices (anilingus, anal intercourse, intercourse followed by fellatio, etc.) Loss of endogenous nutrients caused by diarrhea consequent to parasitical infection is a factor, they wrote.

Dr. Mark Whiteside, of the Institute of Tropical Medicine in Miami, analyzed the Belle Glade AIDS epidemic virtually since its inception.

In addition to the "insect vector" (mosquitoes as possible carriers of an arbovirus) explanation, he added:[9] "We do feel that the tremendous parallel between diseases like tuberculosis and AIDS in these environmental and poor areas are indirect evidence for relation to living conditions and perhaps socioeconomic conditions. And we are seeing the same kind of pattern develop in other areas of South Florida...

"We think that the pattern of disease down here, and in places like Belle Glade, more resembles the pattern of disease in the tropics, i.e., the Caribbean or even Central Africa -- especially the pattern of the disease among our non-risk cases, where the disease manifests multiple opportunistic infections and a high incidence of tuberculosis." (In fact, an increase in TB nationwide has accompanied the

HIV/AIDS explosion).

As Whiteside was quoted by *Time* Magazine[26] concerning the squalid conditions and poverty of Belle Glade within its semitropical setting: "There is raw sewage on the ground and rats running all around."

Low zinc levels were discussed not only by such researchers as Jain and Chandra in regard to general malnutrition among many peoples of the world, but also by those who have stressed how zinc is lost through seminal emissions.[10] There is at least a modest possibility that overactive sexuality, accompanied by abundant orgasms, and this within a setting of prior immunological insult, dietary insufficiency, drug abuse, and the like, plays a role in further lowering body defenses.

The role of zinc in prostaglandin E1 synthesis has become of concern in the last few years to those who connected essential fatty acids (EFA) -- their deficiency, imbalance or synthetic alteration -- to a lowered immune response in humans.

The essential fatty acids problem is of immediate impact on the Western, or developed, world, and may be part of the explanation of how the seemingly affluent West can be undergoing its own unique form of dietary deficiency even while its populations are said to be the best-fed(and most medicated)on earth.

Zinc deficiency and, probably, EFA deficiency, are implicated in thymus atrophy in both animal models and in malnourished human children[12,19,20,21] and can be treated or prevented by these substances. Acrodermatitis enteropathica, a condition in which the zinc absorption mechanism in the intestine is defective, is a dramatic example of zinc deficiency, one reflected by alterations in the T4:T8 ratio.[22,23]

(The thymus gland, so major a role player in immune function, is a target not only for nutritional deficiencies of zinc and EFAs, but also for damage from glucocorticoids, since physiological concentrations inhibit prostaglandin E1 function as well.[24,25])

Research reported by Fabris *et al.* in 1988 in Italy indicated new interest in zinc levels and immune and thymic functions. Studies on 19 LAS or AIDS patients showed decreased levels of zinc and nearly undetectable amounts of circulating thymulin.[50]

The essential fatty acid (EFA) role in nutrition, deficiency and immune disturbance quickly points to *food processing* -- in its totality, the major combination of industrial investment and profit-taking in the U.S.A. -- as a possible factor in overall ill-health in a seemingly healthy population.

This writer, together with the late Harold Harper, M.D., has discussed food processing in detail[2,11] as a major contributor to what may be called "malnutrition of the affluent," a way to explain how Americans and much of the Western world's population can at once be both over-fed and undernourished at the same time.

In such research we have indicated how refinements in the processing of cereals, grains, wheat and raw sugar have led to an over-abundance of essentially nutritionless refined carbohydrates in the standard diets of the West, and how the exponential development and use of synthetic chemicals in the preservation, coloring, buffering and "marketability"-enhancing of foods has introduced a glut of new compounds into the food chain and human metabolism, and how refined sugars, starches and salt are implicated in a staggering variety of chronic, systemic metabolic diseases and challenges.

Another major alteration in the food chain and its effects on human metabolism has been the introduction of hydrogenated fats, particularly in the elaboration of margarine and other vegetable oils, and the interference because of hydrogenation in the relationship between EFAs and prostaglandin E1, the latter involved in immune response.

Horrobin's seminal work in this area[12] notes that: "If PGE1 is important in T-lymphocyte function then it is possible that the immune system could be modulated by nutritional changes which determine PGE1 formation. The nutritional and other factors which can modify the pathway have recently been much more clearly understood. Essential fatty acids, pyridoxine (Vitamin B6), zinc and Vitamin C are all important. There is evidence that in some members of Western societies intake of all four of these agents may be marginal and therefore that a nutritional failure of PGE1 synthesis may be common."

If EFAs are themselves deficient in Western diets and if hydrogenation in food processing further affects them (hydrogenation of vegetable oils converting up to 40 percent of the natural EFA cis-linoleic acid to an altered, or *trans*, form), then by simple dietary and food processing habits alone we are presented with an interference in the immune system independent of all other factors.

Horrobin also notes that "for almost fifty years it has been known that the consequences of zinc deficiency and EFA deficiency are virtually identical," and now that EFAs are linked to prostaglandin E1 synthesis and the latter to immune modulation,[13] these deficiencies take on new and sinister meanings. As we shall see, they also provide a rationale in the metabolic/nutritional therapy of metabolic diseases in general and AIDS in particular for the administration of EFAs, zinc, and Vitamins B6 and C.

Lawrence Burton, Ph.D., a zoologist, is no stranger to controversy. He is best known for developing the IAT, or "immunoaugmentative therapy" (vaccines from blood serum) for cancer, a line of treatment opposed by U.S. medical officialdom. But he also is a researcher who has looked into many aspects of metabolic disease.

In July, 1985, his clinic in the Bahamas was closed by Bahamian officials, allegedly at the behest of U.S. authorities, who were well aware that many Americans had sought treatment, often successfully, at his off-shore facilities.[28] He had earlier been literally driven out of his Long Island, N.Y., quarters, where he pioneered his non-toxic approach to cancer.

Dr. Burton is convinced that the primary reason for his closure in the Bahamas (he subsequently was allowed to reopen) is that he ruffled the feathers of the U.S. pharmaceutical establishment, particularly after he revealed animal experiments in which he was able to produce AIDS-like symptoms by dosing rectal areas with lubricants reflecting the major brands used by sexually active U.S. gays.[29]

The official reason given was that some of the Burton patients had turned out to be seropositive for "the AIDS virus," and statements from U.S. officials suggested that blood from such patients might have been "pooled". Burton hotly denied all charges and as of this writing there has been no confirmation of a single Burton patient coming down with a positive antibody test for "the AIDS virus," let alone a case of AIDS.

His own research, not published in a medical journal

though available for explanation by videotape,[30] involved colonies of mice genetically developed to exhibit differing levels of fragile immune systems. It was on these animals that he tested a theory that he developed after interviews with male homosexual patients, with particular emphasis on their sex acts. The clue was in the question, "What effect does repeated and sustained introduction of lubricants into the anal cavity have upon the immune system?"

"Could it be," he asked, "that these lubricants, commonly used by homosexuals in anal intercourse, are being absorbed into their systems and causing immune depression?"[31] He set up a control group and then segregated the test mice into different categories, and in these he inserted any of several popular lubricants as well as a popular shortening, corn oil, margarine, etc. Immune depression effects were noted in all the test animals, and 10 out of 12 of them died.

It was Burton's conclusion that he had induced AIDS or AIDS-like symptoms into test animals simply by inserting large fatty globules into their systems from petroleum jelly-based and simple large-molecular substances.

This was in 1982, a line of research based on interviewing four anal-receptive male homosexuals who had been diagnosed with AIDS. Burton did a followup study in 1983, reportedly at the request of one of the companies which manufactures such lubricants. This time, AIDS-like symptoms again appeared in virtually all the animals, all but one of the test mice died, and the control mice survived in perfect condition.

In a third set of experiments, Burton tested agar-agar, a derivative of kelp, which the zoologist had found in one of the lubricants. He used the agar-agar alone in rectal penetration of test animals, and they all died. He also footnoted part of the AIDS puzzle: kelp, he later learned, is a favorite food of Haitians, originally placed on the Centers for Disease Control (CDC) list of "risk" groups (and later dropped.)

The Burton research points to a whole new dimension of general concern in establishing nutritional-deficiency links to AIDS, and it was seized upon by William H. Moore, Jr., Burton's attorney (and himself holder of a medical degree.)

Building on earlier research from several quarters

implicating the hydrogenation of polyunsaturated fats with widespread degenerative and metabolic disease, Moore argued that hydrogenated fats, consumed orally over the years and -- in the form of anal lubricants -- inserted rectally are probably involved in immune suppression.

In a letter to the then National Cancer Institute Director Vincent DeVita, Moore wrote:[32] "It is particularly intriguing to note that some of Dr. Burton's animal studies ... have demonstrated that polyunsaturated fats in the form of corn oil margarine are particularly prone to cause both AIDS and cancer in laboratory animals when inserted in the anus or fed to the animals."

Moore was simply adding a voice of concern to others which have been raised in opposition to the hydrogenation processing of polyunsaturated fats, particularly in the production of margarine.

A growing body of research continues to make the connection between this particular food processing and an inhibition of the body's use of prostaglandin E1, a substance which, among other things, has a regulating effect on aspects of the immune system directly bearing on T cells.[33]

While the relationship between essential fatty acids and the immune system is new, complicated and at times contradictory, it does point to a possible long-term nutritional deprivation developed over time in populations dependent on processed foods for sustenance.

Precursors of PGE1 are cis-linoleic acid, an essential fatty acid, which in turn is desaturated into gamma-linolenic acid by delta-6-desaturase enzyme, then converted to dihomogammalinolenic acid, and then to PGE. It is the hydrogenation process which suppresses the availability of cis-linoleic acid by transforming significant amounts of it to trans-linoleic acid. Thus, the latter is an antagonist to cis-linoleic acid and directly inhibits PGE1 synthesis, a major influence on the immune system.

As Moore summarized in his DeVita letter: "Since the mid-1920s the oil seed industry has been producing margarines and vegetable shortening by hydrogenation of polyunsaturated fats and introducing trans-linoleic acid into the human food chain, and may have been introducing a chronic immune suppression along with it, by blocking the conversion of cis-linoleic acid to PGE1 which could well be responsible for widespread immunosuppression, due to interference with lymphocyte regulation."

Much of the pioneering work along this line was done by Horrobin, who called attention to PGE1's major role in the regulation of thymus development and T-lymphocyte function.[34]

He also expostulated, in 1979, that "by careful attention to diet it should be possible to activate T lymphocyte function in the large number of diseases... in which such function is defective." Noting that "it is ... of particular interest that many cancer cells and virally infected cells are unable to make PGE1 because they cannot convert linoleic acid to gamma-linolenic acid," he reasoned that the direct provision of essential fatty acids as a therapeutic tool was worthy of investigation.

Medical writer Wayne Martin is among investigators who have associated the rise in heart attack deaths in the Western world after 1930 to the end results of the change in food processing occurring after 1920 "when the new oil seed industry introduced into our food three greatly harmful lipid substances (including) the unnatural trans-trans isomer of linoleic acid, which had never been in human food prior to 1920 and which entered our food in margarine and refined oils, (blocking) the conversion of natural cis-linoleic acid to prostaglandin E1[35]...

In 1978, Hans Kaunitz pointed out[36] that "consumption of polyunsaturated vegetable oils has dramatically increased in the United States during the last 60 years" and that "the average American consumes in his daily diet two to three times more unsaturated vegetable oils than 20 years ago ... Since 1913, total fat consumption has doubled on account of the increase in the intake of polyunsaturated vegetable oils or of the margarine derived from them."

Three years earlier, it had been estimated[37] that as much as 15 percent of the dietary fat consumed in the U.S.A. was of *trans* fatty acids.

Horrobin's research also points out that the hydrogenation processing of vegetable oils converts as much as 40 percent of the natural essential fatty acid linoleic acid to its "trans" form. "Estimates of EFA {essential fatty acid} intake rarely make allowances for this and so much of our apparent intake is of no value," he stressed.[34]

Earlier research had shown that this "trans" form of linoleic acid is useless since it inhibits the conversion of cis-linoleic acid to the next step (gamma-linolenic acid, GLA) and increases requirements for essential fatty acids. [38,39] Further, saturated -- or "hard" -- fats and cholesterol, increased in Western diets, are effective inhibitors of the enzyme desaturase and reduce GLA formation. [40,41,42]

Ohlrogge has also pointed out [43] that "about 5-8% of the fatty acids in modern Western diets are unusual in the sense that they possess *trans* double bonds and/or double bonds in other positions of the acyl chain. The presence of these unusual structures in our diets is derived from two sources. The first is industrial hydrogenation of vegetable oils ... A secondary source ... arises from foods containing ruminant fats (e.g., butter, cheese, beef fat) which contain *trans* fatty acids as a result of microbial biohydrogenations occurring in the ruminant stomach... The relative contribution of these two sources of *trans* isomers has also shifted in favor of the hydrogenated vegetable oil."

Booyens and van der Merwe are among investigators adding that a chronic imbalance between essential fatty acids (arachidonic acid, gamma-linolenic acid and eicosapentaenoic acid) "appears to be implicated in the etiology of many intractable diseases"[44] and that "optimal dietary manipulation of AA, GLA and EPA may have profound effects on reversing processes believed to be important in these disorders."

They, Horrobin, other investigators and practicing physicians have thus proposed (e.g., Marcus[45]) administration of substances high in essential fatty acids and/or their metabolites, such as evening primrose oil and certain fish oils, as useful adjunctive therapies.

Recent research[41,47,48] has stressed the multifactoriality of lipids (fats) and immune response, with Gurr noting that experiments "illustrate once more the principle that PG [prostaglandin] and EFA [essential fatty acids] may modify immune function according to a bell-shaped dose response relationship and should now be regarded as modulators of immune function rather than as simple inhibitors."

It is now evident from animal research and epidemiological studies that food processing techniques have greatly altered the Western diet, that among many

154

other problems which arise from this reality are the immune depressing effects of certain altered foods and/or deficiencies, and that the actual malevolent effects of the same may be long-term. Certainly earlier voices clamoring against hydrogenation and margarine (such as John H. Tobe[49]) as early as the early 1960s have been partially vindicated.

It is abundantly clear that part of the "substrate" on which an opportunistic new virus might feed would be long-simmering effects of immune depression occasioned by alterations of the food chain and the introducing of unnatural new structures into the human metabolism.

The ingestion of hydrogenated fats -- orally and even rectally -- may thus be one more important piece in the puzzle of the etiology of AIDS, and another reason why so much of the Third World, however impoverished it may be in other ways, has far less likelihood of suffering from actual AIDS (whether substantial portions of its people may ultimately have "the AIDS virus" or a mutated form of it.)

Substantial work[14,15,16,17] has already indicated the deficiency levels of Vitamin C within the human family in general and the Western world in particular, and the increasing importance Vitamin C as ascorbic acid or ascorbate plays in general nutritional health.

The use of megadoses of this substance has been shown[18] to be useful in a wide spectrum of diseases, for anti-viral, antioxidant and other reasons.

Pauling, Stone, Szent-Gyorgyi and other Vitamin C pioneers have pointed to chronic Vitamin C deficiencies and the possibility that there is virtually a "chronic, subclinical scurvy" syndrome (CSS, after Stone) pattern in much of the world, particularly in the West, where food processing let alone addiction to specific "socially sanctioned" drugs (alcohol, nicotine, etc.,) may further rob the body of its already depleted Vitamin C stores.

Compounding the problem of subclinical nutritional deficiencies in the West are estimated lacks of other vital trace minerals (particularly selenium and magnesium) and the industrial toxication of water supplies with chlorine and fluorides (see Chapter Ten). All of these advents of the modern era represent elements of man-made nutritional deficiency and synthetic nutritional alteration in the Western world.

155

REFERENCES

(1)   Sonnabend, J.A., "The etiology of AIDS." Nutrition Research, I:i, 1-12, 1983.

(2)   Culbert, M.L., What the Medical Establishment Won't Tell You that Could Save Your Life. Norfolk, Va: Donning, 1983.

(3)   Jain, V.K., and R.K. Chandra, "Does nutritional deficiency predispose to acquired immune deficiency syndrome?" Nutrition Research, IV: 537-543, 1984.

(4)   Hughes, W.T., et al., "Protein-calorie malnutrition: a host determinant for Pneumocystis carinii infection." Am. J. Dis. Child. 128: 44-52, 1974.

(5)   Baar, H.S., "Interstitial plasmacellular pneumonia due to Pneumocystis carinii." J. Clin. Patho. 8:19-24, 1955.

(6)   Chandra, R.K. and D.H. Dayton, "Trace element regulation of immunity and infection." Nutr. Res. 2: 721-733, 1982.

(7)   Sidhu, Gurdip S., and Wafaa El-Sadr, "Some thoughts on the acquired immunodeficiency syndrome (AIDS)." Nutr. Res., V: 3-7, 1985.

(8)   Archer, Douglas L., and Walter H. Glinsmann, "Intestinal infection and malnutrition initiate acquired immunedeficiency syndrome (AIDS)." Nutr. Res. vol. 5, 8-9, 1985.

(9)   Interview with Dr. John Grauerholz, in special report (AIDS Is More Deadly than Nuclear War), National Democratic Policy Committee, Oct. 1985.

(10)   Weiner, Robert G., letter, J. Am. Assn., 252:11, 1409, Sept. 21, 1984.

(11)   Harper, Harold, and M.L. Culbert, How You can Beat the Killer Diseases. New York: Arlington House, 1977.

(12)   Horrobin, D.F., et al., "The nutritional regulation of T lymphocyte function." Medical Hypotheses V: 969-985, 1979.

(13)   Mertin, J., et al., "Nutrition and immunity: the immunoregulatory effect of n-6 essential fatty acids is mediated through prostaglandin E." Int. Archs. Allergy Appl. Immun. 77:390-395, 1985.

(14)   Stone, I. The Healing Factor: Vitamin C Against Disease. New York: Grosset and Dunlap, 1972.

(15)   Pauling, Linus, Vitamin C and the Common Cold. San Francisco: Freeman, 1970.

(16)   Cameron, Ewan, and Linus Pauling. Vitamin C and Cancer. Menlo Park, CA: Linus Pauling Institute of Science and Medicine, 1979.

(17)   Cathcart, Robert F., "Vitamin C in the treatment of acquired immune deficiency syndrome." Medical Hypotheses 14: 423-433, 1984.

(18)   Cathcart, Robert F., "The method of determining proper doses of Vitamin C for the treatment of disease by titrating to bowel tolerance." J. Orthomol. Psych. 10: 125-132, 1981.

(19)   Golden, M.H.N., et al., "Zinc and immunocompetence in protein-energy malnutrition." Lancet 2: 1226-8, 1978.

(20)   Brummerstedt, E., et al., "Animal model of human disease. Acrodermatitis enteropathica, zinc malabsorption." Am. J. Pathol. 87:725-8, 1977.

(21)   O'Dell, B.L., et al., "Analogous effects of zinc deficiency and aspirin toxicity in the pregnant rat." Nutr. 107: 1222-8, 1977.

(22)   Julius, R., M. et al., "Acrodermatitis enteropathica with immune deficiency." J. Pediatr. 83: 1007-11, 1973.

(23)   Moynahan, E.J., "Acrodermatitis enteropathica: a lethal inherited human zinc deficiency disorder." Lancet 2: 399-400, 1974.

(24)   Manku, M.S., et al., "Prolactin and zinc effects on rat vascular reactivity: possible relationship to dihomo-gammalinolenic acid and to prostaglandin synthesis." Endocrinology 104: 774-9, 1979.

(25)   Horrobin, D.F., et al., "Physiological cortisol levels block the inhibition of vascular activity produced by prolactin." Endocrinology 99: 406-19, 1976.

(26)   "AIDS: a growing threat." Time, 40-47, Aug. 12, 1985.

(27)   Bulletin Today, Manila, Jan. 28, 1986.

(28)   Culbert, Michael L., op. cit.

(29)   Barry, Bill, "Are lubricants killing gays?" Hustler magazine, March 1984.

(30)   Videotape, Immunology Researching Centre, Ltd., Freeport, Bahamas, August 1985.

(31)   Private communication, William H. Moore Jr., Esq., September 1985.

(32)   Letter, William H. Moore, Jr., Esq., to Vincent DaVita, Sept. 25, 1985.

(33)   Mertin, Jurgen, et al., loc. cit.

(34)   Horrobin, D.F., et al., loc. cit.

(35)   Martin, Wayne, "The beriberi analogy to myocardial infarction." Medical Hypotheses 10: 185-198, 1983.

(36)   Kaunitz, Hans, "Toxic effects of polyunsaturated vegetable oils." In Symposium on the Pharmacological Effect of Lipids (ed., Kabara). Champagne, III: American Oil Chemists' Society, 1978.

(37)   Schock, C.G., and W.E. Connor, "Incorporation of the dietary trans fatty acid (C18:1) into serum lipids, the serum lipoproteins, and adipose tissue." Am. J. Clin. Nutr. 28:1020, 1975.

(38)   Holman, R.T., and E. Aes-Jorgensen, "Effects of trans fatty acid isomers upon essential fatty acid deficiency in rats." Proc. Soc. Exp. Biol. Med. 93: 175-9, 1956.

(39)   Anderson, J.T., et al., "Effect on serum cholesterol in man of fatty acids produced by hydrogenation of corn oil." Fed. Proc. 20: 96, 1961.

(40)   Brenner, R.R. and R.O. Peluffo, "Regulation of unsaturated fatty acids biosynthesis. Effect of unsaturated fatty acid of 18 carbons on microsomal desaturation of linoleic into gamma-linolenic acid." Biochim.

Biophys. Acta 176: 471-9, 1966.

(41)   Brenner, R.R., "The desaturation step in the animal biosynthesis of polyunsaturated fatty acids." Lipids 6: 567-75, 1971.

(42)   Brenner, R.R., "The oxidative desaturation of unsaturated fatty acids in animals." Mol. Cell Biochem. 3:41-52, 1974.

(43)   Ohlrogge, J.B., "Distribution in human tissue of fatty acid isomers from hydrogenated oils." Dietary Fats and Health. Champaign, Ill.: American Oil Chemists' Society, 1983.

(44)   Booyens, J., and C.F. van der Merwe, "Chronic arachidonic acid eicosanoid imbalance: a common feature in coronary artery disease, hypercholesterolemia, cancer and other important diseases. Significance of desaturase enzyme inhibition and of the arachidonic acid desaturase-independent pathway." Medical Hypotheses 18: 53-60, 1965.

(45)   Marcus, Stephen G., "Breakdown of PGE1 synthesis is responsible for the acquired immunodeficiency syndrome." Medical Hypotheses 15: 39-46, 1984.

(46)   Gurr, M.I., "The role of lipids in the regulation of the immune system." Prog. Lipid Re., Vol. 22, 257-287, 1983.

(47)   Locniskar, Mary, et. al., "The effect of quality and quantity of dietary fat on the immune system." American Institute of Nutrition report, 1983.

(48)   Gershwin, M. Eric, et. al., Nutrition and Immunity. Chapter 10: Lipids. San Diego, CA: Academic Press, 1985.

(49)   Tobe, John H., Margarine (The Plastic Fat) and Your Heart Attack. St. Catherines, Ont., Canada: Provoker Press, 1962.

(50)   Fabris, N., et al., "AIDS-zinc deficiency, and thymic hormone failure." J. A. Med. Assn., 259:6, 839-840, Feb. 12, 1988.

Chapter Ten

THE FLUORIDATION CONNECTION

For decades, controversy has raged in the U.S.A. over the use of fluorides in municipal water supplies. On the one hand, the American Dental Assn. and the American Medical Assn. have assured the public that fluoridation helps prevents tooth decay in children (though not in adults). On the other hand, anti-fluoridationists say that the chemicals -- byproducts of the aluminum and phosphate fertilizer industries and therefore originating largely as industrial wastes -- are poisons which accelerate aging, cause specific dysfunctions in the body, impair the immune system and may cause death.

By the time the AIDS epidemic was breaking full force in the U.S.A., battles over to fluoridate or not to fluoridate were reaching standoff proportions in the "second round" of battle, largely because of statistical links between higher rates of cancer and fluoridated cities.

The new voices added to the fight were primarily those of Dean Burk, Ph.D., and John Yiamouyiannis, Ph.D. These two biochemists jointly made the statistical and research case[1,2,3,4,5,6,7] linking fluoridation and cancer in the U.S.A.

Dr. Burk, now deceased, was recently retired from the National Cancer Institute, which he helped found, when he devoted himself almost full-time to the fight against fluoridation. Dr. Yiamouyiannis was, like Dr. Burk, already interested in connections between nutrition and disease when he took up the cudgels against fluorides.

At about the same time as he was publishing the major anti-fluoridation book, *The Aging Factor*[8], Dr. Yiamouyiannis began tracking data on AIDS cases along with the earlier statistics on cancer. He made some intriguing findings: in terms of cases per million, there were three to four times more reported AIDS cases in cities with fluoridated water supplies than there were in cities without such toxic chemicals.

His initial survey noted AIDS cases per 1 million population in the major AIDS cities, with figures taken from the 1982 *Morbidity and Mortality Weekly Reports*

159

(Sept. 24) and the status of fluoridation based on Centers
for Disease Control (CDC) statistics in 1975:

New York City	31.6	cases per million
San Francisco	24	" " "
Miami	19.1	" " "
Newark, N.J.	7.6	" " "
Houston	5.2	" " "
Los Angeles	4.9	" " "

The Ohio biochemist would be the first to note all
kinds of variables in any such assessment, and does not
argue that fluoridated water is the *cause* of AIDS. But the
figures are indeed revealing; the first three cities in terms
of AIDS cases are fluoridated; the next three in
prominence are not, even though Houston and Los Angeles
are said to have low levels of some natural fluorides.

Piqued by this seeming disparity between contrasting triples in the top six AIDS reporting cities, I updated
these figures as of February 6, 1984, for *THE CHOICE*, the
publication of the Committee for Freedom of Choice in
Medicine, Inc.[9] At that time, the breakdown was:

New York	153	cases per million
San Francisco	126	" " "
Miami	87	" " "
Newark, N.J.	49	" " "
Los Angeles	36	" " "
Houston	23	" " "

I then followed this in September 1984 with a further breakdown, which I published in a San Francisco
newspaper.[21] The new figures:

New York City	239.1	cases per million
San Francisco	207.7	" " "
Miami	159.3	" " "
Newark, N.J.	83.9	" " "
Los Angeles	62.7	" " "
Houston	59.2	" " "

The only shift was that Los Angeles was now slightly
ahead of Houston; otherwise, the three-to-fourfold increase

of AIDS cases in fluoridated cities over non-fluoridated cities was holding. This has apparently been the situation in selected European cities as well, but data are inconclusive.

In 1985, another investigator checked the same data bases and came up with similar figures (personal communication.)

After 1985, with HIV/AIDS becoming more generalized, the linkage of its early sites to fluoridation became more obscure.

There are a number of vital considerations in any such linkage:

First, it is to be expected that in New York City, one of the first sites where AIDS was identified (if not yet named) in the late 1970s and early 1980s and where a major problem with drug addiction exists, and which also contains a high-profile and visible homosexual community, there would be a higher ratio of AIDS cases, simply based on population alone.

It is *not* expected, however, that San Francisco, a city of miniscule population proportions, should be Number Two, despite San Francisco's fame as a "gay mecca." With a fixed population of slightly over 700,000 in comparison to the millions in the immediate New York metropolitan area, the San Francisco figures are indeed noteworthy.

But they are doubly noteworthy when contrasted with Los Angeles, a city whose metropolitan area population exceeds San Francisco's many times over. By any measurement -- gay bars, bath houses, publications, organized groups, visible political campaigns -- Los Angeles, at the beginning of AIDS, had far more homosexuals than San Francisco even if, by being diluted in a far vaster population base, they might have seemed to have less impact than did San Francisco's *proportionally* higher, more visible gay community.

Nor does anyone seriously dispute that fast-lane gay activities in both places are essentially the same -- that is, the gay community in one is not insulated from the other. Both cities also have whopping drug problems, both in terms of intravenous drug use and in considerable consumption of so-called "recreational" and "street" non-IV drugs.

Variables in food, air pollution, race and age would

seem, at least superficially, unable to account for the disparity in percentage AIDS cases, unless one argued that the more polluted air of the Los Angeles basin somehow confers a certain degree of protection against AIDS!

If indeed the considerable gulf in percentages of AIDS cases between the two cities has to do with *anything*, then surely that remaining element, bound to something citizens in both places do daily, must bear on drinking water or its ingredients.

The database analysis is far from sufficient to make a clinching case for the connection -- but it is, at the very least, highly suggestive.

Suffice it to say that there are fews areas of national policy setting and scientific debate more controversial than the fluoridation fight, replete with charges of political extremism and the involvement of major economic considerations.

I was particularly mindful of the possible fluoride connection when I attended a dental/nutritional conference in Rio de Janeiro in October, 1985. That same month *Time* had reported on data and projections from various AIDS cases[10] and, in terms of total cases, Brazil was in the *second* spot, ahead of France, Haiti, Canada, and West Germany, and ten places ahead of its nearest competitor in Latin America, Mexico.

Out of curiosity, I asked my dental hosts if Brazilian cities were fluoridated, unlike much of Latin America. Indeed, both Rio de Janeiro and Sao Paulo, reporting the largest clusters of cases, are fluoridated, I was told.

Such connections again do not make any firm case: Rio de Janeiro, in particular, is a major world tourist city. Both it and Sao Paulo have both flourishing homosexual communities and drug problems. Yet the prevalence of AIDS in Brazilian cities, while AIDS remains either so unnoticed or underreported in other major cities in Latin America, must be taken into account. And this reality does not overlook the fact that Brazil, alone among Latin American countries, was a recipient of the suspect WHO smallpox vaccine.

Just how would fluorides figure into the AIDS picture?

Among the many negative connections between fluorides and disease, Dr. Yiamouyiannis points to a "disarming the immune system" effect ranging from allergic-type reactions[11,12] to fluoride-affected decreases in the rate of white blood cell migration, a first line of defense in the viability of the body's entire system of immunity.

Several studies have confirmed the white cell migration-decreasing effect of fluorides.[13,14] In another study,[15] D.W. Allman and co-workers from the Indiana University School of Medicine found that by feeding animals 1 part per million fluoride, urinary levels of cyclic AMP (adenosine monophosphate) jumped by more than 100%. This was significant since other research has shown[16,17] that cyclic AMP inhibits the migration rate of white blood cells.

In 1980, a research dentist warned about this same reality, noting that because of the inhibitory effects of fluorides on leukotaxis (white blood cell migration) "I have doubts about the absolute safety of water fluoridation on a long-term basis."[18]

Too, cyclic AMP inhibits the ability of white blood cells to destroy bacteria and viruses, as indicated in research by Weissmann et al.[19]

Dr. Yiamouyiannis has also pointed out that recent research into the "free radical" superoxide indicates that fluoride exposure may also cause the release of such toxic oxygen products from white cells into the blood stream -- and increased superoxides in blood give rise to tissue damage and accelerate ageing.[20]

The superoxide factor constitutes another rationale for the "scavenging" of reactive oxygen toxic species (ROTS) in a general therapy not only for AIDS but all forms of degenerative disease as well.

It is also known that fluoride ion inhibits an enzyme involved in the phosphorylation process. Phosphorylation is part of the regulatory process of the immune system, and any alteration in it will adversely affect that system.

The "over-phosphorylation" of the host has also been linked to cancer inducement and other aspects of health. Manganese apparently blocks this fluoride phosphorylative effect.[22]

Too, fluoride ion and retroviruses themselves may have a synergistic effect in interfering with a major regulatory system whereby they inhibit surface cell receptor sites for epidermal growth factor (EGF). This inhibition

163

in turn interferes with the nutritional status of individual cells (through altered amino acid, glucose and microtubular and protein synthesis activity). These can have profound implications for health in general.

The "transforming" retroviruses, particularly sarcoma viruses, are implied in this EGF binding inhibition in animals.[23] The speculative presence of fluoridation *and*, say, "the AIDS virus" could thus have a doubly damaging effect on a major regulatory function.

Hence, the immune depressing and generally unhealthy elements associated with fluoridation may very well play a role in setting the stage for AIDS and, together with other co-factors, perhaps virtually assure its presence in a given subpopulation.

REFERENCES

(1)   Burk, Dean, and John Yiamouyiannis, "Fluoride and cancer." Congressional Record H7173-6 July 21, 1975.

(2)   Yiamouyiannis, John, and Dean Burk, "Cancer from our drinking water?" Congressional Record H12731-4 Dec. 16, 1975.

(3)   Yiamouyiannis, John, and Dean Burk, "Fluoridation of public water systems and cancer death rate in humans." Paper presented at the 67th Annual Meeting, Amer. Soc. Biol. Chem. Fed. Amer. Soc. Exp. Biol., June, 1976.

(4)   Yiamouyiannis, John, "Fluoridation of drinking water and cancer," Lebensschutz, vol. 3, no. 3, 42-43, 1976.

(5)   Yiamouyiannis, John, "Relationship between fluoridation of drinking water and increase in cancer death rate." Der Naturarzt., vol. 98, no. 7, 216-218, 1976.

(6)   Yiamouyiannis, John, and Dean Burk, "Fluoridation and cancer: age dependence on cancer mortality related to artificial fluoridation." Fluoride, vol. 10, no. 3 102-123, 1977.

(7)   Yiamouyiannis, John, "Fluoridation-linked cancer deaths per 100,000 population corrected for age, race, and sex." Health Action, vol. 2., nos. 11-12, 1981.

(8)   Yiamouyiannis, John, Fluoride, the Aging Factor, Delaware, Ohio: Health Action Press, 1983.

(9)   "AIDS-fluoridation connection noted," The Choice, X:1, 16, 1984.

(10)   "A scourge spreads panic." Time, p. 50, Oct. 26, 1985.

(11)   Saunders, Milton, "Fluoride toothpastes: a cause of acne-like eruption." Arch. Dermatology, vol. III, 793, 1965.

(12)   Beerman, Howard, and Bernard Krishbaum, "Drug eruptions." Dermatology, Moschella-Pillsbury-Hurley, 350-384, 1975.

(13)   Gibson, Sheila, "Inhibition of the immune system with low levels of fluoride (percentage inhibition with MIF assay)." Testimony before the Scottish High Court, Edinburgh, McColl vs. Strathclyde Regional Council, and Exhibit 165, 1981.

(14)   Wilkinson, Peter, "Inhibition of the immune system with low levels of fluoride (percentage inhibition with chemotactic response assay)." Testimony before the Scottish High Court, Edinburgh, McColl vs. Strathclyde Regional Council, and Exhibit 636, 1982.

(15)   Allmann, D.W. and M. Benac, "Effects of inorganic fluoride salts on urine and tissue 3'5' cyclic-AMP concentration in vivo." J. Dental Res., vol. 55 (supplement B), 523, 1976.

(16)   Rivkin, Israel, and Elmer L. Becker, "Possible implication of cyclic 5'3'-adenosine monophosphate in the chemotaxis of rabbit polymorphonuclear leukocytes." Federation Proc., vol. 31, 2492, 1972.

(17)   Estensen, R.D., et al., "Cyclic AMP and cell movement." Nature, vol. 245, 458-460, 1973.

(18)   Gabrovsek, J., "The role of the host in dental caries infection." Hexagon (Roche), vol. 3, no. 3, 17-24, 1980

(19)   Weissmann, Gerald, et al., "Leukocytic proteases and the immunologic release of lysosomal enzymes." Am. J. Path., vol. 68, 539-559, 1972.

(20)   Gablet, W.L. and P.A. Leong, "Fluoride inhibition of polymorphonuclear leukocytes." J. Dental Res., vol. 48, 1933-1939, 1979, cited in Yiamouyiannis, The Aging Factor, 1983.

(21)   Letters to the editor, San Francisco Examiner, Sept. 14, 1984.

(22)   Li, H.-C., "Phosphoprotein phosphatases." Current Topics Cell. Reg., vol. 21:129, 1982.

(23)   Todaro, G.J., et al., "Transformation by murine and feline sarcoma viruses specifically blocks binding of epidermal growth factor to cells." Nature, 264:26, 1984.

165

Chapter Eleven

A BIOLOGICAL WARFARE/VACCINES CONNECTION?

The central mysteries concerning HIV are, in summary, its sudden appearance on a broad scale in three different geographical regions at or about the same time, its ability to hide and change its protein coat, its predilection for wiping out the very system in the human body which would be susceptible of stopping new viral invaders, and its seeming incurability.

All of which has led to many speculations about just where HIV truly came from -- a question apart from whether HIV is the cause, or is part of the cause, or is only a "marker" for, the HIV/AIDS infection curve.

AIDS has thus become a target for use and misuse politically. It is, by any definition, a perfect weapon in the sense that it could be introduced into an unknowing population with very little or no early announcement of its arrival. It aims directly for the immune and nervous systems of the target population.

By the time its presence is known it is too late and substantial numbers of the target population will die. The creation of a vaccine is enormously compromised by the virus' extreme mutability.

It was on December 7, 1985, symbolically enough, that the Soviet Union admitted[1] the existence of 10 cases of AIDS in the U.S.S.R. after earlier denying that the syndrome existed in Communist states, but it promptly blamed the outbreak on U.S. biochemical/biological warfare experimentation. The East Bloc made similar claims at international meetings, and grudgingly admitted to low numbers of HIV carriers.

Are governments involved in clandestine biological warfare in violation of various international agreements? Well, of course they are, though they are not often caught in the act.

Bruce Halstead, MD, a widely published cancer

researcher, marine biologist, plant biotoxicologist and exponent/proponent of "alternative" therapies in degenerative disease, observed[2] that "the Committee for Responsible Genetics says that the overall military spending on biochemical research bearing on germ warfare has increased 400 percent since 1980. Genetic engineering, which deals with the design of new and virulent viruses and bacteria, is estimated for 1985 to be about $27 million. Genetic engineering has the potential of opening up a flood of new and extremely dangerous germ warfare agents. Is AIDS one of these?"

But such speculations are not one-sided:

A classified report prepared for the National Security Council (U.S.) and obtained by *The Washington Times*[3] claimed that the U.S.S.R. was using genetic engineering to create virulent new biological weapons that could be deployed as early as 1989 -- if, in fact, some had not already *been* deployed. Robert H. Kupperman, a chemical warfare expert at Georgetown University's Center for Strategic and International Studies, told the *Times* that "it's like making designer drugs."

The report was prepared by the Central Intelligence Agency and the Arms Control and Disarmament Agency. Outlining extensive violations by the Soviets of two antibiological warfare treaties, the report stressed its concern that "we believe the Soviets are using recent advances in biotechnology, such as genetic engineering, to develop a new class of CBW [chemical, biological warfare] agents that can be rapidly produced for deployment."

In 1986, British venereologist John Seale was the first expert in the field to make the claim that "the AIDS virus" was manmade -- whether by Americans or by the Soviets. He was first quoted[4] by a tabloid called *Weekly World News* as claiming the virus was developed by the Soviet Union for germ warfare and that it was made from the visna virus, which we have seen is a structure which produces AIDS-like conditions in sheep.

Dr. Seale was quoted as claiming that the visna virus had been available for research in biological warfare for more than 35 years, and that it had been evolved upward to lethal levels through guinea pig and mouse experimentation. However, it spread quickly in Africa through the reuse of unsterilized hypodermic needles. It spread through

American and British drug addicts much the same way, he claimed.

That same year, the *London Sunday Express* carried Seale's views, but had him saying that the virus "was artificially created by American scientists during laboratory experiments which went disastrously wrong -- and a massive coverup has kept the secret from the world until today."[19]

Alan Cantwell Jr., MD, who dogged the AIDS story from the perspectives of its causation either by a hidden, shape-changing microbe[20] and/or as the result of a man-made virus, reveals in a followup book[24] that by 1987 Dr. Seale was backtracking on some of his more inflammatory comments, while admitting it was "technically feasible" to manufacture the virus. Seale was said to have complained that he had been frequently misquoted about what he really meant.

No sooner was the Seale furor underway -- and for some time overlooked or underreported in the U.S.A. -- than the possibility that "the AIDS virus" was spread into Africa through the World Health Organization's smallpox eradication vaccine program was reported in England.

Pearce Wright, a science writer for *The London Times*, broke the story May 11, 1987.[5]

Wright cited the recent death of a 19-year-old American soldier three weeks after he had been inoculated for smallpox as ordered by the U.S. Army. He developed AIDS-like symptoms and died after briefly responding to treatment.

The *Times* article was cast in terms of WHO investigating its own suspicions that its 13-year African smallpox campaign might have triggered the dormant HIV, and noted that the vaccine--*Vaccinia*--can activate other viruses. Was this done on purpose? WHO has denied that its smallpox vaccine caused AIDS. Yet the explosion of AIDS in central Africa neatly corresponds with the target areas -- and the timeframe -- of the smallpox vaccine eradication program.

It also dovetails with the fact that Brazil, the only Latin American recipient of the WHO smallpox vaccine, has far and away the greatest number of cases of AIDS in the Americas outside the U.S.A. and is the "number two" country worldwide in AIDS cases.

Oddly enough, American readers went virtually

uninformed about *The London Times* story of May 11, 1987, with none of the major media carrying the story -- a fact that was itself further grist for conspiracy theories.

On March 28, 1986, a strange document was sent to major political and scientific leaders and publications in the United States. It was called "This is a Bio-Attack Alert", and was authored by lawyer Ted Strecker, since deceased, and his brother, Robert Strecker, MD, a Glendale, Calif., gastroenterologist.[6]

The extensively annotated document claimed that AIDS represented a biological attack on the U.S.A. by the U.S.S.R., that the disease was introduced into Africa by the World Health Organization through the connivance of Soviet agents working through international agencies and the U.S.' own National Institutes of Health, and that various diseases had been inoculated by international agencies from research "cell lines" developed in the U.S.A. The overall objective is to inflict Americans with enough immune depression to pave the way for a fast "bio-attack," they asserted.

Utilizing existing documents from the standard literature, the Streckers argued that WHO "asked for" development of "the AIDS virus" and it was supplied, and that it is the bovine visna virus (BVV) in man with "a *trans-acting* transcriptional regulator gene inherited from bovine leukemia virus" (BLV).

While this assessment at first blush seems extreme, the documents the Streckers cite can be construed as making their case: -- Vol. 47 of the Bulletin of the WHO, pp. 257-274 (1972) notes[7] the recommendation that "a systematic evaluation of the effects of viruses on immune functions should be undertaken. A number of viruses should be studied and a standard set of immune functions should be employed ... The effects of virus infection on different cell types ... should be studied ... An attempt should be made to ascertain whether viruses can in fact exert selective effects on immune function ... by affecting T cell function ... The possibility should be looked into that the immune response to the virus itself may be impaired if the infecting virus damages more or less selectively the cells responding to the viral antigens..."

The Streckers developed an extensive literature search to buttress their view that American and interna-

169

tional science was used, wittingly or unwittingly, to "look into" the manufacture (as a human-animal viral combination) of a new virus to selectively wipe out the immune system.

Robert Strecker, in less rhetorically hyperbolic terms, has produced a video study (1988)[8] on this subject. The Streckers and several others believe that mass immunization campaigns (smallpox in Africa, hepatitis B and polio in the USA) may have been vehicles for the spread of a new virus or provirus, whose political aims run from selective murder to mass genocide.

The Streckers doubt that AIDS is exclusively a sex-and-blood-borne disease and, at any event, suspect HIV will mutate to the point where it is contagious in many different ways.

The literature presentation was met with deafening silence at home, and Ted Strecker has since died. Robert Strecker's views were published in a respected British Medical journal.[25]

By November, 1986, the fact that well credentialed scientists could be making claims about the manmade nature of"the AIDS virus" could no longer be completely overlooked by the U.S. media. Even so, the reporting was tepid. That month *Time* gave a brief account of the Seale and Strecker views and added that "AIDS experts" found such assessments "far-fetched."[21] There was no effort whatsoever to reproduce the Streckers' extensive literature citations or to secure from the AIDS officialdom meaningful responses to the detailed charges they laid down.

By 1987, there were rumors floating around in the AIDS underground that while the syndrome might have been introduced into Africa through the WHO smallpox vaccination campaign, it had been clearly introduced into the U.S.A. through the experimental hepatitis B vaccine project, in which a vaccine "for homosexuals only" was provided experimentally. Its utilization in 1978-81 in New York City and later elsewhere neatly matched the presumed early period of AIDS cases (though does not take into account possible ones before that).

The hepatitis vaccine theory fell along two general paths:

First, noted AIDS researcher Mathilde Krim speculated[22] that a biological accident might have occurred

170

in which AIDS developed from HIV-contaminated batches of gamma globulin inoculated into male homosexuals in New York for the purpose of protecting them from hepatitis infection -- a very real part of the modern medical sequelae of homosexual behavior.   Gamma globulin made from pooled human blood from Africa and the Caribbean might have been a possible origin, she speculated.

Second, that same year, medical commentator Gary Null quoted J. Anthony Morris, a virologist who had worked for the National Institutes of Health (NIH) and for the Food and Drug Administration (FDA) in virus vaccine research, as claiming that "the AIDS virus has been around for years."[23]

Noting the possible emergence of HIV in about 1979 or right after the introduction of the first hepatitis B vaccine for male homosexuals in New York City, he reached the conclusion that the experimental hepatitis vaccine, derived exclusively from homosexual carriers of the hepatitis virus, was contaminated with HIV, a virus whose prior existence was inferred by the presence of antibody in blood "taken 40 to 50 years ago, and stored in an icebox."

Cantwell,[34] tracing the various reports[35,36] by Cladd Stevens of the New York City experimental hepatitis vaccine trials with homosexuals, notes how -- while the Centers for Disease Control (CDC) in Atlanta steadfastly refused to make any connection between HIV/AIDS and the vaccine -- followups of the original group of 212 men studied over time since their first vaccine inoculations in 1978 showed an opposite picture: 6.6 percent of that group had anti-HIV antibodies in their blood samples which were collected in 1978 and 1979, or two to three years before the "official" recognition of AIDS. By 1981, 20% of the original 212 had HIV antibodies and by 1984 40% had them.

The minimal assumption one might make from this is that HIV/AIDS was lurking around New York City at least by 1978. The medium assumption would be that it had some connection with the new vaccine program. The maximum assumption would be that it was *placed* there, or by some terrible "biological accident" just happened to be there.

The fate of San Francisco gay men whose blood was stored since the hepatitis B vaccine project started there is also eloquent. As we have seen, some 77 percent of the San

Francisco "cohort" had developed AIDS or AIDS-related diseases by 1989 (the bad news), yet 20 percent remained free of symptoms (the good.)

In his searing and sabre-rattling assessment of AIDS as all-out biological warfare waged by the East Bloc against the West, Dr. William Campbell Douglass traced the incredible story of how a refugee Polish scientist, virtually bereft of American scientific credentials, had been able to move from the New York City Blood Center to "masterminding" the hepatitis B vaccine project.[38]

The early connections between HIV/AIDS and American homosexual males outside New York City and the first studies of Danish males "infected with AIDS" by 1981/82 revealed the startling pattern: most had made trips to, or been in contact with men from, New York.

As we point out elsewhere, there is evidence that there may have been HIV or something like HIV present even 10 years earlier in the U.S.A. But the hepatitis B vaccine project among male homosexuals in New York and the rapid outbreak of what would later be called AIDS provides a series of statistics far too large to be ignored or written off as coincidental. The vaccine connections do not stop there, however.

Eva Lea Snead, MD, an innovative Texas physician who has also been a vocal proponent of "alternative" medicine, added to the vaccines-as-AIDS-causes-or-containers by publishing her monograph on "Immunization Related Syndrome" in 1987.[9]

Her research bore on the similarities between HIV and a particular simian virus (SV-40) which causes a clinical syndrome similar to, if not indistinguishable from, AIDS. She noted that SV-40 is carried by the African green monkey -- and that it was precisely from this monkey that the original polio vaccines were manufactured.

Examining a wealth of documentation on SV-40, a well-studied virus, and the advent of the polio vaccines, Dr. Snead became convinced that the immune-depressing, cancer-causing SV-40 monkey virus contaminated the vaccines at least before 1963, and possibly thereafter, and that the contaminated polio vaccines are the root cause of the explosion of AIDS, childhood leukemias, and a number of other modern-era pathological disasters.

Like the Streckers, Dr. Snead derived her conclusions from extensive published data gleaned from the standard or "orthodox" literature.

The possible contamination of vaccines by viruses capable of causing diseases in humans need not be biological warfare, but gross scientific errors whose participants must desperately cover up the mistakes. And yet...

Perhaps the most bizarre yet well-researched notion as to the origin of AIDS came from Army Lt. Col. Ted Bearden (retired), a nuclear engineer.

Col. Bearden, who is employed by an aerospace company, speculated in a 1988 book[10] that AIDS has been triggered by advanced Soviet electromagnetic technology as well as virus-manufacturing. "Phase conjugate" weapons not only "beam in" diseases of all kinds to destroy humans from within but constitute high-technology weapons capable of bringing civilization as currently understood to a standstill, he argued.

Bearden's thesis is that the U.S.S.R. has far outpaced the United States in the development of "scalar electromagnetic weapons" (as a followup to the energy theories late last century and earlier this century of Tesla and others).

These directed-energy weapons have been deployed many times against U.S. targets, quite aside from the U.S. population, in order to provoke an American response to see how much the U.S. is aware of the technology, he wrote.

Bearden has made a commanding and sweeping review of the theories of directed energy, and his assessments cannot be lightly dismissed. While the Bearden thesis is chilling in the extreme, it has the positive side of proclaiming the existence of a technology (electromagnetic therapy, about which theories and uses abound) which not only can allegedly cure AIDS but virtually everything else.

Both Bearden and the Streckers point to the well-intentioned National Cancer Act of 1971 (President Nixon's "Conquest of Cancer" program) as an all-out effort against cancer which, intentionally or unintentionally, left the door open to fullscale penetration by East Bloc scientists and agents.

It must be borne in mind that the Nixon effort was in response to the growing reality that the most rapidly advancing disease condition in the U.S.A., cancer -- by then the number-two "natural" killer of Americans -- was nowhere close to being stopped after years of public and private research.

In some quarters, the National Cancer Institute (NCI), the repository of federal funds for research on a disease which it seemed neither to understand nor be able to cure, was little more than a laughingstock, a federal agency largely manipulated by outside private interests wrapped around the multi-billion-dollar "cancer industry."[11]

Nixon wished to make the conquest of cancer a hallmark of his administration, spokesmen suggesting that by 1976, the bicentennial of the American republic, somehow the most feared of the diseases would be brought under control. (By 1976, the first five-year assessment of the effort showed how far afield the reality was.)[12]

It must also be noted that the breakthrough for cancer seemed within striking range because of the monumental discovery of the "double helix" (DNA/RNA) genetic code, an explanation of the basic replicative machinery of cells by Watson and Crick, in 1966. The knowledge gleaned from this discovery fueled vast new research in molecular biology, microbiology and any number of overlapping new fields looking at the origins and manipulation of the genetic code.

The advent of HIV/AIDS *must* be set within the politics of the war on cancer in the United States if one is to make some rhyme and reason out of the selection of the federal laboratories used for research on, and indeed the semantical evolution of, an "AIDS virus" which American officialdom attempted to make into a member of the "HTLV" virus family.

It should be understood that the central obsession of American cancer research in the 1960s and 1970s was the viral theory of cancer, that major public and private research money went into virology (as well as into developing toxic chemotherapeutic drugs) and that the viral concept was the dominant passion in oncological research when President Nixon declared the war on cancer.

In the meantime, both controversy and a hint of mystery surround what Alan Cantwell calls "serious virus contamination problems" and Michael Gold called *A Conspiracy of Cells.*[37] These are descriptions of the errors and miscues which may abound at government research labs utilizing "tissue cell culture" techniques.

The ability to grow and study viruses was moved a

174

quantum leap ahead in the 1960s by the advent of the new methods. Viruses could be injected into live cells, grown, studied, traded between laboratories, a move which brought great changes and some chaos into the viral research arena.

That new viruses could seem to be created which were in effect contaminations of old viruses became public with the Essex-Kanki mishap (Chapter Two). Earlier, another "new" human retrovirus (HL 23), allegedly cultured from human leukemia cells, turned out to be neither new nor human but old and simian.

It is an open question to ponder what might have happened had some new viral technique or product "gotten out", by simple error, and contaminated a blood supply or a vaccine or a group of people. What steps would be necessary to cover up the error?

The first virus claimed to cause a very rare form of human leukemia was that described by Robert Gallo, as noted, as the "human T-cell leukemia/lymphoma" virus type 1. As we have seen, the designation was later changed to "T-cell-lymphotropic" or "T-lymphotropic" as HTLV-II and HTLV-III were subsequently "discovered."

The apparent isolation of HTLV-I as a human cancer-causing virus, similar to an allegedly cancer-causing virus in cats, was at least some modest kind of payoff for the American commitment in public money to unravelling the cancer puzzle.

But were several manmade or man-altered "human cancer viruses" already in existence? Were they in effect just sitting around waiting to be used? Did the faltering National Cancer Institute, already under heavy congressional oversight for its manifest failure to do much of anything against the war on cancer, need to pull a new virus out of the air, or a new disease out of the lab?

These are all horrendous and perhaps unfair questions, but they have to be asked given the ever murkier background of the origin of the HIV theory of AIDS, and even of the evolution of AIDS itself as an ever-changing syndrome.

All we know is that the Nixon Conquest of Cancer program, a failure, was in the hands of the NCI, and that this same federal institute became the primary research conduit for the "war on AIDS." It was as if failure was to be amply rewarded with a lot more funding and prestige. At the same time, the Nixon effort literally threw open the American research doors to the whole world, particularly the East Bloc.

Bearden, noting the early history of the 1971 national cancer effort and its sinister international implications, has written:[13]

"Iron Curtain country scientists were invited to participate [in the U.S.-declared war on cancer] and they did so with alacrity. At the time -- ironically -- penetration of our recombinant DNA genetic research was one of the highest priorities of the Soviet KGB. Obviously, many KGB scientists/agents were infiltrated into our labs under this program (some of our research labs at Ft. Detrick, for example, still employ more Communist than American scientists.)

"In these cancer labs, animal viruses were repeatedly injected and reinjected into human cell cultures until new viral strains emerged that preferred human cells. These viruses could then be cultured and the effects (or lack of effects) of various chemicals and drugs against them could be ascertained.

"These new viruses are exactly what one would wish to develop if one were seeking a biological warfare virus to which humans were not resistant, and one which preferred humans as its host.

"Sometime during the early 1970s, KGB agents who had infiltrated U.S. cancer research laboratories may have deliberately contaminated the World Health Organization's smallpox vaccine with one or more of the lethal new viruses available in the Western cancer laboratories. Massive WHO smallpox vaccinations [in the Seventies] then resulted in the appearance and spread of the AIDS disease."

In 1986, a response to a question put to the chief of the National Institute of Health's Laboratory of Central Nervous System Studies and Laboratory of Slow, Latent and Virus Infections came up with a relatively incredible answer:[14]

. "No, emphatically no! There is no defensive or offensive warfare microbiology done at Fort Detrick today. It is the national cancer research facility of NIH. In this facility I have a building where more good and loyal Communist scientists from the USSR and mainland China work -- with full passkeys to all the laboratories -- than

Americans. With night-working U.S. citizens and foreign Communist investigators here, obviously there is no 'secret' biological warfare activity going on. Even the Army's infectious-disease unit is loaded with foreign workers -- not always friendly nationals. It is a valid research unit on worldwide problems of infectious diseases in which no classified or secret activities unfold..."

This statement is susceptible of many interpretations, running from the naive to the sinister.

By 1987, AIDS was clearly a political football for major contenders in the Cold War, and information and disinformation abounded on both sides. The smokescreen of such claims and counterclaims made it difficult to know which side -- if either -- to believe.

In April 1987 a staffer of the Washington Bureau of Intelligence and Research wrote in the *Los Angeles Times*[26] that the worldwide rumors about AIDS' being a manmade virus produced by American scientists were part of a Soviet program of disinformation. Abroad, the Soviets could claim that the presence of "AIDS virus" in Filipino prostitutes outside the U.S. Subic Naval Base clearly showed Americans were spreading "the virus."

There were stories circulating in the underground press and elsewhere that AIDS might have been the result of a CIA plot to infect Cuban pigs with the African swine fever virus(ASFV).[27,28]

While one might recoil in shock over allegations that humans test new viruses on other humans for either scientific or political reasons, the sorry reality is that there is nothing new in such behavior. In the U.S.A. alone:

-- 400 poor black syphilitics were never told they had syphilis and were allowed to develop the disease and remain untreated in an experiment conducted by the U.S. Public Health Service between 1932 and 1972 in Macon County GA. The whole idea was to see what would happen if syphilis were left untreated.[29]

-- The CIA has conducted drug experiments on unwilling, unsuspecting American citizens, in New York, San Francisco and elsewhere, the data available in a shocking tome entitled *A Higher Form of Killing.*[30]

-- The U.S. Army "bioattacked" unsuspecting U.S. civilians and cities in the 1950s and 1960s, the most infamous incident being a six-day "germ fog" experiment in

San Francisco.[31]

— U.S. government biowarfare attacks took place in subways, at airports and on highways in the U.S.A. as well as on U.S. military bases.[32]

— The *Los Angeles Times* cited 239 U.S. Army biowarfare experiments in which unsuspecting civilians and military personnel were the subjects.[33]

In what Scaramouche might describe as a world gone utterly mad, all such experiments might be excused as being in the interest of national security, and the elaboration of human viruses designed to wipe out immune systems might be described as part of sound cancer research.

The salient point is that at least a dozen countries, probably more, have the technology to produce "designer bug", human-adjusted, animal-derived,[15,16,17] spliced-together viruses whose primary targets are hostal immune and nervous systems. The question of who did what to whom for what reason is less vital than the possibility that such a thing could have been done, and is probably being done.

In 1973, Danish cancer researcher J. Clemmesen may have predicted far more than she knew when she gave the summation address of an international symposium on comparative leukemia research. The talk at the time was of viral associations with leukemia, and the elucidation of the genetic code had occurred only seven years prior. Prescient, sensitive scientists were asking philosophical questions.

Observed Clemmesen:[18]

"..With regard to the risk of virus-spread, conditions are even worse, and this is not only the case among postmortem pathologists, but also among clinical pathologists handling blood samples as if they were sterile and never would contain contaminations... Also in everyday life we are gradually packing people closer together in buses and on planes and in greater numbers than in the days when lice and fleas would give a warning. In addition blood transfusions and vaccinations are increasing the intimacy of contact with biological surroundings.

"We are in fact establishing conditions for a possible pandemic of an oncogenic virus variant on the scale of the influenza epidemic of 1918.

"... We have increased the world's population of creatures ... by artificial breeding of practically identical individuals which increases the chance for any virus to travel far and for a long time under identical conditions, and their mutants will have equal chances to survive...

"We have in tissue cultures created conditions for propagation of virus in cells from a host different from the original. This will tend to increase enormously the chance of mutation into variants acceptable to new hosts and by their heterogenic qualities they may have neoplasticity in a new host.

"So it is possible to visualize a mutation of a virus into a variety of high contagiosity to man, resulting in a pandemic of neoplastic disease, before we could develop a vaccine...

"What are the risks involved if some RNA virus or some template would happen to infest some of the production [of industrially produced proteins]?...

"It is... possible to visualize the risk of some desperate persons or nations coming into possession of some virus -- and perhaps even of some vaccine -- so they could threaten to spread their virus unless some request were fulfilled...

"It seems as if we should not leave too much of such ideas to science fiction writers, who by profession are optimists. We may have to study such problems before too long."

"Orthodoxy's" continually switching signals over the company-line theories as to the implied origin of "the AIDS virus" from African green monkeys have never been logical, reasonable answers as to just how a massive epidemic got underway simultaneously in three separate geographic areas at about the same time, even allowing for the more rapid proliferation of viruses among humans due to air travel.

The minimal realities would seem to be that such advanced technological development of man-engineered viruses has been, and is being, carried out, and that perhaps some of the results somehow leaked or got into the population. The more chilling possibility is that the viruses were deliberately placed in human populations either as an experiment or as an attack.

The possibilities of who did what to whom and for what reason are relatively endless. As of 1989, people I personally hold to be intellectually honest, and believing in what they say, had variously described for me the following AIDS conspiracy scenarios, ranging from the most to least common: a secret Soviet biological warfare attack on the West; a plot by world bankers and international conspirators to carry out a presumed population-limiting mandate by a project called Global 2000; a series of laboratory mistakes made in the interest of science, followed by a massive coverup; a botched effort by the U.S. to weaken the Castro regime; a U.S. plot against Communists; a U.S. establishment conspiracy by moralists against homosexuals; one part of an involved effort by extraterrestrials to either absorb, control, take over or otherwise utilize the human population on earth for reasons not yet fully elucidated.

The scientific importance of any or all these speculations, of course, still dangles tantalizingly from the concept of "the AIDS virus" as the sole cause of the HIV/AIDS infection curve.

Other than some suggestions that the U.S. start fullscale war against the East Bloc, none of these speculations gives the slightest hint about what to *do* about the HIV/AIDS problem.

Wherever HIV came from, whatever it is, what to do about the syndrome with which it is rightly or wrongly associated must be the first order of business.

Meanwhile, the old-boy network in AIDS/cancer research in the U.S.A. rolls along -- the scientist who helped remove the failed cancer drug AZT from the shelf and push it into prominence as the first anti-HIV drug in 1989 became the head of the National Cancer Institute (NCI.) The former NCI head, in harness as the war against cancer flopped, went on to become a major executive at a major cancer research facility at a reported quadrupling of his federal salary. The band really *did* play on.

REFERENCES

(1)   Chung, Connie, "NBC Nightly News," Dec. 7, 1985.

(2)   Halstead, B.W., AIDS and Nutrition. Colton, CA: Golden Quill, 1985.

(3)   Diaz, Tom, "Soviets create 'designer bugs'." The Washington Times, August 6, 1985.

(4)   "AIDS is secret Soviet weapon." Weekly World News, Jan. 21, 1986.

(5)   Wright, Pearce, "Smallpox vaccine 'triggered' AIDS virus." The London Times, May 11, 1987.

(6)   Strecker, T., Strecker, R., "This is a bio-attack alert." Privately published and circulated, March 28, 1986.

(7)   Allison, A.C., et al., "Virus-associated immunopathology: animal models and implications for human disease." Bulletin of the World Health Organization, 47: 257-274, 1972.

(8)   Strecker, R., "The Strecker Memorandum." Glendale, CA, 1988.

(9)   Snead, E.L., Immunization Related Syndrome. (Privately published) San Antonio TX, 1987.

(10)   Bearden, T.E., AIDS: Biological Warfare. (Book in press) 1988.

(11)   Culbert, M.L., What the Medical Establishment Won't Tell You That Could Save Your Life. Norfolk VA: Donning, 1983.

(12)   Culbert, op. cit.

(13)   Bearden, T.E., "Soviet phase conjugate weapons (weapons that use time-reversed electromagnetic waves.)" Bulletin of the Committee to Restore the Constitution, January 1988.

(14)   Mosely, B., Interview of D. Carlton Gadjusek. Omni magazine, March 1986.

(15)   Alizon, M., and Montagnier, L., "Lymphadenopathy/AIDS virus: genetic organization and relationship to animal lentiviruses." Cancer Research 6: 403-214, 1986.

(16)   Burny, A., et al., "Bovine leukemia virus, a distinguished member of the human T-lymphotropic virus family." Retroviruses in Human Lympholeukemia. Tokyo: Japan Sci. Soc. Press, 1985.

(17)   Corneo, G., et al., "Could bovine leukemia virus be a possible agent of some human lymphatic leukemias?" Acta Haemat 72: 65-6, 1984.

(18)   Clemmesen, J., "Summation." Comparative Leukemia Research 1973. Tokyo: Univ. Tokyo Press, 1973.

(19)   "AIDS made in lab shock." London Sunday Express, Oct. 26, 1986.

(20)   Cantwell, A.J., in AIDS: the Mystery and the Solution. Los Angeles CA: Aries Rising, 1986.

(21)   "Infectious propaganda." Time, Nov. 17, 1986.

(22)   Interview Magazine, February 1987.

(23)   Null, Gary, "Medical genocide: the AIDS panic." Penthouse, April 1987.

(24)   Cantwell, A. J., in AIDS and the Doctors of Death. Los Angeles CA: Aries Rising, 1988.

(25)   Strecker, R.B., "AIDS virus infection." J.Royal Soc. Med. 79: September 1986.

(26)   Bailey, Kathleen, "Soviets sponsor spread of AIDS disinformation." Los Angeles Times, April 19, 1987.

(27)   Rappoport, Jon. AIDS Inc. San Bruno CA: Human Energy Press, 1988.

181

(28)   Rappoport, Jon. "African swine fever, Fidel and the CIA." San Jose Metro, June 4, 1987.

(29)   Jones, J.H., Bad Blood: The Tuskegee Syphilis Experiments. New York: The Free Press, 1981.

(30)   Harris, Robert, and Jeremy Paxman. A Higher Form of Killing. New York: Hill and Wang, 1972.

(31)   "Army germ fog blanketed S.F. for 6 days in '50 test." Los Angeles Times, Sept. 17, 1979.

(32)   "Army used live bacteria in tests on U.S. civilians." Los Angeles Times, March 9, 1977.

(33)   Los Angeles Times, Dec. 4, 1984.

(34)   Cantwell, AIDS and the Doctors of Death, op. cit.

(35)   Stevens, C.E., "No increased incidence of AIDS in recipients of hepatitis B vaccine." New Eng. J. Med. 308: 1983.

(36)   Stevens, C.E., et al., "Human T-cell lymphotropic virus type III infection in a cohort of homosexual men in New York City." J. Am. Med. Assn., 255: 1986.

(37)   Gold, Michael, A Conspiracy of Cells. Albany NY: State University of New York Press, 1986.

(38)   Douglass, W.C., AIDS: The End of Civilization. Clayton GA: Valet Publishers, 1989.

AIDS—other voices, other views...

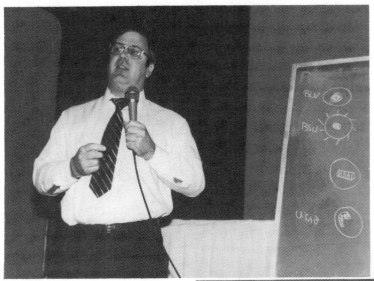

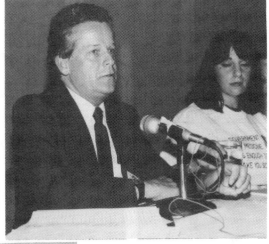

Above, Glendale physician Robert Strecker in a chalk-talk points out how "the AIDS virus" may be produced by splicing together two animal viruses—designed to "evolve upward" in humans. At right, Mike Culbert (left) and Eva Lea Snead, M.D., at a Chicago conference where both called into doubt the basic premises regarding HIV/AIDS. Dr. Snead has strongly linked AIDS with the SV-40 simian virus and the polio vaccine.

—PHOTOS FROM THE CHOICE

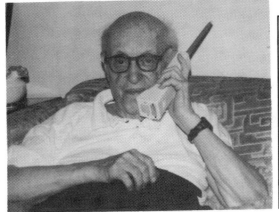

At left, Emanuel Revici, M.D., the pioneering New York researcher/physician who has used "guided lipid" therapy in managing the HIV/AIDS infection curve, as well as many other degenerative diseases. A medical maverick to whom many patients feel they owe their lives, Dr. Revici, 92, in 1988 won a major court decision allowing him to continue practicing.

—PHOTO FROM THE CHOICE

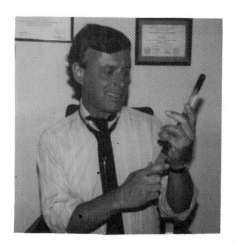

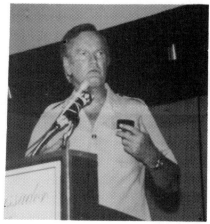

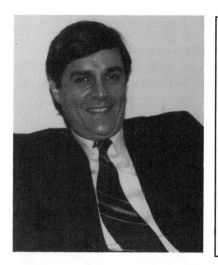

Above, left, New York's Steve Calazza, M.D. who has connected AIDS with syphilis and treated hundreds of patients with penicillin and antibiotics with heartening results. Above, right, Bruce Halstead, M.D., a world-famed researcher and spokesman for medical freedom of choice, was among the first Americans to alert the world to the possible chemical, biological warfare (CBW) aspects of AIDS. At left, Laurence Badgley, M.D., Northern California physician who helped pioneer natural and metabolic approaches to HIV/AIDS. Below, left, Rodrigo Rodriguez, M.D., and Dr. Robert Bradford of the Bradford Research Institutes, who introduced eclectic AIDS protocols in Mexico.

—PHOTOS FROM *THE CHOICE*

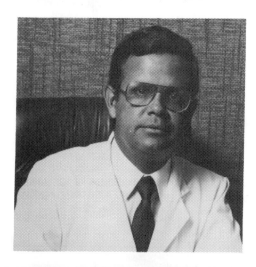

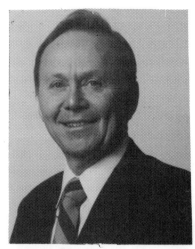

Chapter Twelve

IS IT REALLY ONLY SYPHILIS?

"He who knows syphilis, knows medicine." --
Sir William Osler

It was an aphorism at the turn of the century that to know syphilis was to know, essentially, the whole of medicine:

Syphilis, "the great imitator" (or "masquerader") which had laid waste to parts of Europe centuries before and is still endemic today in some Third World populations, had become the great "shadow on the land" even by the 19th and 20th centuries.

Here was a condition of many manifestations, phases and lifelong "carrier states," capable of being passed from mother to child as effectively as from lover to lover, transmissible essentially, but by no means uniquely, through sexual intercourse.

Syphilis, particularly in its secondary and tertiary stages, can mimic hundreds of other conditions, ranging from simple flu-like symptoms and swollen glands to general wasting, dermatological involvements, serious complications of internal organs, general weakness and malaise, dementia and severe immune depression. Reactivated parasites, widespread respiratory and other (opportunistic) involvements used to be, and still can be, part of the picture.

The difference is that today Western physicians, educated as to how the mass proliferation of penicillin, and other antibiotics, essentially brought syphilis to its knees in the immediate post-World War II years, rarely ever see "classical" syphilis.

In the 19th and early 20th century a clinician interviewing a young, sexually active male (or female) with wasting symptoms, rashes, swollen glands, and general malaise might make the early clinical assumption (observation only) that he was seeing a syphilitic, and he was apt to be correct.

As knowledge of syphilis grew, any of several blood tests to find the spirochetal causative agent, *Treponema*

183

pallidum -- or simply reactions to *T. pallidum* -- would only confirm what the clinician suspected.

Centuries before, many physicians thought that The Great Pox was a skin disease, and that treatment to make pustules vanish (with gold and other heavy metals and minerals) was the equivalent of "curing" syphilis.

It took many years to recognize that syphilis was a generalized, constitutional disease of many phases and manifestations of which skin eruptions, however prevalent, were only one set. (This typically allopathic error, we might add, is redolent of the 20th-century fixation by orthodox oncology on the assumption that cancer is tumor disease -- that to treat tumors, which really are only the more notorious symptoms of the underlying metabolic disease, is somehow the equivalent of treating the disease, and that whatever happens to the tumor is a fair monitor of the course of the disease itself.)

The "imitator" was thought to lurk behind virtually every conceivable pathological sign of the patient earlier in this century, particularly if that patient was thought to be part of a "high-risk group" as socially delineated: in this case, any sexually active and usually unmarried young person.

The study of syphilis, its etiology, multiple manifestations, its various experimental treatments, its abundant sequelae and its transgenerational effects, was dominant in Western medicine up until the advent of the "wonder drugs." Suddenly, the world was told, The Great Pox had met its match--primarily penicillin, provided in millions of units.

And descending syphilis rates in this country from the mid-1940s onward, with occasional starts and stops, seemed to confirm this. The older massive aqueous penicillin treatments provided in enormous doses and the more complicated blood tests were eventually swapped for a form of penicillin called benzathine and the common U.S. Public Health Service-endorsed VDRL blood test.

Armed with this simple, easily interpretable test for reactions to *T. pallidum* and mass-produced benzathine penicillin, it was thought, syphilis was now, finally, under control: a disturbing relic from the past which had finally yielded to the technology of evolving human science.

In the meantime, other diseases came along to take

the place of syphilis in terms of multiple manifestations. Increasingly common in the postwar era was infectious mononucleosis, later attributed to the Epstein-Barr virus (EBV). "IM" became "the kissing disease," primarily among teenagers, since B-cell and saliva-inhabiting EBV could easily spread though necking sessions.

The resultant syndrome, ranging from mild bouts of flu-like symptoms, general fatigue, etc.to -- rarely -- fatal outcomes, now became itself, on a smaller scale, a "great masquerader" which could be mistaken for many other conditions.

American clinicians in the 1940s/1950s might be just as apt to observe the features of "IM" and make the correct diagnosis purely on intelligent speculation as were their counterparts of the 19th and early 20th centuries apt to diagnose correctly secondary syphilis simply on the basis of signs and symptoms.

We are now faced with yet another "great imitator." A vast range of symptomata common to secondary, dormant and even tertiary syphilis, and to infectious mononucleosis, is now part of the ever-expanding HIV/LAS/ARC/AIDS infection curve.

Young clinicians now are likely to be correct when they diagnose, by physical symptoms and signs alone, the LAS or ARC level when they see before them wasting, flu-stricken, chronically fatigued sexually active young people with swollen glands, "thrush" in the mouth, etc. Now that HIV antibodies with several tests can confirm what the clinician can visually detect, masses of people are being diagnosed as "AIDS-positive."

In the modern pre-AIDS era, failure to detect actual syphilis came to be relatively commonplace simply because so few young medics were schooled in the guises and devices of the disease they had been told had been all but obliterated thanks to mass prophylaxis with benzathine penicillin.

As a writer in *The Atlantic* recounted[23] in 1988, of 241 patients with neurosyphilis seen between 1965 and 1970 at the Medical College of Virginia, 115 had never been diagnosed with any kind of syphilis. And a study of 20 syphilitics seen in the 1970s at two major New York City hospitals found that the patients had been misdiagnosed with everything from hernias to leukemia to multiple sclerosis.

That, now, syphilis might be mistaken for AIDS and vice-versa was a point most eloquently made in a 1984 article ("Secondary syphilis masquerading as AIDS in a young gay male."[1]) in a medical journal. Involved was a man who admitted to over 5,000 sex partners in 16 years and who had "constitutional complaints, diffuse lymph node enlargement, and widespread skin lesions...mistakenly attributed to AIDS by both the patient and medical staff upon admission."

Only followup investigation revealed that it was old-time syphilis that had caused these conditions, not the HIV/AIDS infection curve.

What if AIDS isn't really AIDS but is indeed syphilis? If in fact the young patient's major complaint is really the spread of *T. pallidum* though the tissues, however deadly it may be, he at least has an altogether *curable* disease -- and curable without recourse to designer drugs, human-engineered interferon or any modern-era gimmick.

A small but growing body of researchers and doctors believes essentially that the HIV/LAS/ARC/AIDS infection curve is either syphilis or something very much like it -- dressed up with some new names and disguises -- or that what is being called AIDS is an infection in which syphilis, or at least a spirochete, has played the major role.

These researchers note there is *no* single symptom or sign attributable to the whole infection curve let alone to full-blown AIDS itself, very much including Kaposi's sarcoma and *Pneumocystis carinii* pneumonia, which has *not* been seen in syphilis! Not one.

Among these and other scientists there is also a second school of thought: that the HIV/AIDS infection curve may not be exclusively syphilis, but that somehow the new mystery virus HIV is either a "co-factor", somehow working synergistically with syphilis, or simply a common "marker" for an advanced syphilitic infection -- particularly of *neurosyphilis*, the form of advanced syphilis lurking in the brain, cerebral spinal fluid, and nerve tissues known to be difficult to diagnose and, by implication, more difficult to treat.

Neurosyphilis is something modern clinicians, if they encounter the disease at all, would be more likely to see in older syphilitic patients than in young people.

The dissenting voices on the nature of syphilis, let alone of AIDS, began earlier in this century, primarily with Bergel,[2] who proposed that syphilis-like infections may occur as a result of a virus-like variant of the syphilis spirochete.

In recent times, Salvatore Catapano in New York followed to some extent the same idea in seeing manifestations of AIDS, particularly Kaposi's sarcoma, as syphilitic, and advocating immune stimulation (through typhoid vaccine) before treatment with penicillin.[3] He has seen reversals of numerous HIV/AIDS symptoms.[24]

(By late 1988 Catapano, a laboratory researcher, had secured a U.S. patent on the typhoid vaccine-immune enhancing protocol and several U.S. physicians were reporting highly encouraging results. Luke Olmstead, MD, San Diego, noted rapid improvement in six patients. A Los Angeles doctor had seen some kind of immune enhancing in 30 patients.[28])

(In July 1989, Southern California physician Valentine Birds, MD, told me he was "quite excited" about his results with the typoid vaccine-followed-by-aqueous penicillin approach, both in terms of therapeutic results and research.

(He had found that a whopping *85 percent* of AIDS patients, 9 out of 10 in effect, turned positive for syphilis on blood tests after receiving the typhoid vaccine. Of all AIDS patients, 60 percent responded to the treatment, which was largely 15 million units of aqueous penicillin daily over 15 days, and sometimes low doses of the cancer therapeutic agent Oncovin.

(The "failure group", he said, were those still on AZT or with a prior history of AZT, and those who had been "compromised" by pentamidine.)

In Berkeley, California, researcher Joan McKenna and her group began studying immunosuppression in San Francisco Bay Area homosexuals and data on AIDS cases in Africa.[4] She found epidemic syphilis in both groups, even though the syphilis might have been regarded as cured because blood was now "seronegative" on VDRL tests and/or undertreated.

She matched signs and symptoms of syphilis and full-blown AIDS and found virtually 1:1 correlations. Out-

187

break of symptoms, however, followed years of "chemical immunosuppression" not only by illegal drugs but by the persistent overuse of antibiotics and other substances to treat the continuing infections and inflammations present in such "high-risk" people.

Noting, as we had in our earlier monograph, that a linkage of "illegal" drug use of *all* kinds (not only intravenous) brought the drug/AIDS connection to 79 percent, she added chemical immunosuppression by "legal" drugs. This kind of research would suggest that chemically induced suppression of the immune system might approach 100 percent in people in the HIV/AIDS infection curve.

McKenna, Harris Coulter,[5] German researchers[6] and the late Dr. Stephen S. Caiazza,[7,16] in New York City, a heroic physician with a mostly-gay, mostly-HIV/AIDS patient load, and a few other doctors, reached some similar if not identical conclusions:

-- There is massive underdiagnosed or misdiagnosed syphilis in America and the Western world, despite (or because of) the proliferation of benzathine penicillin as a treatment of choice. Benzathine penicillin may be adequate to assuage symptoms in primary and secondary syphilis, but syphilis may move swiftly to the central nervous system.

-- A great deal of the spread of misdiagnosed or underdiagnosed syphilis is among very sexually active homosexuals, where it is epidemic. It is also epidemic among central Africans in the same countries and areas where HIV/AIDS is thought to have broken out with the worst numbers.[9,10,11,12]

-- The VDRL test may be adequate for diagnosing early syphilis but turns in many "false negatives" serologically for advanced syphilis, particularly syphilis in the central nervous system and brain. Hence, reliance on the VDRL and benzathine penicillin as the primary arms against syphilis is the equivalent of spreading false hope: there is much more syphilis around than has been either diagnosed or treated.

-- Benzathine penicillin apparently does not cross the "blood-brain barrier" so is useless against neurosyphilis.

-- An adequate therapy, if not *the* adequate therapy, for advanced syphilis is other forms of penicillin and certain antibiotics.

188

-- The symptoms of HIV/AIDS suggest that the real disease is syphilis, or a kind of spirochete, not a brand-new pathology.

-- An adequate therapy, if not *the* adequate therapy, for HIV/AIDS ought to be forms of non-benzathine penicillin and also benzathine penicillin itself.

These same researchers have noted that syphilis is well-known as an immune depressant in and of itself even though such depression may not occur until the "latent" and tertiary (advanced) stages. As syphilis historically entered these stages, it left its victims open to invasion by -- or reactivation of -- opportunistic infections, be they bacterial, viral or fungal.

It is likely that the presence of HIV and/or other immune-depressing co-factors undercut the commonly used "serological" (in distinction to the more complicated treponemal) tests for syphilis, primarily because the former rely on immune reactions. If the immune system is under attack -- the hallmark of HIV/AIDS -- then a blood test dependent on immune reactions to prove the existence of another germ or disease is, at the very least, compromised.

Should HIV and syphilis turn out to be fellow travellers -- an epidemiologically logical conclusion based on the prevalence of both in the very same populations -- then the activity of the one (HIV and co-factors) could obscure the presence of the other (syphilis) at least in tests dependent on immune reactions.

The first treatments of the HIV/AIDS infection curve with penicillin were reported by two West German physicians, Klaus-Uwe Dierig and Urban Waldthaler, the first case having been a kind of fluke: guessing that a patient's gonorrhea-caused endocarditis might be the reason for his confusion, shortness of breath, considerable weight loss and spiking fevers, they treated him with huge doses of penicillin daily for three weeks. His symptoms disappeared.

This was in 1981 or on the eve of the arrival of AIDS as a new syndrome.[15]

They later found that this same patient "tested positive" for HIV, and a review of his 1981 laboratory tests revealed abnormalities consistent with HIV infection. They then used superdose penicillin treatments on six diagnosed AIDS and ARC patients and claimed clinical remission of all symptoms.

Dierig began finding that serological tests on sera from deceased AIDS patients were revealing unexpected syphilis, even when various non-treponemal-specific tests were still "negative" for the bacterium. Independently, Dr. Caiazza in New York began finding the same thing: "hordes of syphilis treponemes" from the sera of 20 AIDS patients who had died, most of them "negative" for syphilis.

These independent and parallel discoveries in 1986 led to collaborative research between the American and Germans as they jointly realized that:

-- Much syphilis exists among AIDS patients, most of it unsuspected.

-- Standard syphilis blood tests in immune-suppressed AIDS patients may be, and usually are, highly misleading, turning in many false negatives.

-- Benzathine penicillin has done an inadequate job of syphilis prophylaxis over the years.

-- The classical signs/symptoms of HIV/AIDS may only be those of syphilis.

-- AIDS patients, particularly those with neurological elements, should be treated by heavy and long-term penicillin doses.

-- At the very least, syphilis, or at least treponemes (also causing such infections as yaws and pinta) is playing an unexpectedly important role in AIDS.

In 1986, Dr. Caiazza engaged in an act most people would find heroic: checking positive for HIV himself -- the product, he believes, of far too many needlestick injuries from treating his own caseload of AIDS/ARC patients in New York, so many of whom had died -- and deciding that his own sera would be a good "negative control" for the hypothesis that syphilis was inducing many AIDS symptoms, and finding that he was negative for syphilis, he inoculated himself with the syphilis germ.

His violent reactions, and treatment, are recounted in detail in his own, riveting account.[29] Risking his health, and possibly his life, he learned what he had set out to learn.

He told me he had literally gone from being an early-ARC-type patient to developing devastating full-blown symptoms in a single weekend ("I could hardly crawl across the room.")

From that point on, Dr. Caiazza began treating HIV/AIDS patients with long-term penicillin therapy.

It is essential to note that Dr. Caiazza and the Germans are not holistic medical practitioners but men cut from the allopathic mold. They are honest, pioneering, willing to think new thoughts. (See *NOTE*, pg.196).

(Caiazza believed that two attempts on his life in West Germany may have been prompted by his own research. A German attorney, he told Coulter, had mentioned that "if what you are telling me is true [about syphilis and AIDS, particularly as to the curability of AIDS with standard versions of old-time penicillin] -- then you're both in great danger."

(The attorney had noted that "forty percent of all pharmaceuticals for the Western world are produced in West Germany.")[17]

In the U.S.A. Dr. Caiazza could not get his early results and theories published in the standard medical journals, and his requests for state aid to bolster his research went unheeded. But he did become known to the rapidly expanding "underground" of AIDS research and sufferers, and the AIDS-syphilis links did receive attention, though only in a peripheral way.

In the June 18, 1987, *New England Journal of Medicine*, Boston and Seattle researchers reported previously unsuspected syphilis in the central nervous systems of AIDS patients.[19,20]

The same year, the Centers for Disease Control assessed (in January 1988,)[21] the incidence of secondary syphilis to be the highest since 1950, and reported that it had increased 32 percent over 1986. But AMA medicine was not going to abandon the VDRL nor yield to the AIDS-is-syphilis (or AIDS-is-caused-by-a-spirochete) line of reasoning.

Fears of a widespread recrudescence of syphilis paralleling the geometrically spiralling HIV/AIDS caseload, and continual prodding by Caiazza, the New York Committee of Concerned Physicians, and others kept adding to the debate.

Recent research pointed to concurrent neurosyphilis/AIDS infections, and failure of benzathine penicillin therapy in persons with HIV infection. It also underscored the reality that there were persons with AIDS and syphilis in whom syphilis blood tests were "seronegative."

An assessment by Kenneth G. Jordan, MD, in the *Western Journal of Medicine* of "modern neurosyphilis" claimed that "most current data do not currently support the view that concurrent HIV infection produces accelerated or resistant neurosyphilis."[22]

Even so, a number of metabolic/eclectic physicians have added aqueous penicillin to multifactorial treatment protocols for ARC/AIDS patients. Among the first group so treated in the Bradford Research Institute-Mexico experimental cluster a faster resolution of opportunistic infections was noted. But in a many-faceted treatment program -- including that during which three BRI patients became negative for HIV in peripheral blood -- it is impossible to tell what single substance may be working.

In analyzing responses to questions put to several hundred patients, including those who entered the Mexican program, we found that a common element in HIV infection among individuals who otherwise did not fit profiles for HIV/AIDS (little promiscuity, no prior history of substance abuse) was a relatively recent secondary syphilis diagnosis.

By late 1988, Dr. Caiazza had treated about 150 patients with HIV/AIDS over a 2-year period "beginning with patient number one -- myself," he told me in an interview. And by 1990, right before he died, he was into a fourth year of essential control of HIV and syphilis himself, admitting he did not know "when to stop treatment," and eschewing metabolic or "natural" therapies.

Like many full-time AIDS-treating practitioners, he had become frustrated with the results of standard or orthodox therapy and even more frustrated when he tried to do something different, albeit within the allopathic mode. He was so cheered at the disappearance of or mitigation in clinical symptoms that he exulted: "We're at the beginning of the end," and he did not mean this negatively.

Because under New York statutes a doctor doing something out of the ordinary cannot admit patients to the hospital for an unapproved therapy (in this case, aqueous penicillin for AIDS), Dr. Caiazza had, by 1988, developed an in-office program of starting with procaine penicillin daily, or more often benzathine penicillin at 2.4 million units once a week over six weeks, and then switching to a version of tetracycline indefinitely. "I don't know when to stop, but as long as those symptoms stay down we keep treating," he said.

He recalled the case of a 77-year-old transfusion-associated AIDS case, a man in an incoherent, practically vegetative state ("squash rot", as he described it) literally carried into his office by his son. After several rounds of penicillin treatment the man was back in command of his faculties and able to drive himself to Dr. Caiazza's New York office.

The young physician notes that the penicillin treatment cannot yet be considered a "cure" for full-blown AIDS, that "I can't raise a dead body," but that pre-AIDS patients in the main respond beautifully to the treatments. "I'm saying that the healthy stay healthy despite the fact their T cells may go up, down or sideways."

In fact, Dr. Caiazza had little faith in the T-cell immune panel, opting -- as have some others -- for measurements of neopterin levels as a better sign of progress. He was particularly upset over the obsession with T4 cells, he said, when he sent two samples of blood "from the same puncture from the same arm of the same patient the same day to the same laboratory but with separate names" -- and found a difference in T4 cells of several hundred!

Dr. Caiazza and other exponents of the syphilis-AIDS link could only stand up and cheer when the Centers for Disease Control (CDC) announced in their *Morbidity and Mortality Weekly Report*[26] the results of an extraordinary two-day conference of experts held in March 1988. Their consensus findings and recommendations stopped short of stating that AIDS is syphilis or even that HIV and spirochetes are AIDS. But they found:

-- "The clinical manifestations, serologic responses, efficacy of treatment, and occurrence of complications of syphilis may be altered in patients coinfected with human immunodeficiency virus (HIV)."

-- In "some" HIV-infected patients with confirmed syphilis, *both* nontreponemal (e.g., the standard VDRL) *and* treponemal (e.g., DFA-TP or any assay which locates the actual spirochete, not the body's response to it) tests *may be negative* -- that is, in terms of laboratory response the syphilis may be masked ("masquerading").

-- "Case reports have suggested that [syphilis] treatment failures, including progression to neurosyphilis, may occur more frequently in patients coinfected with HIV than in those with syphilis alone."

-- Even more strikingly, the CDC recommendations were that "persons with HIV infection acquired through sexual contact or intravenous drug abuse should be treated for syphilis" and that "all sexually active persons with syphilis should be tested for HIV." The recommendations note that "HIV test results are clinically important in managing persons with syphilis..." and that "neurosyphilis should be considered in the differential diagnosis of neurologic disease in HIV-infected persons."

-- "Benzathine penicillin regimens should not be used to treat either asymptomatic or symptomatic neurosyphilis in HIV-infected patients"; rather, aqueous crystalline or procaine penicillin should be used.

Implicit, though not stated, is the rhetorical question: "Is HIV simply a marker for masquerading syphilis?" (as suggested by the AIDS-syphilis researchers) or "is syphilis simply a marker for HIV?"

Dr. Caiazza could only consider as a gift from Olympus this tardy recognition of the HIV-syphilis connection from American orthodoxy.

He was, of course, not the only American physician who has made the connection, but he was certainly a pioneer in the field. In California, Dr. Kerby Stewart reported some heartening results,[25] and the use of injectable penicillin was added to various multifactorial programs, including those at the Bradford Research Institute-Mexico.

Since dementia has been noted in HIV/AIDS patients almost from the beginning of the epidemic, the revised Centers for Disease Control (CDC) parameters for

AIDS diagnoses now make dementia an indicator for AIDS. Yet, mental aspects of syphilis have been noted in the literature for centuries. Widespread mental disturbances ranging from confusion to outright paresis were part of the syphilitic sequelae, and of course still are.

The difference is, now, the depressed states, mood swings and mental confusion which may be observed in a sexually active young person may be ascribed to AIDS (particularly if he or she is "positive" for HIV) rather than to syphilis.

Caiazza, clamoring for recognition of the syphilitic connection in AIDS, argued:[27]

"In the HIV-positive individual with even subtle neurologic findings, it is impossible -- given present-day technology -- to rule out neurosyphilis. Therefore, in such a patient, unless another medically acceptable explanation can be found that accounts for the observed neurologic deficit, a presumptive diagnosis of neurosyphilis must be made and, barring any contraindications, appropriate therapy instituted. This becomes especially pertinent if it is remembered that ... the therapy for neurosyphilis is relatively easy, benign and harmless ...

"We are told that AIDS ultimately has a mortality approaching 100%. Given this harsh reality, and given the easy reversibility of neurosyphilis in the AIDS patient, do we not owe our patients the benefit of the doubt? In my opinion, it is remiss of the physician attending an AIDS patient with neurologic dysfunction not to aggressively look for and aggressively treat neurosyphilis."

Under a best-case scenario, syphilis would turn out to be AIDS, a point of view with which few scientists concur. In the worst-case scenario, syphilis would turn out to have a great deal to do with the HIV/AIDS infection curve -- a connection, indeed a likelihood, that simply cannot be overlooked.

Should that be the case, then untold human suffering would have been induced by the suggestion that HIV, a new virus, is the single cause of an incurable, supposedly always-fatal disease.

Along the way, as is now developing, a vast new multi-billion-dollar industry would have grown up around HIV/AIDS in the mass proliferation of inconclusive and possibly irrelevant blood tests and in the long-term manage-

195

ment of many opportunistic infections and the short-term treatment of full-blown conditions. A situation analogous to the cancer industry in the U.S.A. would arise -- and is, in fact, arising.

Scientist Joan McKenna is fully aware of the primacy of the allopathic model in American medicine and what it means to dissent therefrom (as is Dr. Caiazza, recalling the strange apparent attempts on his life.) As Dr. McKenna told Harris Coulter:[18]

"The medical profession is pretty much locked in to the viral theory of AIDS. There is a lot of politics there. You have to understand that the only new money into biological research in recent years ... has been for Legionnaire's Disease and AIDS. As a result, laboratories are being built and careers are being made on this money.

"And the money is earmarked for research on the virus, not for the investigation of syphilis or of chemical immune suppression. Doctors who do not accept the official line on AIDS can find themselves in a lot of trouble."

REFERENCES

(1)   Smego, Raymond A., et al., "Secondary syphilis masquerading as AIDS in a young gay male." N. Caroline Med. J. 45: 253-254, 1984.

(2)   Syphilis im Lichte neuer Untersuchungen (1925) cited in Townsend Letter for Doctors, June 1988.

(3)   Townsend Letter for Doctors, June 1988.

(4)   McKenna, J.J., et al., "Unmasking AIDS: chemical immunosuppression and seronegative syphilis." Med. Hypotheses 21: 421-30, 1986.

(5)   Coulter, Harris, Aids and Syphilis: The Hidden Link. Berkeley CA: North Atlantic Books, 1987.

(6)   "Clinical improvement noted in AIDS/ARC patients given antitreponemal agents." CDC AIDS Weekly, Feb. 16, 1987.

(7)   "Possible link between syphilis and AIDS." New Scientist (New Zealand), 1558, April 30, 1987.

(8)   New York Committee of Concerned Physicians (letter, press release) 1987.

(9)   Masawe, A.E.J., "Serological tests for syphilis in Uganda." E. African Med. J. 47: 12, 673-680, 1970.

(10)   Quinn, Thomas C., et al., "Serologic and immunologic studies in patients with AIDS in North America and Africa." J. Am. Med. Assn. 257: 19,

2617-2621, 1987.

(11)   Mason, P.R., et al., "The serological diagnosis of syphilis." Cent. African J. Med. 31: 10, 192-193, 1985.

(12)   Ahmed, S.A., et al., "Prevalence of syphilis in South Sudan." J. Com. Dis. 17:3, 251, 1985.

(13)   Coulter, op. cit.

(14)   Thompson, Lloyd. Syphilis. Philadelphia and New York: Lea and Feiger, 1920, 1929, 1931.

(15)   Townsend Letter for Doctors, June 1988.

(16)   Scythes, J.B., "Primum non nocere." Hologram (Canadian Holistic Med. Assn.), VI:6, September 1988.

(17)   Coulter, op. cit.

(18)   Coulter, op. cit.

(19)   Johns, D.R., et al., "Alteration in the natural history of neurosyphilis by concurrent infection with the human immunodeficiency virus." N. Engl. J. Med. 316: 1569-72, 1987.

(20)   Berry, C.D. et. al., "Neurologic relapse after benzathine penicillin therapy for secondary syphilis in a person with HIV infection." N. Engl. J. Med. 316: 1587-9, 1987.

(21)   "Continuing increases in infectious syphilis -- United States." Centers for Disease Control (MMWR) 37: 35-38, 1988.

(22)   Jordan, K.G., "Modern neurosyphilis -- a critical analysis." West. J. Med. 149:1, 47-57, July 1988.

(23)   Leishman, Katie, "AIDS and syphilis." The Atlantic, January 1988.

(24)   Ibid.

(25)   Ibid.

(26)   Morbidity and Mortality Weekly Report, Centers for Disease Control, Atlanta GA, 27:39, Oct. 7, 1988.

(27)   Caiazza, S.S., "Neuropsychiatric AIDS and neurosyphilis: overlap." J. Ortho. Med., Third Quarter 1988.

(28)   "Treatment with typhoid vaccine shows startling results; begins in SD." San Diego Gay Times, Dec. 16, 1988.

(29)   Caiazza, Stephen S., AIDS: One Doctor's Personal Struggle. New York: Caiazza, 1989.

Chapter Thirteen

THE CLASH OF PARADIGMS: TOWARD ECLECTIC AND HOLISTIC THERAPY FOR HIV/AIDS

By 1990, standard or Western medicine, captained by that of the U.S.A., and therefore allopathic in tone, outlook and content, had made inroads against the HIV/AIDS infection curve, but so minimal that the diagnosis of full-blown AIDS was still described by the American Medical Assn. as an inevitably fatal condition. (Even so, the mortality rate stayed at or around 60 percent -- it was only the *presumption* that full-blown cases would die that led to the sweeping assessment.)

Perhaps the best orthodox results were being turned in against *Pneumocystis carinii* pneumonia, the form of lung disease appearing in at least 60 percent of AIDS cases and originally having the poorest prognosis.

The general feeling of medical orthodoxy was that with both new and old drugs this particular expression of AIDS might be prevented entirely (though this was not convincingly demonstrated) and even when it occurred some prolongation of life might occur with the use of the aerosol version of pentamide and other more toxic drugs.

Unfortunately, the possible inhibiting of PCP or slowing down of its progress can only be accomplished at great metabolic cost, for the various drug therapies now used experimentally or artificially in the U.S.A. and elsewhere exact a tremendous toll on the immune system, the very system which the syndrome is attacking in the first place.

Some people cannot tolerate AZT (azidothymidine, zidovudine, Retrovir, touted as the only drug which as of 1990 could "slow down" HIV) or a number of other experimental compounds and as we note in the HIV/AIDS infection curve (see Appendix I) diseases, conditions, and infections are simply waiting in line like dominoes ready to strike the immune-depressed AIDS patient.

As of summer 1988, the labyrinthine processes of the Food and Drug Administration (FDA), while faced by the greatest calamity in modern American medical history, had only come up with the authorization of two drugs, AZT and trimetrexate, and use of a few other older drugs, as "legal" treatments for the various manifestations of AIDS. Alpha-interferon was added in Fall 1988. By mid-1989, aerosol pentamidine and Ganciclovir had been approved.

FDA Commissioner Dr. Frank Young, his department assailed by dying AIDS patients and freedom-of-choicers on the one hand demanding access to anything which might be of benefit, and on the other by establishment hardheads opposing any change in the FDA's chronically slow drug-approval process, had loosened some FDA regulations out of both compassion and political awareness. By 1988, he said, 178 substances were in some stage of human testing, including 39 antiviral drugs, 34 drugs to treat opportunistic infections, three vaccines, and various other substances thought to be of some benefit. More are being worked on. (See Appendix II)[13]

The Western orthodox medical model (we call it the allopathic paradigm) is based on the assumption that medicine largely consists of detecting the pathogen, or cause, finding a drug to destroy the pathogen, and then attacking the pathogen.

Allopathy needs a set of symptoms, and a demonstrable pathogen, in order to do battle. In HIV/AIDS, this has largely meant that when a presumed HIV/AIDS patient "tests positive" for "the AIDS virus", even if he is showing no symptoms at all, allopathy has little for him to do. In effect, he is told to come back "to doctor" when he has symptoms of something -- that is, there is "something to treat." This is usually called "expectant observation" in medical jargon.

There is little the Western or allopathic physician can do to stop something before it happens, since in HIV/AIDS this would mean boosting or improving the human immune system -- and at this late date Western or allopathic medicine still does *not* believe anything like that can be done outside of some extremely expensive and unproven manmade techniques.

To quote John Renner, MD, a distinguished spokesman of supposed anti-quackery (Midwest Council Against Health Fraud, National Council Against Health Fraud), voicing the common allopathic view: "I know of nothing that 'boosts' the immune system .. this (offering substances, usually nutrients and food substances to help modulate immune response) is just a sales gimmick because the immune system has had so much media coverage in the past four years."[7]

Hence, the worried HIV/AIDS asymptomatic is likely apt to do nothing unless and until symptoms develop -- that is, when it may either be too late or disease is grossly advanced. Since standard Western medicine knows of little or nothing to do between the advent of presumed infection and the outbreak (if any) of symptoms, the patient is truly left fending for himself.

Some physicians, even of the allopathic mode, by 1987 and 1988 were beginning to advocate the *early* rather than the last-minute use of toxic drugs, figuring that if indeed HIV/AIDS is caused by "the AIDS virus" then the earlier one starts attacking the virus with a drug, the better. Indeed, in terms of HIV, it makes sense to use an anti-HIV drug earlier rather than later -- unless, by so doing, the patient's overall immunity (or total host defense) is so further compromised that he will become fatally ill anyway.

(And there was enough research, by 1989, to suggest that AZT could actually "slow down" disease progression in early phases -- yet not cure the condition.)

The allopathic armamentarium is now composed of experimental toxic drugs to attempt to halt the "replication" of HIV, or to interfere with the enzyme it must utilize for such replication, reverse transcriptase (RT), or to interfere with its capacity to "bind to" target cells or to deflect its capacity to target certain cells. Allopathic research is also attempting to find synthetic ways to enhance or modulate immunity, while almost entirely ignoring the abundant evidence that a vast variety of natural substances at least anecdotally and empirically have such capability.

There were voices of caution within standard medicine as early as 1984 advising that "aggressive chemotherapy is not the way to go" in managing AIDS' myriad infections.

Efforts to utilize recombinant interferons and interleukin II in attempts to restore immune capacity were mixed at best, with the *Journal of the American Medical Assn.* (JAMA) noting in 1984[1] that "there is no evidence that alpha-interferon stimulates the immune system and the side effects of the agent (aesthenia, fever, headaches, peripheral neuropathy, modest neutropenia, thrombocytopenia, and possible hepatic toxicity) may well outweigh the benefits of this therapy over other chemotherapies." Even so, it is now an "authorized" treatment.

French researchers observed[2] in August 1985 that "these studies suggest that treatment of AIDS patients with a combination of HTLV-III/LAV replication inhibitors and immune regulatory agents may be more effective than either treatment alone" -- though the results referred to were spotty at best.

In 1984, Poulsen *et al.,* reported[3] a regression of a case of AIDS-connected Kaposi's sarcoma with Dapsone, a pre-existing drug (such success could not be repeated).

The French pioneered HPA-23 as a viral replication inhibitor (and made sadly famous as the drug which failed to save the life of American film star Rock Hudson).

Suramin, used for years in the treatment of African sleeping sickness, for a time was trumpeted as a useful antiviral-AIDS agent until its side effects were observed to far outweigh any benefit.

In vitro studies by fall 1985 had shown[4] inhibition of HIV by trisodium phosphonoformate (Foscarnet), known to be an inhibitor of herpes simplex I and II, cytomegalovirus and the animal retrovirus visna, but virus production increased upon withdrawal of the drug. *In vitro* studies in 1985[5] showed it to have a dose-related inhibitory effect on HIV.

In 1985, ribavirin (virazole), already well-known in the "gay underground" as an anti-viral drug legally obtainable in Mexico, was cleared by the U.S. Food Drug Administration (FDA) for use against respiratory syncytial virus in infants and young children. This seemed to bring it closer to possible use against AIDS in the U.S.A. even though oral ribavirin had reportedly produced side effects.[8,9] It was still not a "legal" AIDS treatment in 1990, and results in AIDS were mixed at best.

In fall 1985 French researchers first jubilantly announced short-term successes in AIDS with cyclosporine-A, but rapidly muted their enthusiasm after three patients died.[12]

Immune-enhancement treatment with thymic

humoral factor (THF) was tried[14] and led researchers to conclude that "it might be hypothesized that if immunomodulation is to offer some hope to AIDS patients, it should be attempted."

D.R. Hicks *et al.*, reported[32] the inactivation of HIV by nonoxynol-9, a non-ionic surfactant in several spermicides in *in vitro* studies.

Pompidou *et al.* showed[33] that low concentrations of both isoprinosine and sodium diethyldithiocarbamate (Imuthiol) inhibited HIV expression and reverse transcriptase activity in HIV infected H9 cells and normal peripheral blood lymphocytes *in vitro)*. All of these were early attempts to mount a challenge to HIV and its presumed everexpanding disease syndrome.

As doctors face problems of recurrent fungal, parasitic, viral and bacteriological infections in AIDS patients, they rely on antibiotics and other drugs, virtually all of which are involved at some level either in immune depression or actually exacerbate parts of the problem (as in the spread of *Candida albicans*, a frequent common denominator in AIDS patients).

Hence, HIV/AIDS represents one of the most complicated medical nightmares ever to face Western medicine, a challenge made all the more difficult by the dominance in Western medicine of a single school of thought in its obsessive hunt for the single therapy for the presumptive single cause.

In the meantime, patients whose cases are generally *not* reported in standard medical literature but nonetheless appear in the media and elsewhere have shown that a general approach to AIDS many call "holistic" is prolonging lives, diminishing symptoms, and holds out a better hope than drug and antibiotic modalities.

The rise of the holistic paradigm has largely been fueled by the desperation caused by a disease Western orthodoxy regards as incurable and it is swiftly beginning to make inroads into the whole of medicine.

An outgrowth of several social and scientific currents -- the anti-establishmentarianism of the 1960s, the resurgence of homeopathy and naturopathy, a blending of ancient Oriental and indigenous American medical traditions, the "New Age" movement in self-awareness and spiritual inquiry of the 1960s and 1970s, the health-consciousness of the 1980s, the rapid growth of nutrition as a science and medical subspecialty, the restating of various Eastern philosophies -- "holism" is claiming to find answers where "orthodoxy" fails.

Briefly stated, the holistic doctrine in health and disease holds that man is the union of mind, spirit and body, that both "ease" and "disease" must be understood within this triad, that no disease or metabolic condition is standing alone, that physically man is the sum of his parts. Disease, then, is seen as spiritual and mental as well as physical. No therapy can succeed without taking into account all these parts.

It is also a restatement in the 1990s of the debates which wracked French medicine exactly a century before -- which is more important, the germ (microbe, virus, bacterium, fungus) or the terrain (the natural condition of the host)?

History has dictated that the Koch-Pasteur Germ Theory of Disease, just coming into prominence then, at least temporarily won the debate. But the collapse of immune systems, the myriad assaults on host defense through man-made and natural pollutants, toxins and lifestyle changes, are causing a resurrection of the debate.

The controversy has never been sharper than as it relates to the HIV/AIDS infection curve when perceived in its *multifactoriality* both as to cause and management. The conclusion that assumes thunderous proportions in this clash of paradigms as it relates to HIV/AIDS is simple:

The terrain (the natural condition of the host) is more important than the germ (HIV)!

The matching reality is that Western science, propounded on the "scientific" model of rationalism, double-blinded tests, animal models and repeated experiments, has developed vast information on the nature of disease while virtually ignoring or remaining oblivious to the actual total metabolic condition of the *host*, the patient in whose natural terrain a disease state is developing.

The first flicker of "establishment" medical interest in this other approach -- which tends to focus on natural nutrients and positive thinking -- was in the *Lancet*, which reported in July 1985[15] that a group of U.S. physicians was following 10 AIDS patients with Kaposi's sarcoma who had "chosen not to enter conventional treatment protocols."

They added that "eight are still alive an average of 21.5 months after diagnosis (range 13-37 months)" and that "these men seem to be surviving at least as well as patients who have been treated," inasmuch as the average survival rate for KS alone in New York was 29 months, and that for KS plus *P. carinii* and/or other opportunistic infections was 14 months.

The researchers observed: "These men in our study may not be representative of KS patients in general. Their choice to forego conventional medical therapy may indicate a strong, independent psychological make-up which could enhance survival. They are all following a vegetarian (macrobiotic) diet and have strong social support systems ... The survival of men with KS for longer than three years with no medical intervention indicates that occasional 'successes' in uncontrolled treatment protocols may in part reflect part of the spectrum of the natural course of the disease that is favored by as yet undefined host and/or extrinsic factors rather than an effect of a particular drug."

Yet the reverse assessment could be made; namely, that standard or orthodox therapy is mostly a failure and that opting to reject it, let alone favoring natural methods of immune enhancement, could in fact be better choices.

By 1990, some of these macrobiotic patients had added years of existence to their lives.[54]

By 1985, clusters of patients involved either in "holistic" programs alone or in mixed therapies, combining elements of standard medicine and holism, began to be reported in the major media and presented cases of survivors from advanced AIDS achieving survival intervals as high as 5 or more years, or even longer than the syndrome had been officially named.

Since the average lifespan after a patient was first hospitalized with AIDS had been estimated at 224 days, virtually all these cases were remarkable in many aspects.

Illustrative cases include that of Louie Nassaney, diagnosed in May 1983 with Kaposi's sarcoma, and found to be free of KS by October 1984, and by late 1989 a visible, physical-fitness exponent of positive thought.[17] He underwent seven months of interferon treatment, found no improvement, rejected chemotherapy and radiation, and switched to a program of physical fitness, nutrition, vitamins, holistic healing, and metaphysics in December

1983.

In the same group of Los Angeles patients, Steven Stucker claimed good health after being an AIDS patient for five years during which he had multiple bouts of AIDS-related diseases. He went through interferon and radiation treatments as well as dietary change, vitamin administration and cessation of smoking.

A San Francisco Bay Area patient, Stuart Anderson, came to the attention of the Bradford Research Institute in April 1983 or a year after his Kaposi's sarcoma was diagnosed (April, 1982) and many months after giving up chemotherapy treatments at a Veterans Administration hospital.

Anderson met several times with this writer to describe the various changes he made monthly in his nutrition and eating habits. He utilized up to 35 vitamins, minerals and other natural substances daily, though his ingestion of oral vitamin C was by far the major element.

For several years, Anderson made his story available to the print and electronic media, only frustrated that so few people actually believed his seeming visible victory over KS (lesions were gone though some signs and symptoms persisted.) In an oxidative blood test advanced by the B.R.I., Anderson showed no trace of oxidative damage from any pathological condition as of March, 1984.

It was self-education in reading about diet and nutrition which had sent Anderson into the realm of metabolic/nutritional therapy, he said. He eventually became a patient of Robert F. Cathcart III, M.D., Los Altos, California, who was at the time beginning to treat AIDS patients with megadoses of Vitamin C backed by other natural substances.

At one point Anderson was able to build tolerance to 120 grams daily orally of the substance, a level he maintained for two months. It was his own investigation into parasitical connections with KS and AIDS in general that helped stimulate the B.R.I.'s interest in the same.

Anderson died Oct. 29, 1985, though not directly of AIDS[18] and also after a round of antibiotic treatments.

By 1987 and 1988, it was clear that increasing numbers of patients were surviving full-blown AIDS and LAS/ARC levels by many years. Expected to be dead within a few months to, at the outside, two years of diagnosis, depending on the various diseases and infections, long-term survivors began to be noticed by the media.

These were in distinction to those who simply were noted statistically or by retrospective review as having had HIV/AIDS as early as 1974 and who were presumably still alive in the late 1980s.

In 1987, the *New York Times* reported[46] on a happier side to the controversial hepatitis vaccine study group: 13 men "already infected with the AIDS virus had lived nine years without developing AIDS" and had "perfectly normal" immune systems.

That is, homosexuals provided the hepatitis B vaccine in 1978, and whose stored blood, on retrospect, had HIV antibodies, were alive and well nine years later.

As we have seen, a re-evaluation in 1989 of San Francisco gay men enrolled in the hepatitis B vaccine project and whose blood on retrospect had been found positive for HIV as early as 1978 showed that at least 20 percent had remained symptom-free going on 11 years.

This writer was in touch with one of the San Francisco patients, who had since moved elsewhere. His longtime battle with HIV and AIDS-related symptoms is related in the Prologue. By 1990 he was, at the least, a 12-year "survivor." He may have been infected in the mid-1970s.

In 1988, the Centers for Disease Control (CDC) reported[10] that at least 20 percent of people diagnosed with AIDS (apparently full-blown AIDS as by prior CDC definition) in 1985 were still alive -- and that from 3 to 8 percent of all cases diagnosed by 1983 were also still alive.

These figures would suggest that there are several hundred to several thousand long-term survivors of a syndrome which one major study suggested is fatal within one year for 50 percent of those afflicted.

Epidemiologist Ann Hardy reached the obvious conclusion: "AIDS may not be 100% fatal." She had been tracking a group of 45 men diagnosed with AIDS in 1983 or before through the CDC.

Another group of long-term survivors has been followed[11] by innovative physician Jay Levy at the University of California-San Francisco, one of the first establishment researchers to espouse the multifactoriality of HIV/AIDS and delineator of the "ARV" virus. One of his patients is a Kaposi's sarcoma (KS) case who by 1989 had been in remission since 1982. In 10 patients he has followed HIV virus can no longer be found in the blood, and some of these were 5-year survivors by 1989.

Writer Denise Grady in 1988[10] found KS patient Dan Turner (the Levy patient diagnosed in 1982), Elizabeth Ramos of Boston (recovered from PCP that had been diagnosed in 1985), and Michael Callen, New York, who learned he had AIDS in 1982.

Bernard Gavzer in 1988[47] found Steve Callahan, San Francisco (diagnosed in 1983), Cristofer Shihar, Los Angeles (KS in remission since 1984), Mark Fotopoulos, New York (diagnosed in 1985), Michael Leonard, New York (diagnosed in 1985), Gary Brown, Wichita (diagnosed in 1984 -- who shunned all orthodox medications entirely), Kenny Taub, New York (diagnosed in 1985), Ron Glenn, Atlanta (diagnosed in 1985), George Kish, Atlanta (recovered from various AIDS conditions, diagnosed first in 1982), and Tom O'Connor, a writer who was in good health in 1988, or 8 years following his diagnosis in 1980 with what would later be described as ARC.

These are individuals who chose to "go public." But there are now many other survivors beating the odds -- none considered "cured" in the fullest sense of the word, yet people who are ordinarily healthy, back at work or school even while "seropositive," and having been so for years.

The recovery of a physician from full-blown AIDS through fasting and diet under the care of an open-minded brother medic is movingly recorded in the 1987 book *Roger's Recovery From AIDS.*[50]   Scott Gregory has described the "unorthodox" and "eclectic" therapies followed by other long-term survivors.[50]

The patients referred to here, in the main, have two things in common aside from long-term survival: they have either combined orthodox medications with any number of "unorthodox" approaches, or they have abandoned orthodoxy altogether AND they have the unquantifiable element of "positive mental attitude," which increasing numbers of clinicians are coming to view as the single most important component of the holistic paradigm. (See Chapter Fifteen).

Barrie Cassileth *et al.,* found that up to 13 percent of hospitalized U.S. cancer patients use some from of "alternative" or" unapproved" therapy.[51] A 1989 survey by

Roger Hand, MD, at the University of Illinois-Chicago College of Medicine (18 of 50 AIDS patients using one or more alternative therapies vs. 2 of 30 cancer patients) suggested that "the use of alternative therapies may be much higher in patients with AIDS".[52]

This is a natural consequence of the realities: orthodox medicine has at least a minimal "cure" rate in cancer, if all sides agree on the meaning of the word "cure" -- it has *none* against AIDS. The only mystery here is that even *more* AIDS patients do not turn to "unorthodoxy."

All kinds of foreign research suggesting certain benefits in HIV/AIDS patients was snarled in the FDA's hoary machinery of old-boy networking with giant pharmaceutical companies and spin-off medical industries.

A growing number of new compounds or old drugs with new applications were not able to be applied in the U.S.A. because of the suffocating provisions of the Food, Drug and Cosmetic Act as amended in 1962 with the progress-thwarting "Kefauver amendments" regarding "efficacy."

Dextran sulfate, for two decades an essentially non-toxic drug used in Japan in arteriosclerosis, and reported in various countries as useful as an antiviral,[45] was blocked in the U.S.A. (as of this writing) for general use for lack of sufficient data.

The use of ozone gas, an oxidative agent, shown promising in European research as another essentially non-toxic use of a non-patentable natural thing, was regarded as illegitimate therapy.

(The ozone gas debacle is reflective of U.S. orthodoxy at its worst. Although work by various German researchers over several years had indicated the usefulness of ozone -- and, by implication, any agent capable of releasing nascent atomic oxygen -- against viruses in general let alone HIV in particular, it was not until Fall 1988 that U.S. researchers indicated interest in its further study. Preliminary findings at the Bethesda, MD, Naval Hospital and the Veterans Administration Medical Center in San Francisco had "suggested" that ozone "might be used to reduce symptoms in AIDS patients" as well as help cleanse donated blood. [44]

(That the U.S. would wait several years to give a modest nod to the use in an incurable, deadly disease of a natural gas which is essentially a form of non-toxic oxidative treatment when used appropriately was among many of the outrageous realities which sent "gay activists" into the streets demanding a change in American drug-approval policies.)

Even AL-721, a combination of fatty acids to be consumed much as one puts butter on a cracker and which counts as a food product, was left in legal limbo in the U.S.A. despite Israeli research indicating some usefulness of the combination as an antiviral and immune enhancer.

The controversial chelating agent EDTA (ethylene-diamine-tetraacetic acid), at the heart of an ongoing storm over efficacy in circulatory and heart conditions, and legally available for lead poisoning treatment, was "disallowed" for use against HIV/AIDS despite East German research strongly suggesting antiviral efficacy.[30]

HIV/AIDS sufferers, told by their medical/governmental establishment that they might have months to years to live with an incurable disease and that scientific progress required years of careful testing on rats, mice, rabbits and primates before the laborious process of utilizing humans could be attempted, were aghast: "If you have no cure, if we are going to die anyway, what possible reason can there be to keep us from anything with only a whisper of possible efficacy?"

This was the collective rhetorical question hurled at the FDA, AMA and the interlocking directorate of pharmaceutical giants and device-manufacturers that control American medicine.

Frustrated and angry, AIDS patients began developing "underground" pipelines for forbidden drugs ranging from Europe to Asia to Latin America, began concocting AL-721 "workalikes", began "networking" with underground newsletters, "guerrilla clinics," information centers, buyers' clubs, and procuring imported herbs, other plants and concoctions of every kind and variety.

By late 1988, the testing and bureaucratic logjam was beginning to break, if only a little. FDA Commissioner Frank Young, beset by an outraged, victimized minority more vocal and better organized than even the freedom-of-choice cancer patients battling over access to FDA-disapproved laetrile just a few years before, thrice loosened FDA restrictions as to the importation of foreign drugs, however "unapproved" in the U.S.A., and announced a cutback in red tape for the development of new AIDS drugs.

A "parallel track" had been set up by the FDA by 1989 to allow the "compassionate" use of experimental AIDS drugs while they were still under investigation.

The precedent had already been set, perhaps unintentionally, by the development of azidothymidine (AZT), but the fact that corners were cut on a "compassionate" basis to rush this synthetic, toxic drug onto the market at an estimated cost of up to $12,000 per patient per year (while other drugs much less expensive and of proven value were left twisting in the wind of bureaucratic limbo) hardly led the HIV/AIDS-stricken community into a burst of charitable feelings toward the government.

In the U.S., standard or orthodox physicians with foresight and courage are from time to time stepping out ahead of the crowd and are doing innovative things, even at some risk to their careers or persons.

The essentially 100 percent failure of allopathic medicine to stem the HIV/AIDS tide began leading a number of conscientious physicians into a consideration of at least parts of the holistic paradigm, particularly those having to do with diet and supplements.

One of the earlier approaches to HIV/AIDS which earned the wrath of the American medical establishment was -- and is -- the use of Vitamin C, already at the forefront of major controversies concerning cancer and other diseases.

California orthopedic surgeon Robert Cathcart has been the doctor of several of California's long-term HIV/AIDS survivors. His major therapies: enormous oral and intravenous doses of ascorbate or ascorbic acid (Vitamin C) and special diets. It was his patient, Stuart Anderson, who at one point had reached the incredible oral level of 120 grams daily of the vitamin.

Cathcart reached national attention in 1985 with his Vitamin C/dietary approach.

The Anderson case highlighted the growing caseload of AIDS patients treated by Dr. Cathcart[19], almost to the point of Vitamin C's being considered a "cure" of the disease.

He already had noted since 1983[20,21] that "preliminary clinical evidence is that large doses of ascorbate (50-200 grams per 24 hours) can suppress the symptoms of the disease and can markedly reduce the tendency for secondary infections." He found clinical remission even while laboratory evidence of helper T-cell suppression continued.

But by 1986, as Dr. Cathcart told me in the first of two interviews, he had seen mildly depressed T4:T8 ratios restored to normal in two ARC patients.

"Vitamin C in tremendous doses is extremely effective in *Pneumocystis carinii*," he said. "It knocks down the patients' malaise and prevents problems of allergic reactions to drugs. It is also effective against Kaposi lesions. Enormous doses seem to affect the lesions, reduce their numbers and reverse them in some cases."

It is necessary to maintain the daily discipline of taking megadoses of Vitamin C. In one case, Dr. Cathcart said, he had provided 7.5 *lbs.* of Vitamin C in oral and intravenous form over a 14-day period to a single patient. Symptoms subsided yet they returned after the heavy ascorbate administration was withdrawn.

Dr. Cathcart, who by 1988 had seen about 250 HIV/AIDS patients in more than five years' experience utilizing Vitamin C with the syndrome, believes the vitamin's best use is in early ARC (let alone prevention). He has seen several long-term patients reaching four-year survivals.

The California physician emphasized that an "anti-yeast" diet including acidophilus, garlic, horseradish, etc., is almost as important as Vitamin C therapy. The yeast problem, he noted, is the "number-one killer" in many AIDS patients.

Dr. Cathcart is also a fervent believer in the necessity of marshaling a strong positive attitude. "We've got to shut down the oxidative catecholamines," he avers -- a reference to substances associated with depressed mental states.

In our second interview (1988), Dr. Cathcart was as frustrated and exasperated at medical orthodoxy and the politics of the "gay community" as he was steadfast in his advocacy of Vitamin C and diet. He was quite candid: "Of these 250 patients the bottom line is that most are dead, but I have some 4- and 5-year survivors, people who will continue to do well as long as they behave themselves."

He had administered up to 300 grams of Vitamin C over 24 hours, finding that not only HIV/AIDS patients responded, but also sufferers of Epstein-Barr Virus (EBV), *Candida albicans* yeast infection (both often prime players in HIV/AIDS), chronic fatigue syndrome and teenage mononucleosis did well on the program. He had never seen the blood of an HIV/AIDS patient turn seronegative or a complete restoration of immune panels.

Like many a maverick doctor in the HIV/AIDS era, he had doubts both about the meaning of the immune panels and the nature of HIV, yet he has seen people remain completely healthy with altered immunity and HIV seropositivity as long as they adhere to his program.

"I'm convinced HIV is not the Lone Ranger, that something else has to trigger it off. Something makes the immune system just go to pieces," he said.

He also found that megadoses of Vitamin C could help offset the side effects of the drugs used in PC pneumonia.

In AIDS cases, "the right diet and Vitamin C can double life expectancy," he said. "I never claimed a cure."

In an interview in early 1985, the operator of an allergy-testing laboratory in Vienna, VA., claimed to have seen one year's AIDS remissions in 18 of 19 male volunteers through administrations of vitamin megadoses (particularly Vitamin C), minerals and stress-reduction techniques.

Dr. Russell M. Jaffe was quoted[23] as saying that "as far as we know, we have the first systematic data that shows we can improve immune function" in AIDS patients, with T-cell ratios climbing in all cases after starting at below 0.2. He was waiting for publication in medical journals before commenting further on what appeared to be a promising lead, he told me. He published his own expanded protocols in 1987.[24]

The Jaffe approach, and that of others, points to the need to enhance the body's natural immune system to ward off infections rather than simply to inhibit viruses, even though the anti-viral, anti-free radical activity of Vitamin C and other natural substances has been demonstrated.[27]

Dr. Jaffe's overview of HIV/AIDS therapy is that AIDS is simply the most recent in a spate of autoimmune syndromes, the early diagnoses of which are usually lacking. He recommends a number of positive-thought tech-

212

niques and treatment with Vitamin C, fatty acids, AL-721, D-penicillamine, monolaurin, Naltrexone, herbs, sauna, nutrients and various "anti-cortisol/ anti-estrogen" strategies, plus lithium, DMSO, BHT, glucose, insulin, potassium and zinc.

Peter R. Rothschild, MD, Ph.D., and others have shown an immune-modulating effect for antioxidant enzymes, an activity which might be of greater biological significance than their free radical-fighting capabilities.[53]

However, the utilization of vitamins, minerals, enzymes and other natural substances runs afoul not only of standard allopathic medical thought in the U.S.A., but frequently involves its proponents in administrative and statutory proceedings within the United States.

Even so, several U.S. practitioners have suggested metabolic/nutritional modalities for AIDS treatment.

DaPrato and J. Rothschild, viewing AIDS as "the final expression of a maladaptive, unremitting stress response secondary to polymicrobial enteric infections, malabsorption, nutrient deficiencies and subsequent colonization by the AIDS virus" exacerbated by drugs, seminal plasma and "the institutionalized fostering of a death expectation," suggested[25,40] a treatment program based on nutritional supplementation and the use of immunologic adjuvants and "stress hormone antagonists" together with treatment for parasites and viruses. Zinc and Vitamin C were among substances suggested.

In the area of cortisol antagonists, Dr. Orm Bergold, working in Costa Rica and West Germany, implemented experimentally a treatment model involving various aspects of metabolic therapy and natural substances to reduce cortisol levels, holding that cortisol is the "co-factor" in HIV/AIDS development. He observed great successes at early HIV/AIDS levels, claiming in some cases to have seen patients "turn negative" for HIV. [41,42]

Stephen G. Marcus, who pointed to prostaglandin E1 synthesis interruption as being responsible for AIDS, as noted in earlier chapters, proposed[26] a treatment including administration of gamma-linolenic acid (GLA), pyridoxine, niacin, Vitamin C, L-lysine, zinc, eicosapentaenoic acid and anti-oxidants (including Vitamins A,C,E, pantothenic acid, para-aminobenzoic acid, inositol, selenium, glutathione, cysteine and methionine.)

Such forward-thinking holistic and eclectic physicians as Laurence Badgley, MD,[28] in California and Leon Chaitow, ND, in Great Britain[29] have proposed and implemented to the extent possible broad-spectrum multifactorial programs based on natural therapies, nutrients and positive thought.

In Fall 1988, reporting on a six-month followup of 38 HIV/AIDS patients treated with as extensive a metabolic program as could be managed in the U.S.A., Dr. Badgley found[39] that 83 percent had experienced overall health improvements, average T4 helper cell increases were 13 percent, two persons developed KS lesions, one throat cancer, none developed PC pneumonia.

In addition to average daily supplements of Vitamins A,C,E and most of the Vitamin B complex, plus iron, zinc, selenium, germanium, Coenzyme Q10, 25 percent used garlic, 36 percent used the herb echinacea, 82 percent used acupuncture, 81 percent used homeopathic remedies, 56 percent in general used herbs and mushrooms, 72 percent physically exercised -- and 72 percent meditated 4.2 hours per week. Significantly, too, 85 percent said their orthodox doctors supported their nutritional programs.

The John Bastyr College of Naturopathic Medicine, one of two in the U.S. to be granted official accreditation, developed a limited metabolic treatment program in February 1986 for HIV/AIDS patients. Reporting in Fall 1988[31] on 15 patients, including cases of shingles, thrush, bronchitis and pharyngitis in five patients, four of the 15 showed decreased lymphadenopathy, and virtually all reported subjective feelings of feeling better, happier, more energetic and more hopeful.

In New York, consistently embattled nonagenarian Emanuel Revici, MD, a Rumanian-born physician and research scientist who has devoted much of his life to the riddle of cancer, was reporting impressive improvements in immune systems of HIV/AIDS patients with his "guided lipid" therapy and diet.[34]

Dr. Revici, who has proposed a metabolic model of health and disease built around a foundation of cosmic dualism, anabolic-catabolic forces and the utilization of fatty acids by the body, has used lipids in combination with minerals in the non-toxic management of the HIV/AIDS infection curve.[34,35]

Also in New York, a limited "alternative" program utilizing acupuncture, special diet and other natural methods was said by 1988 to have slowed down symptoms or disease progression in 60 percent of 200 patients (mostly ARC level) at Lincoln Hospital since 1984.[48]

In Massachusetts, nutritional consultant Ann Wigmore, long an exponent of good health through proper diet, came under attack[36] by state officials for promoting "live" foods, "energy soup" and eating plans as useful in rebuilding immune systems in HIV/AIDS patients. A magistrate did not agree with health officials who sought to punish her for advocating medicinal uses of food since, he argued, in the absence of any known cure by orthodoxy, how could she be guilty of leading anyone astray from "recognized therapy" by insisting on a vegetarian diet?[37]

Virtually all doctors who, publicly or privately, are attempting new treatment models for a many-faceted disease are reporting considerable increases in longevity, decline in clinical symptoms, and overall improvements both mentally and physically. Broad-minded, allopathically educated physicians, mindful of the first injunction of the Hippocratic Oath ("first, do no harm") and having seen dozens of their patients die under standard or orthodox approaches, are increasingly open-minded.

Dr. Robert Brooks, who by August of 1987 had treated some 300 HIV/AIDS cases in Los Angeles, combined some "alternative" practices with traditional Western approaches. He was quoted as saying: "We hear a lot about vitamins and supplements. I have patients bring in what they want and take a look at some of the things to make sure they're doing nothing harmful. And some go to a nutritionist."[38]

The physical aspects of the holistic paradigm are usually those which are described by the Europeans as "biological" medicine and by the Americans as "metabolic" therapy. They include a broad spectrum of nutrients which standard or allopathic physicians, while not agreeing as to their importance, might accept into a treatment design, or protocol: for example, Vitamins A and C for their various suggested capabilities as enhancers of immune function and possible nonspecific antiviral effects.

They might accept Vitamin E along with these as antioxidants (destroyers of free radicals, or toxic oxygen

215

by-products) and for wound-healing and possibly chelating (the making soluble of heavy minerals and metals) properties. Both sides would agree that zinc has a number of essential properties, that it may be an immune booster, along with selenium.

They might agree on the need for a patient to consume fewer refined carbohydrates and animal proteins and ingest more natural fruits and vegetables.

They might also agree on the need for exercise. Anywhere beyond that, however, any divergences would be extremely sharp, and any reliance on any of these metabolic or biological features in lieu of toxic synthetic drugs and antibiotics would essentially be regarded as quackery.

The more committed metabolic physicians would see the necessity of specific fatty acids as possible immune system modulators and antiviral agents, and would accord certain amino acids, certainly L-cysteine and L-methionine, as well as antioxidant enzymes, immune enhancement status.

Metabolic physicians would see in Vitamin B6 and folic acid non-specific immune modulators, and would liberally use a wide range of oral enzymes for protein-digesting and antioxidant properties.

They would use many food factors and herbs for immune modulation, antiviral properties, detoxification, energy building. Some of them would use cortisol antagonists and hormone balancers.

Most of them would use any or all of these substances in lieu of toxic drugs, antibiotics, steroids, synthetic hormones and radiation -- all these latter being harmful to the human body even though they might have short-term relevance against specific bacteria, viruses and fungi.

For, in the holistic paradigm, the therapeutic effort is primarily aimed first at building up the sum total of all aspects of body health (immunity, or the various factors which go into the immune system; endocrine balance; nutrient balance) to promote what may generally be called *host resistance*, the "terrain" of the body.

For the holistic, metabolic, biological or even eclectic practitioner, the general health of the host is of greater overall importance than knowledge of which pathogenic microbes are present to do harm.

Detoxifying the body, with everything from herbal teas to coffee enemas and "high colonics", is seen as essential to any such program, for so much of ill health simply seems to begin with putrefaction and decay, not only of the lengthy, serpentine gastrointestinal tract but of other organs and tissues as well. Removing toxins from the body through diet, enemas, sweats, saunas, exercise is a natural part of a total program.

Exercising properly, sleeping well, forcing the body to take in and utilize oxygen and natural sugar (not sucrose), are vital to the program. In time, the control of diet and eating habits become the central features of a biological program: making certain the body has enough natural, necessary nutrients in proper amounts is held to be the beginning of good physical health and the key to its maintenance.

Combining the holistic paradigm with eclecticism -- using methods from "orthodoxy" as well as the "alternatives" -- was the hallmark of the HIV/AIDS treatment program followed by the Bradford Research Institute-Mexico, which reported in 1988 its considerable success in 66 patients seen since 1983. (See Chapter Sixteen).

To the eclecticist, even though the primary goal of therapy is enhancing overall host defense, the current status of viral, bacterial and fungal infection cannot be overlooked.

As our medical group learned years ago in dealing with terminal cancer, it is well and good to allow time to pass while a total metabolic program of vitamins, minerals, enzymes, amino acids and hormone balancing can begin to take over; it is quite another thing to utilize a "heroic" measure -- be it a toxic drug, a blast of radiation, a surgical procedure -- in order to save a life which has only hours to days of probable survival.

In the physical saving of a life, an eclecticist will not disavow any life-saving modality, even if the means utilized to save a life can mean a metabolic problem later on.

Resurgent homeopathy, representing a medical school of thought which was once paramount even in the United States, may play a certain role in HIV/AIDS. It is the use of minute dilutions, usually of herbal or mineral origins, to apply "the law of similars" and look for "the essence of the medicine" as applied to HIV/AIDS.

Since homeopathy is basically the utilization of such dilutions in precise symptom-matching, the multiplicity of

217

HIV/AIDS infections thus presents both a considerable challenge to, and opportunity for, homeopathic remedies, and some of the long-term survivors have blended the use of homeopathics with their other programs.

In 1989, a Greek homeopathic organization reported the normalizing of blood profiles and symptoms in 12 HIV/AIDS patients treated with homeopathics alone.[55] All were still HIV antibody-positive.

In the holistic and eclectic paradigms there is room for chiropractic manipulation, massage, acupressure, and acupuncture from Oriental concepts of energy flow, pain control and the holistic oneness of the body. There is room for yoga, meditation, biofeedback, self-hypnosis.

The great majority of these things is now far removed from the allopathic model because they represent individualized, personalized, ever-changing protocols, mixtures of therapies and approaches not susceptible to "controlled, randomized, double-blind" studies in animals and man, the hallmark of Western medical research.

Their lack of perfect predictability or reproducibility from one person to another let alone one group to another means that they are not "scientific" or even "responsible," as this era's major spokesmen for the allopathic industrial complex like to say.

The armamentarium of the physical part of the holistic treatment approach is vast (see Appendix III).

But so intense has the examination of surviving patients from a great number of terminal diseases been that both the "orthodox" and "unorthodox" medical communities have unavoidably had to examine the awesomely important yet unmeasurable aspects of mind and attitude.[16]

And HIV/AIDS has provided the unexpectedly perfect model for just such considerations.

REFERENCES

(1)   Cole, Helen, "AIDS associated disorders pose complex therapeutic challenges." J. Am. Med. Assn. 252: 15, 1987-1988, Oct. 19, 1984.

(2)   Zagury, Daniel, et al., "Repairing the T-cell defect in AIDS." Lancet, August 24, 1985.

(3)   Poulsen, Asmus, et al., "Regression of Kaposi's sarcoma in AIDS after treatment with Dapsone." Lancet, March 10, 1984.

(4)   "Foscarnet," Lancet, Sept. 21, 1985.

(5)   Sandstrom, Eric G., et al., "Inhibition of human T-cell lymphotropic virus type III in vitro by phosphonoformate." Lancet, June 29, 1985.

(6)   Hruza, George, et al., "Dapsone for AIDS-associated Kaposi's sarcoma." Lancet, March 16, 1985.

(7)   Scott, J., and Lynn Simross, "AIDS: underground options -- the search for hope." Los Angeles Times, Aug. 16, 1987.

(8)   "Possible AIDS drug OK'd to treat another disease." Associated Press, in San Francisco Examiner, Jan. 2, 1986.

(9)   "AIDS drug closer to use in U.S." Associated Press, in San Francisco Examiner, Dec. 18, 1985.

(10)   Grady, Denise, "AIDS survivors," American Health, September 1988.

(11)   Krieger, L.M., "Battling AIDS: a report from the front lines," San Francisco Examiner, May 21, 1987.

(12)   "AIDS drug fails to save a 3rd patient." United Press, in San Francisco Chronicle, Nov. 13, 1985.

(13)   Cimons, Marlene, "FDA chief warns of false hope on AIDS drugs." Los Angeles Times, July 14, 1988.

(14)   Berner, Y., et al., "Attempted treatment of acquired immunodeficiency syndrome (AIDS) with thymic humoral factor." Israel J. Med. Sci., 20: 1195-1196, Dec. 1984.

(15)   Levy, Elinor M., et al., "Patients with Kaposi's sarcoma who opt for no treatment." Lancet, July 27, 1985.

(16)   Solomon, G., "The emerging field of psychoneuroimmunology with a special note on AIDS." Advances 2: 6-19, 1984.

(17)   Simross, Lynn, "AIDS victim runs to beat the odds." Los Angeles Times, Nov. 14, 1985.

(18)   Private communication.

(19)   Null, Gary, "Medical genocide; part four: the AIDS coverup," Penthouse, December 1985.

(20)   Cathcart, Robert F., "Vitamin C in the treatment of acquired immune deficiency syndrome (AIDS)." Medical Hypotheses 14: 423-433, 1984.

(21)   Cathcart, Robert F., "Vitamin C function in AIDS." Medical Tribune, July 13, 1983.

(22)   Mansell, P., et al., "The use of isoprinosine in an attempt to improve immune function in AIDS and AIDS related complex." Proc. ASCO, vol. 4, March 1985.

(23)   Harris, Richard F., "AIDS work uses stress therapy, vitamins." San Francisco Chronicle/Examiner, Jan. 1985.

(24)   Jaffe, Russell, "Prospects for immune reconstitution. "Privately Published, 1987.

(25)   DaPrato, Robert A., and Jonathan Rothschild, "The AIDS virus as an opportunistic infection: therapeutic implications." Privately published,

219

1985.

(26) Marcus, Stephen G., "Breakdown of PGE1 synthesis is responsible for the acquired immunodeficiency syndrome." Medical Hypotheses L15: 39-46, 1984.

(27) Dahl, Helen, and Miklos Degre, "The effect of ascorbic acid production of human interferon and the antiviral activity in vitro." Acta Path. Microbiol. Scand. Sect. B., 84:280-284, 1976.

(28) Badgley, Laurence, Healing Aids Naturally. San Bruno CA: Human Energy Press, 1986.

(29) Chaitow, Leon, and Simon Martin, A World without AIDS. Great Britain: Thorsons Publishers Ltd, 1988.

(30) Wunderlich, V., and G. Sydow, "Disintegration of retroviruses by chelating agents." Arch. Virol., 73: 171-183, 1982.

(31) Standish, L. J., "Evaluating natural therapeutic treatment of AIDS and ARC." Townsend Letter for Doctors, October 1988.

(32) Hicks, Donald R., et al., "Inactivation of HTL-III/LAV infected cultures of normal human lymphocytes by nonoxynol-9 in vitro." Lancet, Dec. 21/28, 1985.

(33) Pompidou, Alain, et al., "In-vitro inhibition of LAV/HTLV-III infected lymphocytes by Dithiocarb and inosine pranobex." Lancet, Dec. 21/28, 1985.

(34) Revici, E., "Research and theoretical background for treatment of the acquired immunodeficiency syndrome (AIDS)", Townsend Letter for Doctors, March 1987.

(35) Culbert, M.L., "Emanuel Revici: the dualistic, anabolic-catabolic world of a 91-year-old genius." The Choice, Fall 1987.

(36) Wigmore, Ann, Overcoming AIDS and other Incurable Diseases the Attunitive Way through Nature. Boston MA: Wigmore Foundation, 1986.

(37) "Ann Wigmore digs in." The Choice, Fall 1988.

(38) Simross, Lynn, "The doctors: they're not saying 'no' to alternative remedies." Los Angeles Times, August 16, 1987.

(39) Badgley, L. E., "Natural therapies for AIDS." Townsend Letter for Doctors, October 1988.

(40) DaPrato, R. A., and J. Rothschild, "The AIDS virus as an opportunistic organism inducing a state of chronic relative cortisol excess." Med. Hypoth., November 1986.

(41) Bergold, Orm, "Stress, cortisol and 'stress diseases.'" Privately published, 1987.

(42) Personal communication, 1988.

(43) Grady, D., loc. cit.

(44) "Studies say ozone may combat AIDS." (Associated Press) San Diego Union, Oct. 27, 1988.

(45) Mitsuya, H., et al., "Dextran sulfate suppression of viruses in the HIV

family: inhibition of virion binding to CD4 cells." Science, 240, April 1988.

(46)   Altman, Lawrence, "AIDS mystery: why do some infected men stay healthy?" New York Times, June 30, 1987.

(47)   Gavzer, Bernard, "Why do some people survive AIDS?" Parade, Sept. 18, 1988.

(48)   "Nuevo tratamiento contra el SIDA." Vitalidad (Madrid, Spain), May 1988.

(49)   Owen, Bob, Roger's Recovery from AIDS. Malibu CA: DAVAR, 1989.

(50)   Gregory, Scott, and Bianca Leonardo, They Conquered AIDS! Palm Spring CA: Tree of Life, 1989.

(51)   Cassileth, B.R., et al., "Contemporary unorthodox treatments in cancer medicine: a study of patients, treatments and practitioners." Ann. Intern. Med. 101:105 - 12, 1984.

(52)   Hand, Roger, "Alternative therapies used by patients with AIDS." New Eng. J. Med., March 9, 1989.

(53)   Rothschild, Peter R., The Biochemical Relations Between Stress, Mind and Immune System. Honolulu, HI: University Labs Press, 1988.

(54)   Monte, Tom, The Way of Hope. New York: Warner Books, 1989.

(55)   The Choice, Fall-Winter, 1989.

Chapter Fourteen

THE BIOELECTRICAL CONNECTION

Homeopathy, while 200 years old and firmly established as a "Western" school of medicine (though denounced as "crackpot" by American spokesmen for the rapacious synthetic drug industry), is having a vast resurgence of interest in the U.S.A., where at one time it was a recognized school of medical thought. It was, in fact, the primary opponent of "allopathy", which became the monopoly form of medicine and virtually all medical thought in the U.S.A.

Strangely enough, this older form of medicine provides a leap into the possible medicine of the future -- primarily because homeopathy in a certain way may be a bridge between biology and quantum mechanics.

Placed into a modern format, homeopathy, Samuel Hahnemann's science wrapped around "the law of similars," is an effort to treat symptoms of disease with minute dilutions of natural substances which, if given to a healthy person, would actually cause symptoms of the same disease or condition.

This concept is so alien to the allopathic notion and indeed sufficiently hard to grasp at the area of pure logic that it may be dismissed with a laugh.

That is, if it did not have an honorable pedigree. Homeopathy has been known to help cure whole epidemics of infection quite aside from a wide variety of personal human ills. It is a legitimate school of medical thought in many countries, and particularly revered as an accepted medical approach by the British royal family.

"Non-invasive", "non-toxic", the use of homeopathy as a benign medicine which in the 19th century was favored by the upper classes in many countries, was anathema to surgeons and toxic mineral peddlers and later the drug dispensing allopaths. It collided with Solidist "rationalism" in medicine and, in the U.S.A., was almost entirely devastated by the advent of synthetic drugs.

The basic physical tenet of homeopathy, in crude terms, is that by diluting down a substance one eventually will arrive at its "essence" or "nature" -- its *vis medicatrix naturae.* For many decades this was interesting theory, but not demonstrated fact except that so many people seemed cured or healed by homeopathic tinctures. How does one capture an "essence" or a "nature", particularly in the microscope? The answer was always: one doesn't.

In the present century, various experiments have been mounted by the allopathic orthodoxy to discredit homeopathy, primarily by demonstrating that the minute dilutions of substances that are claimed by homeopaths to be effective are so insignificant that they cannot even be recovered in a test tube or seen by a microscope. If there is not enough of the substance to be seen or measured, then surely it does not exist.

But homeopathy opens the door to new meanings of the word "exist" -- very possibly homeopathy is dealing with *pure energy*, something above and beyond, or through and around, the third dimensionally perceptible.

The speculation that homeopathic elements may indeed be elements of energy rather than third-dimensional objects is at the heart of one of the more recent controversies within the annals of Western medicine:

In 1988, French researcher Jacques Benveniste and 11 colleagues in research labs in France, Italy, Israel and Canada demonstrated that an antibody solution so dilute that not a single molecule of the substance could be present seemed to alter the chemistry and internal structure of white blood cells.

While this immunological experiment was not strictly undertaken as a homeopathic one, the American medical monopolists quickly read into it a genuine threat, particularly since it was published in a prestigious British journal *(Nature)* which saw fit to add an editorial disclaimer.

Perhaps the American response was triggered by a *Washington Post* assessment of the experiments: "If taken at face value, the research shows that the immune system's antibodies can work even when the solution they are in is so diluted that no antibody molecules are left in it. There is no known physical basis for such action. It would mean there is some bizarre way that the solution could 'remember' the presence of the antibody molecules and act as if they were still there."[2]

In an extraordinary move, medical orthodoxy dispatched a team of scientists and, oddly enough, a professional magician (usually a star performer at "quack-buster" meetings) to attempt to disprove what Benveniste and associates had reported.

The Americans spent a week going over lab notes and the results of many experiments which had been carefully conducted by the research group and attempted to dismiss this considerable amount of work by claiming it was "filled with inaccuracies and distortions." The French team stood by the results.

But while homeopathy is rising in popularity once again, with New Age thinkers and researchers finding much of merit in Hahnemann's approach, there is also a renewal of interest, if on a lesser scale, in the very field to which homeopathy may ultimately be pointing:

Bioelectrical therapy -- the use of electricity and/or irradiation and/or "directed energy" in the treatment and prevention of disease. Intimately bound up in this renewal of interest are new techniques of microscopy and fresh interest in lines of research attacked, and sometimes attacked viciously, by the orthodox scientific establishments of the Western world, primarily those of the U.S.A. and France.

The bridge between homeopathy and electromagnetics is evident in the combination approach by Dr. Victor Bortot in South Africa: MORA, defined as an electromagnetic system which allows the measurement of precise frequencies and hence enhances homeopathic diagnosis, is coupled with homeopathic treatments and herbal detoxification.

Bortot has claimed the successful treatment of HIV/AIDS, though up to now the evidence is anecdotal and it is not clear what successful treatment really means, particularly if HIV is only a co-factor anyway. German physicist Wolfgang Ludwig developed MORA, a system of treatment/ diagnosis said to involve interactions with one's own "electromagnetic resonances."[12,13,14]

The use of electromagnetic fields, electricity, bioelectricity, and magnetism is a composite new field drawing on both old-time remedies and high-tech science.

These approaches range from certain old-fashioned folk-medicine uses of magnets as curative treatments to the quirky, bizarre, and difficult-to-delineate claims made by the promoters of radionics ("directed energy," or both diagnosing and healing at a distance through the medium of an observer, a machine, a photograph or some representation of the target) in Europe and the U.S.A.

These have been paralleled by a great resurgence of interest in the work and theories of Croatian-born American genius Nikola Tesla, the turn-of-the-century inventor who is best known in the electrical orthodoxy as the developer of the alternating current motor and the high-frequency coil. Tesla was after nothing less than "wireless transmission of energy at a distance with no losses."

Modern reviewers of Tesla's work and theories vacillate between calling him a madman and a genius, and by the middle of this century most of his efforts had been ignored or forgotten -- or, as Teslaites might claim, stamped out by the energy monopolies which perceived a threat in Tesla's ideas.[3]

In the current era, both in Europe and the U.S.A., several promoters utilizing "oscillating waves" and "bioelectricity" are variously claiming to be able to measure the electromagnetic fields of everything from the body itself to its minutest cell, and also claim they can interfere with these fields in such a way as to promote healing. While the ideas may have some modern names and champions they are also echoes of the not-too-distant past:

-- Wilhelm Reich, scientist and mystic, earlier in this century claimed an understanding of energy at variance with theories of the day and the discovery of "bions", minute particles of energy. Reich developed the concept of "orgone energy" and believed he had described the authentic relationship between physiological and mental disturbances.

-- Royal R. Rife, a San Diego scientist, claimed both microscopic advances so refined that live viruses could actually be seen with the "Rife microscope", and the ability to cure terminally ill cancer patients with a "ray tube" tuned to specific electronic frequencies which allegedly killed what he, and later others, believed to be the "cancer virus."

-- Antoine Priore, an Italian-born electrical genius, in the 1950s and 1960s demonstrated in France that he could overcome cancer with the "Priore ray" which allegedly altered magnetic fields.

The history of the harassment and persecution of Reich, Rife and Priore as well as the attacks on Tesla's theories is a lengthy, sad, and at times disgusting litany of jealousy, perverted science and vested interests.

If Reich, Rife and Priore in general may have something in common besides a threat to vested interests, it would seem to be their demonstration of the real nature of all matter: that this nature may be understood in electromagnetic terms, that all energy is, or comes from, electromagnetism, that both disease induction and healing may be derived from such an understanding.

At the extreme end the implications are obvious: if everything is energy and each individual can learn to manipulate energy then there is suddenly an answer to problems of both energy in general and medicine in particular. Were even a figment of this true, then enormous industrial cartels would come acropper.

But while Reich, Rife and Priore have been consigned to history's museum of interesting relics by the "rationalists", interest in the electromagnetic field and how it relates to health and healing keeps growing and flourishing.

Radionics, for example, is a legal treatment for disease in England, France and Germany if neither well understood nor widely accepted. "Oscillating wave" generators have made their appearance in the U.S.A. with underground claims of cures of everything from cancer to HIV/AIDS, and so far not even the FDA has been particularly vigorous in suppressing the unwanted information.

Various people claim to have either the Rife microscope, the "Rife instrument" or parts thereof. Others have other devices and machines which, they say, can cure everything by electrical and/or electromagnetic interference.

By 1990, several U.S. HIV/AIDS patients were claiming some efficacy from small, lightweight "frequency machines" allegedly based on Rife's work.

Along similar lines, there is renewed interest in the work of physiologist E.K. Knott, the probable father of ultraviolet irradiation of blood. In his splendid tome on a "trizoid" look at the medical monolith, physician and cancer researcher Raymond K. Brown noted[4] that Knott's UV approach, beginning in the 1920s, was demonstrated to be useful against viral and bacterial infections and inflammatory processes.

Wrote Brown: "For approximately twenty-five years,

observations and results from several thousand patients were summarized and presented at medical meetings and in major medical journals; blood irradiation as a part of medical practice gradually died out when antibiotics and other products of modern technology appeared. Despite the formation of the Foundation for Irradiation, established by patients whose lives had been saved by the process and the physicians who had used it, irradiation of blood completely faded from the medical scene by the 1970s. At this time, the FDA was given the power to control all medical equipment and devices, so the possibility of a revival of blood irradiation in this country dissolved."

On both a terrifying and scientifically absorbing scale, Army Lt. Col. T.E. Bearden (Ret.), a nuclear scientist, claimed in 1988,[5,6] as we have seen, that AIDS, aside from the manmade viral connection thereto, was actually "beamed into" the U.S.A. through time-reversed "phase conjugate" weapons by the U.S.S.R., that the Soviets have greatly increased knowledge of and developments in "scalar electromagnetic" weapons. As horrifying as his extensive research into this area is, it also points to a projected cure of HIV/AIDS through bioelectrical means.

Bearden also relayed the hidden history of competing theories of energy and the nature of matter, stretching back to the 19th century, and indicated that many useful approaches and theories were simply left unresolved or were squelched by establishment science.

(He is not the only scientist associated directly or indirectly with the space program who has made contributions to a deeper understanding of energy and matter. In 1968, Adrian V. Clark, a researcher associated with the Saturn V Moon Vehicle project of the National Aeronautics and Space Administration (NASA), adduced[7] that the ultimate capability of man may be the controlling of matter through thought energy ["intellectual control of molecular motion."] Like Bearden, he was enamored of the suggestions of new understandings of energy and existence posed by the unidentified flying object (UFO) phenomena as well as by scientific clues in the Bible as to the nature of energy and the universe.

(Bearden, Clark and others are modern-age thinkers with credible backgrounds who have seen energy and nature-of-all-matter concepts from angles at variance with the scientific orthodoxy of our day. Cosmological concepts in general and quantum mechanics in particular are conceptually racing well ahead of Western rationalist science and have opened new vistas as to what may be the very nature of existence.)

At this juncture, the writer has to point out that up to now he has seen no evidence of any cure of any cancer patient, let alone any cure of any AIDS patient, by bioelectrical or magnetic means. But the potentials are clearly there. The fact I have not seen any of these cures does not mean there haven't been any. The work of Rife, in particular, has considerable backup by witnesses and patients.[8,9]

His experience in coming up with a "cancer virus" decades before any such virus was ever demonstrated, a high-resolution microscope that allegedly could "see" viruses, and an energy approach to killing cancer, met with the grossest kind of suppression by U.S. authorities -- who were just as assiduous at attempting to bury any form of cancer therapy developed outside the "old boy network" of pharmaceutical firms and established orthodoxy (the protean struggles of Hoxsey, Krebiozen, Glyoxylide, Coley's toxins, Lincoln bacteriophages, laetrile, etc., all come to mind.)

In Mexico, our research group began using "accelerated charge neutralization" (ACN) in the destruction or partial reduction of tumors and in benign hyperplasias (as well as pain, in some instances) in 1987. Some of the work along this line had been suggested both by Sweden's Bjorn Nordenstrom, a radiologist, and by the Bradford Research Institute's founder, Robert Bradford, by training an electronics engineer.

Bradford had already determined that cancer cells carry a negative electric charge, an element which confers avoidance of immune surveillance. If the negative charge could be replaced by a positive one, then the immune elements -- providing they were essentially intact -- would be drawn to the area and could attack the cancer. Nordenstrom had demonstrated that by adjusting electric frequencies he could destroy or significantly alter tumors. The B.R.I. work, which led to the development of ACN machines, confirmed and expanded on this approach.

Nordenstrom[10] and others have essentially

described the human body as a closed electrical circuit. To such theorists the body may be seen virtually as wiring and conductors. There is, as one researcher calls it, truly a "body electric."[11] Everything that goes on within this electrical body consists of minute exchanges of energy -- bioelectricity, in a word.

Folk-medicine practitioners who use magnets to cure headaches and many other conditions are in their way practicing a form of energy manipulation which exploits electromagnetic fields.

If the body is perceived electrically, then elements of ancient Chinese and Indian medicine, with their emphasis on energy points and energy flows, become palpable and understandable in modern semantics. For ancient medicine and some modern thinkers, all disease (or dis-ease) is a disturbance in energy fields.

Healing consists of righting these fields. The correcting of energy fields may be approached through everything from touch, massage and spinal manipulation to the appropriate nutrients, given as actual doses of food factors or as microdoses (homeopathy). The therapeutic uses of sound, light, color -- all expressions of energy, or waves of energy -- become logical and even feasible, as does "energized crystal therapy."

Just as cancer has provided the opportunity for earlier evidence of cure or healing through "rays" and directed energy, the devastating HIV/AIDS infection curve may do so in an even more dramatic way in the current era. HIV/AIDS may become a model for the "intellectual control of molecular motion" -- mind as healer.

REFERENCES

(1)   Coulter, Harris L. Divided Legacy: the Conflict between Homeopathy and the American Medical Association. Richmond CA: North Atlantic Books, 1982.

(2)   Quoted in "Lab tests' 'homeopathic' result stuns the monopoly." The Choice, 14:3, Fall 1988.

(3)   Lawren, Bill, "Rediscovering Tesla." Omni magazine, March 1988.

(4)   Brown, Raymond K., AIDS, Cancer and the Medical Establishment. New York: Speller, 1986.

(5)   Bearden, T.E. AIDS, Biological Warfare. Book in Press, 1988.

(6)   Bearden, T.E., "Soviet phase conjugate weapons (weapons that use time-reversed electromagnetic waves.)" Bulletin of the Committee to Restore the Constitution, January 1988.

(7)   Clark, Adrian V., Cosmic Mysteries of the Universe. West Nyack, N.Y.: Parker, 1968.

(8)   Lynes, Barry, with John Crane, The Cancer Cure that Worked: Fifty Years of Suppression. Marcus Books, Canada, 1987.

(9)   "San Diegan's cancer work may make cure possible." San Diego Union, July 31, 1949.

(10)   Nordenstrom, B. E.W., Biologically Closed Electrical Circuits. Stockholm: Nordic Publishers, 1983.

(11)   Becker, R., and G. Selden, The Body Electric. New York: Morrow, 1985.

(12)   Chaitow, Leon, and Simon Martin, A World without AIDS. United Kingdom: Thorsons, 1988.

(13)   Foulkes, G., and A. Scott-Morley, "MORA therapy: a revolution in electromagnetic medicine?" J. Alt. Med., July 1984.

(14)   Kenyon, J., "'Tuning in' to subtle energies." J. Alt. and Comp. Med., October 1987.

Chapter Fifteen

THE MIND-BODY-SOUL-CONNECTION

It is true that an impressive, ever-growing arsenal of self-help physical techniques is helping keep HIV/AIDS people living longer, and that these elements range from proper diet and a gaggle of nutritional supplements to herbs of all kinds and combinations, acupuncture, and proper relaxation and exercise.

But above and beyond all of these is the very element referred to in the earlier study (Chapter Thirteen) of long-term Kaposi's sarcoma survivors: something in their attitude which simply does not accept what some researchers have properly called "the institutionalized fostering of a death expectation."

Whether it was Fred M. in our American Biologics group (Chapter Sixteen) turning toward hours of meditation per day above and beyond his eclectic physical program, or a 4-year HIV "asymptomatic" who turned deeply to religion, or several full-blown AIDS cases who expressed themselves simply not yet ready to die while being deeply involved not only in helping themselves but others as well, it early became obvious that attitude alone is a control factor in the infection curve.

This does not surprise investigators who have worked, as our group has, with cancer patients for so many years. Years before the physical scientific aspects of attitude began to be pinned down, the "cancer profile" of personality and attitude had taught us all lessons: some people had obviously "thought themselves into" cancer (as noted semantically in such expressions as "it was just growing on me" or "it kept eating at me") just as others were "thinking themselves out of" cancer.

In fact, a personality profile of cancer patients was among the earlier attempts at linking attitude and pathology: the passive, inward-looking, rules-obeying person seemed more likely to "contract" the disease than did his opposite number.[1,2]

These of course were and are generalities, for so many elements are at play. But the overriding role of attitude in disease induction, management, control and cure has been guessed at by doctors for centuries.

In terms of AIDS, the mental/emotional/attitudinal element must account for a considerable portion of long-term survival.

"Attitude is probably 90 percent of where I am now," according to Manhattan decorator Bruce Zachar in 1988, four years after an AIDS diagnosis and $2^1/_2$ years after statistics suggested he should be dead.[3]

Niro Asistent, of New York, in 1989 told a Baltimore positive-thinking group that although she was diagnosed with ARC in 1985 at age 39 she was now free of antibodies to HIV and attributed this success to meditation, exercise, diet, and learning to love herself. "Love is the only real healing power, the only real healing force," she said.[23] Added Baltimore infectious disease specialist Dr. Donald Pachuta: "The problem with AIDS is that we have an epidemic of AIDS and we have an epidemic of fear -- which is causing a lot of negativity, and I think this negativity is killing people."

Indeed, "imaging", mental exercises, positive-thinking approaches, Western and Eastern varieties of controlled meditation and, simply, a "fighting attitude" ripple through the lives of the long-term HIV/AIDS survivors like new viruses waiting to be analyzed.

They scream for attention but there is no medical model which can absolutely pin them down. Hence, allopathic medicine can only either recoil in horror or break out in laughter when a California certified hypnotherapist asserts (as in Pennsylvania in 1988) that "there's a possibility that 100 percent of people with AIDS could heal themselves."[4]

By then, the self-help, mental-gymnastic, attitude-building seminars of Louise Hay had become well-known. A growing number of California long-term survivors were enrolled in the informal programs the dynamic exponent of changed attitudes and positive thought served up at her weekly meetings.[5,6]

Aspects of healing bearing on the mind, attitudes and simply the intimacy of touch and feeling were highlighted in the best-selling *Love, Medicine and Miracles*[7] by Bernie Siegel, MD, who has recounted his transition from standard allopathic practitioner to exponent of a much broader-based kind of therapy.

Since cancer has, up to now, provided the best model for noting the mind-body-immunity connection, it is within the vastness of cancer cases that the relationships have been studied the most, ranging from the personality profiles of the cancer-prone to the feistiness of cancer survivors -- very much including those patients who break with orthodoxy, and often family and friends, to trek south of the border to try to save their lives.

"Physicians must realize that the patients they consider difficult or uncooperative are those who are most likely to get well," Bernie Siegel has written.[7] The statement echoes the day-to-day experience of "alternative" physicians who are more apt to be faced by questioning, irritating, take-charge, even obnoxious patients than by docile, compliant, unquestioning, passive people who believe the healing process is up to physicians and medicine.

Siegel notes two cancer-attitude studies: psychologist Leonard Derogatis, in a review of 35 women with metastatic breast cancer, found that the long-term survivors ordinarily had bad relationships with their doctors.

And the National Cancer Institute's Sandra Levy and other researchers have shown that aggressive, uncooperative patients tend to have more "killer" immune system cells to attack cancer than do passive, docile ones.

The operative word here, for cancer or AIDS patients, is *control*. The patient who feels he understands what is going on, and believes he can do something about it, is the most likely person to be in control of the patient-physician relationship and, in so doing, the more likely to bring the condition under genuine control. In our Mexican caseloads, be they of cancer, AIDS or any other allegedly terminal disorder, we have seen this time after time.

None of this should really surprise: for centuries, religious exaltation, the power of prayer and belief have demonstrably cured people of their ills. The techniques range from simple belief in the curative power of a forgiving, personalized God to a whole stylized doctrine which rejects the importance of the physical world itself (Buddhism in the Orient, Christian Science in the West.)

Western medicine, obsessed by the rationalist doctrine and the need for reproducibility of results, early in its development and primarily based on the thinking of Rene Descartes, adopted "dualism" as a catch-all thought receptacle -- it admitted there is the mind, or mental self, however poorly understood; and there is the body, about which all can be known.

It was not until the present century that the appropriate connections between mind and body, attitudes and hormones (or the endocrine system) were made, together with growing awareness of how the endocrine system impacts on everything else, very much including the multiple components of "the immune system."

It has been in recent times that it has been demonstrated that attitudes alone can influence behavior in a physical, biochemical way: the brain produces opiate-mimicking substances, endorphins, literally on command from attitudes.

The autonomic nervous system, over whose second-to-second functions it was long supposed "the mind" had no real control, will deliver on order from attitudes, starch will be converted to sugar for energy in the liver as challenge or danger is perceived (the "fight or flight mechanism.")

To the ancients and students of the occult since Renaissance times in Europe, the endocrine glands have always been a source of great power and mystery. It is still believed in some circles that the pineal gland, whose real function in human physiology is little understood, is "the third eye", receptacle of the soul.

The ancient Greeks held that the thymus gland, later to be defined as a regulator of much of the entire immune system, was actually a second mind. The ancients knew that the brain and the tiny structures near it had something to do with behavior, attitudes, emotional drives, growth and development.

Animal experiments, dating back to Pavlov's dogs, had demonstrated the occasional primacy of attitudes over physical behavior.

Can simply forcing yourself to feel better or be happier help overcome disease? Norman Cousins in *Anatomy of an Illness*[8] would argue that this is so -- and a gathering body of researchers would agree.

An American Assn. for the Advancement of Science (AAAS) meeting in San Francisco in 1989 heard from psychiatrist Karl Goodkin that in a study of 40 homosexual men at the University of Texas Southwestern Medical Center, Dallas, it was found that positive thinking, social support and stress reduction might at least delay the time between HIV infection actual development of AIDS.[24]

Since immune system improvements have been noted simply by change in attitude, and because far too many people survive allegedly terminal illnesses against all known physical odds, and because such victories cannot be explained by any physical aspect including known genetic factors, and because mental-imagery proponents since the 1960s have been increasingly proving their point that attitudes can be marshalled to influence, if not control, the course of disease, Western medicine had to respond.

It did so by creating a new word which ultimately would be acceptable for inclusion in insurance company medical treatment computer printouts -- a new discipline which could be fitted into the Western medical paradigm and described with a hodgepodge linguistic structure relatively free of emotional baggage.

The new word, the expressed concept, is *psychoneuroimmunology,* or PNI for short. The polysyllabic description says it all -- mind to nerves to immunity. PNI is now a science. It is as palpable, if still only in infancy, as the concept of the mostly-round Earth. It describes a continent for which only time and application will fill in the mountains, valleys and other features.[9,10]

The PNI-associated work with HIV/AIDS is going on in several areas, including the work of Dr. Lydia Temoshek at the University of California-San Francisco, who in reviewing the cases of long-term survivors said that what they were mentally doing "may affect the immune system and survival."[11]

The major proponent of PNI is Dr. George Solomon, psychiatry professor at the University of California-Los Angeles, who suggests that personality and emotions, especially one's ability to cope with adversity, may help the immune system respond to illness.

Drs. Solomon and Temoshek have found that long-term AIDS survivors share some common mental/emotional features: among them, assertiveness and a sense of purpose, a desire to be in control, ability to ventilate their feelings, and often involvement in helping other patients.

PNI researchers have focused a good deal on

neuropeptides, substances which affect nerve system function and, by implication, immunity, and where and how they are produced and their seeming connection to attitudes and emotion.

The breakthrough linkage was achieved by the University of Alabama's J. Edwin Blalock, who discovered that the immune system also produces neuropeptides, originally thought only to be secretions of the brain -- among the few hundred understood of the possibly thousands of substances produced by what some consider the master endocrine gland of all. The ties between the mind and immunity can now be considered fully established.[12,13,14,15,16]

As if to celebrate PNI's coming of age, *Newsweek* in November 1988[17] dedicated its cover story to "body and soul" and the elucidation, by the major spokemen for PNI, of the discovery of the "feedback loop" -- an intricate interplay of multi-system communication in which not only the brain seems to speak to the immune system, as earlier guessed by researchers, but the immune system also speaks to the brain.

There is suggested here a language of hormones, hormone-like substances and nerve signals, in which two parallel systems are talking to, and talking back to, each other.

It was that same month that researchers reported in Toronto a major breakthrough -- the first evidence suggesting how the brain can physically interact with the immune system to alter the course of disease.

The research, wrote *Los Angeles Times* science writer Thomas H. Maugh II,[22] came from the University of Rochester and University of Chicago and involved discoveries which "provide experimental support of previous observations that stress and depression can make individuals more succeptible to disease, whereas a positive attitude can help fight disease."

The Rochester group showed that some neurons in the central nervous system make direct contact with white blood cells through special receptors in immune system-connected organs. The Chicago team reported that some brain cells can produce interleukin-I (IL-1), an important chemical mediator of immune function. It had been known for years that brain cells respond to IL-1, but it remained to be demonstrated that they actually can produce it.

Rochester neurobiologist David L. Felten was quoted as saying, "We now have a whole new class of drugs -- neuroactive agents -- that can be explored to suppress the immune system."

He and his neurobiologist wife Suzanne and colleagues discovered receptors in bone marrow, lymph nodes, spleen and blood vessels (parts of, or related to, the immune system) that are directly connected to the central nervous system -- the physical evidence of two-way communication in which not only the brain stimulates the immune system, but the immune system actually "reports back" to the brain. Il-2 also suggests two-way communication between the immune system and the brain, Chicago pharmacologist Clifford B. Saper indicated. In Mexico, Peter Rothschild had demonstrated elements of the same.[25]

These studies have given an enormous boost to PNI.

PNI research has helped to establish connections between thoughts, attitudes, emotions, endocrinology and the immune system. Some studies have already shown the connection between incidents of great mental stress and the onset of disease, particularly cancer.

The most beneficial dimension of PNI, however, is in the development of techniques and strategies for applying the mind-body connection to therapy:

If negative thoughts and emotions help induce disease, then surely positive ones must help resolve it.

Outside of the realms of pure faith and religion, the Simontons, and now numerous others, have pioneered ways and means to "visualize" disease and its control through mental images. Some Kaposi's sarcoma patients, for example, now report they may achieve a reduction in symptoms (lesions) simply by forcing themselves to think daily of "erasing" such lesions with a mental eraser.

The Louise Hay group-support techniques go deeply into primary feelings: the facing and assuaging of guilt and shame, fear and rejection.

These are elements of particular concern to homosexuality in America, the first of the two great "reservoirs of infection" of HIV/AIDS.

Psychiatrist Casper S. Schmidt even defined[18] a "group-fantasy origin of AIDS" psychosocial model to explain the rise of epidemic AIDS in a closed population, a model which lies "on the cusp between immunology, pathology and psychology." He noted fantasy complex group psychology, the "scapegoating" ritual (parallel to societal thoughts about lepers in the Middle Ages), "sacrificial witch hunt" and an "epidemic of depression" leading inexorably to "reduction of cell-mediated immunity."

Farfetched as it may sound, the internalizing of social hatred, fear and guilt in an entire subpopulation may indeed, within the dynamics of psychoneuroimmunology, help explain the mental co-factor in the origin of AIDS.

For above and beyond the knowledge that thoughts and attitudes influence body and immunity, the practitioner must often wonder just what the patient really wants. A certain percentage of cancer patients, for example, are known to exhibit through their malignancy a self-fulfilling death wish -- a socially acceptable way to commit suicide.

The homosexual HIV/AIDS sufferer in the U.S.A. (as very distinct in mental make-up from the HIV-infected individual in Africa) often has an extremely low self-image, is often laden with guilt, and may actually believe the wrath-of-God doctrine which suggests he is being punished for unspeakable sins.

If so, he may be mentally articulating a readiness for punishment and death and therefore not be a candidate for self-healing. Self-healing, after all, only begins with the capacity to love and accept one's own self.

So now, biofeedback, Silva mind control, mental imaging, Yoga exercises, deep breathing, meditation of all kinds have been marshalled to attempt to overcome the mental co-factor.[19,20,21]

Yet there are numerous unstructured approaches which over time seem to work just as well, and one of them is a simple semantic trick.

We saw this best epitomized during a lengthy national television town forum in 1987 on the AIDS epidemic. One noted AIDS patient stated his name and observed that "I know I am dying of AIDS." And a long-term survivor was there, from another city, to say, "I am living with AIDS." The earlier speaker is long since dead, the latter still alive.

We have seen the relevance of this simple measure among our terminal cancer and other end-stage patients in Mexico. The swapping of the thought-phrase "I am dying from ..." to "I am living with..." and really *believing* the difference between the two can make all the difference in the world.

We have also seen that there is no specific "how-to" in this area; there is no single ritual, mental exercise, mantra, belief system or imaging technique which can be collectively applied to all people. Mind therapy is as multifactorial as is medical therapy, and what clearly seems to work for Mrs. Smith may fail utterly for Mr. Jones.

There is doctrine arising in all of this to attempt to explain everything in an orderly philosophical way: the insistence, for example, that all attitudes and emotions ultimately evolve from love or fear. It is suggested that all that is "positive" somehow relates to love, and is therefore a good; that all that may seem negative springs from fear, and is bad.

(I am not so sure: I recall the case of one of our melanoma patients who was literally exuding tumorous tissue and staying alive against all odds virtually on sheer gall -- the desire to "wreak revenge" on the husband who had divorced her, and she intended somehow to stay alive simply to spite him.)

Regardless of the wellspring of emotions it is essentially clear that the generally perceived negative attitudes are immune depressing and disease-inducing, while the more generally accepted positive ones are immune enhancing and disease-thwarting. Ultimately, we are dealing here simply with energy, and ways to channel it in semantical thought-forms which are expressable in a third-dimensional, human setting.

To the holistic practitioner, a survey of what mentally happened to a patient months before diagnosis may turn out to be as important as any single item of physical importance referred to in a questionnaire.

With metastatic adenocarcinoma of the bowel, for example, it may be as vital to know that the individual lost his job, or a wife, or a child six months prior to diagnosis as it is to know he had a lifelong predilection for too much animal protein. To the holistically oriented clinician the attitudes and belief systems of the patient, how he mentally and attitudinally sees himself and how he relates to those around him, may be every bit as important as a "SMAC-24" blood test.

If the cancer calamity provided the model to prove the mind-body-immunity connection, then the HIV/AIDS infection curve has provided the opportunity to demonstrate just how this knowledge can be part of a multi-factorial program of healing.

REFERENCES

(1) LeShan, L., "An emotional life history pattern associated with neoplastic disease." Ann. N.Y. Acad. Sci., Jan. 21, 1966.

(2) LeShan, L., You Can Fight For Your Life: Emotional Factors in the Causation of Cancer. New York: Evans, 1977.

(3) Grady, Denise, "AIDS survivors." American Health. September 1988.

(4) Gernerd, Bill, "Self-healing theory on AIDS draws skeptical response." Allentown PA Morning Call, May 25, 1988.

(5) Gavzer, Bernard, "Why do some people survive AIDS?" Parade, Sept. 18, 1988.

(6) Hay, Louise, You Can Heal your Life. Santa Monica, CA: Hay House, 1986.

(7) Siegel, B.S., Love, Medicine and Miracles. New York: Harper & Row, 1986.

(8) Cousins, Norman, Anatomy of an Illness. New York: Bantam, 1981.

(9) Solomon, G.E., Psychoneuroimmunology, New York: Academic Press, 1987.

(10) Solomon, G.E.,"The emerging field of psychoneuroimmunology." Advances, 2:1, Winter 1985.

(11) Grady, loc. Cit.

(12) Benson, Herbert, The Mind-body Effect. New York: Berkeley, 1980.

(13) Lewis, H., and Martha E. Lewis, Psychosomatics: How Your Emotions Can Damage Your Health. New York: Viking, 1972.

(14) Riley, V., "Psychoneuroendocrine influences on immuno-competence and neoplasia." Science, 202: 1981.

(15) Locke, S., Mind and Immunity. Institute for the Advancement of Health, New York, 1982.

(16) Hall, J.G., "Emotion and immunity." Lancet, Aug. 10, 1985.

(17) Gelman, David, and Mary Hager, "Body and Soul." Newsweek, Nov. 7, 1988.

(18) Schmidt, C.G., "The group-fantasy origins of AIDS." J. of Psychohistory, Summer 1984.

(19) Simonton, Carl., et al., Getting Well Again. New York: Bantam, 1986.

(20) Locke, Steven, and Douglas Colligan. The Healer Within. New York: E.P. Dutton, 1986.

(21)   Cyle, Irving, <u>The</u> <u>Healing</u> <u>Mind</u>. New York: Simon and Schuster, 1976.

(22)   Maugh, T.H.II, "New light shed on brain-immune system link." Los Angeles Times, Nov. 15, 1988.

(23)   Painter, Kim, "Positive thinking in treating AIDS." USA Today, FEb. 23, 1989.

(24)   Staver, Sari, "Stress' role in HIV progression to AIDS probed." American Medical News, Jan. 27, 1989.

(25)   Rothschild, Peter R., <u>The</u> <u>Biochemical</u> <u>Relations</u> <u>Between</u> <u>Stress</u>, <u>Mind</u> <u>and</u> <u>Immune</u> <u>System</u>. Honolulu: University Labs Press, 1988.

241

Chapter Sixteen

A FOREIGN CLINIC EXPERIENCE

It has been seen that the same American medical monopoly which failed in the Conquest of Cancer program is the same one, almost lock, stock and laboratory, now in charge of the "war on AIDS."

The corollary to this is that, just as American cancer patients found themselves literally having to flee their own country for "unapproved" or "unorthodox" therapies in cancer, they have had to do the same in terms of HIV/AIDS, at least if they are to have any real clinical environment while they are being treated.

There is this difference between "alternative" cancer treatments and "alternative" HIV/AIDS treatments, however: U.S. orthodoxy claims a limited amount of actual "cure" in cancer (about 10 percent if we delete non-melanoma skin cancer,localized tumors, and the numbers are honest and we agree on the meaning of "cure") but admits to a 0 cure rate in AIDS.

So, at least in terms of cancer, U.S. orthodoxy could make a faintly legitimate claim that Americans "going underground" or seeking "unapproved" therapies abroad might sometimes (though rarely) be doing themselves a disservice. And, in terms of non-melanoma skin cancer, certain localized and non-metastatic tumors and some rare "forms" of cancer, that might be correct.

But in terms of AIDS, there was no reason an American patient should not turn to "alternatives" from Day One, particularly when his own country's medical establishment and surgeon general had told him he had an invariably fatal, incurable disease.

The Bradford Research Institute, particularly its Mexican division, was already deeply involved in developing metabolic and eclectic protocols for cancer, and often for other conditions as well. (Since, officially, lupus, Alzheimer's, Parkinson's, multiple sclerosis and rheumatoid arthritis are, along with most of terminal cancer and all of AIDS, regarded as irreversible or incurable even if they are, at times, manageable through the nostrums and devices of allopathic, or "standard" medicine.)

242

In 1983, the B.R.I.-Mexican division began accepting HIV/AIDS patients on a limited, intermittent basis -- and not through solicitation. Our Mexican medical group had plenty to do exclusive of the AIDS disaster, and the Mexican government played cat-and-mouse as to whether foreign AIDS patients could or should be treated there.

But doctors and patients who already knew of the B.R.I. program in cancer and degenerative diseases in general thought that the same basic approaches might be useful for the new killer disease -- the syndrome was, after all, literally tailor-made for a *multifactorial*, rather than an allopathic, strategy.

The B.R.I., which has some scientific representation in more than a dozen countries, had already evolved the concept of "individualized, integrated metabolic programs" (IIMP) in cancer, built largely around the multifactorial paradigm discussed earlier: concentrating more on the terrain of the host than on the nature of the condition, and bringing to bear all those elements (detoxification, nutrient management, endocrine balancing, immune modulation) which could enhance "host defense", and only thereafter greatly concerned about the cancer cells or their most visible expressions (tumors) themselves.

We were now presented with a syndrome which by its very name suggested the need for just such an approach: "immunodeficiency." By and large, what many of the U.S.-damned "holistic" or "metabolic" or "biological" practitioners had been doing really was, in allopathic terms, "immunotherapy," even if it had not usually been called that.

As in all other disease states, the B.R.I.-Mexico approach did not set out to "cure" something -- but rather to bring it under "control." No one at this time knows exactly what a "cure" for AIDS would truly mean, anyway.

The AIDS challenge was hurled just as the research group, captained by the controversial Robert W. Bradford, an electronics engineer, physicist and laetrile entrepreneur, best known as the latter in many circles, was making headway in various areas of medical research quite aside from the balancing of nutrients (vitamins, minerals, enzymes, amino acids) and diet in developing protocols for diseases and metabolic challenges.

Aside from literally rescuing research on laetrile and

other areas of nutritional therapy, the B.R.I. and its innovative if originally uncredentialed leader (now holder of three honorary doctorates and a bevy of medals, citations and certificates for his research work) had advanced an entirely new discipline as a subspecialty in medicine deserving of its own name, which we jointly baptized *oxidology.*

The latter is "the study of reactive oxygen toxic species" -- or, ROTS, a singularly descriptive acronym for the actual effect of these species on the body -- "and their metabolism in health and disease." Or, in words at the time more familiar to biochemistry and medicine, "the manipulation of free radicals" (although not all ROTS are free radicals, though all oxygen-derived free radicals are ROTS.) This was not a singular discovery by B.R.I.: earlier work by Harman, Schrauzer, Pryor, McCord and others had helped bring the term "free radical" to public attention.

This line of research had connected breakdown toxic products of the metabolism of oxygen with cancer, aging, obesity and, by implication, much of pathology. The cellular damage wrought by ROTS produced in excess of the body's ability to "scavenge" or destroy them through natural, or endogenous, enzymes, was seen as a striking element of many disease conditions. Indeed, B.R.I. now feels there is no area of pathology in which ROTS metabolism does not play at least some role.[1]

The ROTS-scavenging (or "free radical"-attacking) capabilities of certain vitamins, minerals and enzymes provided a new rationale for nutritional or metabolic therapies.

The growing research on the syndrome of aging and its link to ROTS production, increasingly accepted by Western scientific orthodoxy, began to elevate various lines of research into toxic oxygen breakdown products into positions of responsible scientific inquiry, let alone application.

The Bradford group began examining both the "ROTS scavengers" (compounds which would destroy or inhibit the action of such toxic byproducts) as well as the "oxidative compounds" -- in a sense, free radicals or free radical-like substances themselves, or any compound which would release nascent atomic oxygen at the site of an "insult" or pathogenic disturbance.

This line of research drew it into the development of a microscopy technique to examine the effects of ROTS in dried blood (the HLB Blood Test), the delineation of how ROTS-connected morphological changes in dried blood could indicate specific pathologies, and the designing of therapeutic strategies to utilize either ROTS-scavenging or oxidative compounds.

Along the way, Bradford researchers, particularly California biochemist Henry W. Allen, in assessing the world literature on oxidative compounds, found that nascent atomic oxygen is a natural blocker of viral reproduction, certain bacteria and fungi -- and that research suggesting this goes back to the second decade of this century. That is to say, compounds capable of releasing nascent atomic oxygen are natural anti-virals, anti-bacterials, and anti-fungals.

The manipulation of oxidative compounds as therapies, then, is only one more medical discipline or subspecialty literally overlooked or "left on the shelf" primarily because it is not a creature of the petrochemically based synthetic drug industry whose influence over (and often outright control of) Western medicine is, to many, obvious.

Following up on this ongoing research, B.R.I. scientists turned their attention to natural oxidative compounds, including "endogenous" hydrogen peroxide, "exogenous" but natural ozone gas, and industrial chemicals, particularly chlorine dioxide. B.R.I. physicians early in the present decade utilized ozone gas for intratumoral injection.

Later, the B.R.I. published a well researched monograph[2] opposing the faddish hyperadministration of hydrogen peroxide as an all-purpose elixir, even while noting H2O2's utility at extremely low levels as an oxidative agent.

It was from the industrial oxidative compounds that B.R.I. developed Dioxychlor, the name for a family of products whose major *modus operandi* is the release of atomic oxygen. By the end of the decade, B.R.I. had developed Dioxychlor compounds for topical, oral and intravenous use and also homeopathic-dilution drops.

The research group believes Dioxychlor to be the safest and the premiere of the oxidative compounds -- one avoiding the "free radical cascade" outcome of hydrogen peroxide administered in abnormal concentrations and the possible lung-tissue damage of overuse of ozone.

In vitro research at a major American university

showed Dioxychlor could inhibit or destroy HIV, Epstein-Barr, CMV and other agents in a matter of seconds. Just how this would work *in vivo* would remain to be seen.[3]

Hence, for the B.R.I., Dioxychlor became a "safe" antiviral, antibacterial and antifungal agent, and it has been used successfully against all of these in now thousands of cases.

To some extent, Dioxychlor recalls a product called "chlorozone", patented in the 1960s as an effective method of water purification and as a disinfectant.

In his book assailing "scientism" in orthodox thinking, physician-researcher Raymond K. Brown, MD, described[8] how the developers of chlorozone ("the active ingredients ... are presumably ozone, chlorine ions and other oxidizing products of the saline solution"), noting how chlorozone added to the water supply of a Greek village had dramatically reduced an epidemic of infectious hepatitis, used the compound medically and sought medical patents for it. It was administered to over 200 volunteers who suffered from various degenerative conditions and showed documented therapeutic efficacy in topical, oral and intravenous forms.

Full records were kept and reputable physicians (including a University of Athens Medical School professor of orthopedics) attested to the results. Chlorozone had also been shown effective in Viet Nam for almost 10 years in the treatment of civilian war casualties on the basis of the Greek work. Yet, despite affidavits from physicians and patients, patents for the medical uses of this compound were never issued in the U.S.A.

It has been up to independent organizations like the B.R.I. to "rescue" from obscurity avenues of therapeutics -- including the natural and industrial oxidative compounds which have been known about since at least the second decade of this century. Failure of scientific orthodoxy in the Western world to develop research on these simple and potentially inexpensive chemicals while bestowing billions of research funds on the synthetic drug industry speaks for itself.

The minimum reality here is that oxidative compounds are excellent inhibitors of viruses, and should be routinely available.

At the same time, the B.R.I.'s affiliated Mexican

hospital became the only treatment center in North America where a form of European therapy in existence for almost five decades, yet ignored or spurned in the U.S.A., could also be used in its original theoretical setting and combined with "individualized, integrated metabolic programs."

This other research rivulet was that of live-cell -- or cellular -- therapy. While there is a rich history of this kind of medicine in Europe, whose roots go back to ancient medicine in various countries, it remains almost unknown in the U.S.A. except in a limited (and to some, laughable) research setting in which fetal human cells are injected into animals and described as "tissue transfer therapy", or Orwellian Newspeak for "live-cell therapy."

In essence, live-cell therapy is the subcutaneous injection of suspensions of animal fetal or embryonic cells. They must be fetal or embryonic so that the cellular material, held in saline solution, is "immunologically silent" -- that is, it will not excite an immune response in the host (just as pregnancy does not) which would lead to rejection of the cells.

For many years, European physicians, and particularly this century's major live-cell pioneer, the late Paul Niehans, MD, of Switzerland, had known of the incredible potency of live cells -- they seemed to stimulate hostal organs in man matching those of the animal (heart cells to heart, spleen to spleen, etc.), they seemed to rejuvenate and possibly regenerate certain tissue, and, most of all, they "harmonize" hormones -- that is, they balance the little-understood endocrine system.

The effects of this latter capability, especially in rejuvenation, and stimulation of sexual prowess among the elderly, were used in the U.S.A. to besmirch live-cell therapy as the "monkey-gland" or "goat gonad" approach to rejuvenation and immortality.

Even though famous American statesmen and others in the public light (Bernard Baruch, Joseph Kennedy, Charlie Chaplin, etc.) made the trek to Switzerland for such treatments, the thought that cellular extracts from animal embryos, usually of the endocrine organs, could have any real therapeutic value was derided by drug-pushing American medicine.

It was not until 1975 that radioactive tagging of

embryonic animal material injected into humans did in fact demonstrate what many hundreds of European doctors had empirically assumed -- that liver tissue *does* go to human liver, etc. -- though the actual way this occurred was not described, and then only partially (by the Bradford group), until 1986.[4]

It has been seen that the endocrine and immune systems are involved in the mental "feedback loop" of the human "double mind" and it is strongly indicated that the endocrine system is the mediator of emotions (and thus responds to thoughts and attitudes). Inasmuch as the endocrine system, through its mass production of hormones, many of which are not understood, impacts virtually on every other system, very much including cellular and humoral immunity, its balancing should be considered of extreme importance in any therapeutic program. This is specifically what live-cell therapists believe this form of treatment does.

Wolfram W. Kuhnau, MD, an endocrinologist, disciple of Dr. Niehans and head of the live-cell program in Mexico, has explained[5] that the feedback mechanism of the endocrine system allows one gland to make up for the deficits, or excesses, of another. Therefore, any condition in which endocrine imbalance is a major feature (obesity, sexual dysfunction, hyper-and hypo-thyroid problems) will find a resolution or at least strong palliation through live-cell therapy.

In HIV/AIDS patients, the immune system in general is unbalanced. While various organs and systems are involved in this imbalance, it is the thymus gland, once thought to be the "regulator" of the system, which is the primary target of cellular therapy.

The HIV/AIDS patient, as is the case of the multi-allergy, universal-reactor or chronic fatigue syndrome patient, and/or the patient suffering from any form of "autoimmune" disease, is in effect being immunologically whipsawed between chronic immune depression (the alleged hallmark of AIDS through depletion of T4 cells and increase in T8 cells) and acute immune excitation (autoimmune disease.)

What would be theoretically indicated would be the balancing or modulation of immunity -- a theoretical job for live-cell therapy as well as the rationale for injections of thymus glandulars.

In the area of "stress hormone management," a dimension of AIDS therapy already suggested by other researchers (excess cortisol as presumed co-factor to HIV, in the thinking of several) live-cell therapy also becomes a worthwhile tool.

Despite the fears of some that HIV is a manufactured virus derived from animal origins and that one of these may be the "bovine leukemia virus" or something like it, there is no evidence that any such virus may be transferred to humans through live-cell therapy. (There is no ironclad proof that this cannot happen, either.) The utilization of any available matching tissue from any available animal (usually mammalian, including shark) avoids the only presumptive therapeutic complication from this form of treatment: no *human* viruses are transferred.

Many thousands of live-cell injections have been given by the B.R.I.-Mexico collaborators with no known serious toxic side effects or more than transient fatigue reactions.

In Europe, many millions of injections have been given over the years. In 1987, the West German health authorities suspended for a year the use of freeze-dried cellular products made by several companies following the death of a female athlete apparently from excessive injections of the material. However, this proscription did not bear on the traditional use of live-cell therapy -- the selective, conservative (rarely more than six injections in any one treatment) subcutaneous administration of "fresh" (that is, from recently sacrificed animals) cellular material.

This form of therapy, now found effective in a wide variety of ills, carries with it the moral attack by animal-rights advocates. The usual defense of the use of the treatment in Mexico has always been that (with the exception of sharks caught specifically for the purpose of embryonic cell extraction) the cattle from whose embryos cells are extracted were on the way to slaughter for beef sales anyway -- that is, they were not slain with the specific intention of contributing fetal cells for human use.

So, by the time B.R.I.-Mexico began seeing HIV/AIDS patients and developing metabolic protocols for them, both live-cell therapy (for endocrine balancing, immune modulation, tissue strengthening and repair) and oxidative compounds were available to be used as part of an overall protocol.

Together with them, the B.R.I.-Mexico drew on the rapidly accumulating knowledge of metabolic physicians from around the world as to the immune-boosting potentials of many other nutrients (Vitamins A,C,E, several of the B vitamins; zinc; selenium; iron; other minerals; specific amino acids) as well as to the implied antiviral effects of some of these in megadoses.

Minerals, ROTS-scavenging enzymes (superoxide dismutase, catalase), ROTS-scavenging vitamins and even laetrile (as putative Vitamin B17, found -- embarrassingly, it would seem -- in a Rutgers study[6] to be a scavenger of the most toxic of the ROTS, hydroxyl radical) were part of the experimental protocol.

To these were added various essential and non-essential fatty acids, building on the work of other researchers who found relationships between the immune system (and health in general) with these compounds and with the knowledge that the hydrogenation of polyun-saturated fatty acids (PUFA) in food processing had altered the levels and nature of certain fatty acids in the body.

Staphage lysate, butyric acid, a growing list of herbs (as teas, tablets, capsules, foods) were added to the program. Dietary control (reduction in animal fats and proteins, proscription of refined carbohydrates, stimulants, alcohol, etc; emphasis on more fresh fruits and vegetables in as raw or sprouting a stage as possible or as soups and juices) for general health, energy and detoxification; yeast-free foods; and detoxification of the gastrointestinal tract (lactobacillus bifidus, acidophilus, yogurt, dietary change, herbal and coffee enemas, bowel cleansers) and the treat-ment for parasites usually found there, have been essential parts of the program.

Inasmuch as it was our assumption that HIV has something to do with AIDS, even if it is probably neither the cause nor can it be working alone even if it may be a major contributor, and also because almost invariably the viral panels of HIV/AIDS patients will turn up other active viruses, usually cytomegalovirus, Epstein-Barr virus, fre-quently other herpesviruses and hepatitis, then clearly an arsenal of antivirals was called for.

In addition to the possible antiviral capabilities of

some vitamins in megadoses and in addition to Dioxychlor given intravenously and orally, the B.R.I. program began using oral ribavirin (Virazole, Vilona) in all cases of HIV/AIDS and injectable and oral acyclovir in many.

It also included the products isoprinosine and levamisol for presumptive immune-boosting or possible antiviral activity. And, following the optimistic results in Japan utilizing a form of germanium, it also began using this substance, orally and injectably.

The chelating agent EDTA (which, as we have noted, is suggested in some research as an inhibitor of retroviruses) has been given not only because of its chelating properties but because of its ability to "potentiate" live cells.

Dextran sulfate and the fatty acid combination AL-721 were occasionally added to the HIV/AIDS protocols together with (in some cases) aqueous penicillin, a nod to the concept that probably much of what is now being ascribed to "full-blown AIDS" is actually neurosyphilis.

Hence, at the physical level of the program, we had developed ever-changing eclectic protocols consisting of many parts. While we could treat patients in a hospital setting with the full program (though some of them were provided only with an oral protocol) we could control neither prior therapies nor what they would do after they left their treatments in Mexico.

Such is the ever-shifting state of the art in HIV/AIDS concepts and therapies that it is a rare patient who does not continually try any new therapy, vitamin, diet or herb which has a suggestion of efficacy.

Taking into account the nature of our program and of the patients, we reported in fall 1988[7] (see Appendix IV) on our first five dozen cases. We were cheered by what we found:

Our 1988 review referred to three patients in whom, as of 1988, circulating HIV virus could no longer be found, as well as the apparent eradication of cases of immunoblastic lymphoma (a cancer connected directly with a faltering immune system), cryptococcal meningitis,and "walking pneumonia."

Well over two dozen ARC-level patients (by earlier CDC definition) had achieved significant reduction in clinical signs and symptoms and the near-normalization of immune panels (T4, T8 cells, and their ratios). The bulk of patients had been seen since 3 years prior and all but 6 of these had survived in ordinarily good health, none considered "cured" and all presumed to be still "positive" for HIV antibodies.

We had seen the transient and sometimes persistent eradication of KS lesions with such experimental remedies as Dioxychlor, but by no means in every case, and increases in energy, weight gain and immune improvement in practically all patients.

One of our earliest patients, a KS case, was treated intermittently for $4^1/2$ years, yet he would neither give up a drug habit nor visits for chemotherapy sessions in Northern California. Despite his long-term improvements, he died.

Another classic case survived 21 months with full-blown AIDS (PCP and opportunistic infections) combining our program with toxic AZT but was able to work 5-day weeks most of the time and never needed a blood transfusion. He never fully abandoned such habits as cigarettes and cocktails, and went into heavy chemotherapy after a second relapse. He, too, expired, yet by PCP standards had defied most of the odds.

Fred M. of Los Angeles (like many HIV/AIDS patients he does not want his full name used) was the immunoblastic lymphoma patient who was seen at AB-Mexico in 1987. HIV-positive and showing characteristic signs of immune depression, his major symptom was the cancer. His California physicians told him that without chemotherapy treatments he would have no chance at all to live, and even with them he would have a 50 percent survival chance (of up to 5 years.)

Instead, Fred, 53, did the entire program at AB-Mexico and stayed on the maintenace therapy for a full year thereafter. But he added a total vegetarian diet plus herbal bowel cleansers and meditation. A half-year after his return from Mexico his doubting allopathic physicians were still certain he would need chemotherapy treatments and had him come into a local hospital for analysis.

"One of the doctors came into the waiting room and had a long face," Fred told me. "He said, 'The doctors in there are talking about your case.' I asked, 'Why?' He said, 'The tests show you don't need any chemotherapy treatments. You're cured. I don't mean just in remission.

You're cured.'"

One of the more spectacular cases occurred in spring 1989:

Federico I., 30-year-old a Mexican charity case literally referred to our facilities in order to have a place to die, presented with HIV positivity, a cerebral lesion (actual pathology unknown), a semicomatose condition, weight loss and fatigue, a debilitated appearance, *Pneumocystis carinii* pneumonia and extensive candidiasis on the mucosal surfaces. Death seemed immirent.

He was placed on a program essentially consisting of 200 million units of aqueous penicillin (over 5 days), daily Vitamin C and Dioxychlor infusions, together with another infusion of an herbal immune-stimulating combination developed in southern Mexico. Startlingly, by the sixth day he was restored to full cognitive capacity, the brain lesion had healed, the PCP had subsided and yeast infection was down by at least 80 percent. His energy and normal weight rapidly returned, and he remained under weekly observation. There was no visual correlation between the Federico seen in a semicomatose state and the young carpenter able to return to work in a week's time.

Had we managed AIDS -- or treated syphilis? We didn't know. Federico remained stable for the better of a year, yet still died of AIDS complications.

Even some of the earliest "stretcher cases" we saw had evidence of immune system improvement and general energy gain. We were seeing in "terminal AIDS" a situation analogous to "terminal cancer" -- in some cases survival could not be guaranteed, but adding both quality and quantity to life was possible.

In several cases, early-ARC or pre-ARC patients either simply stabilized and remained healthy or so improved that they reported more vitality than ever before, and in some instances looked younger than before.

What we began seeing with this first group of 66 patients, then, were these realities:

-- Immune systems are susceptible of being improved or rebuilt.

-- The HIV/AIDS infection curve may be slowed or halted.

-- Disease expression may be postponed or prevented entirely.

--   Pre-AIDS patients need not advance to full-blown AIDS.

--   Life may be extended in full-blown AIDS patients.

The advantage of the B.R.I.-Mexico program is that it could/can be implemented and escape the obfuscation, intimidation, foot-dragging and police-state tactics of the American Food and Drug Administration and the innovation-quenching activities of American Medical Assn.-controlled licensing and peer review boards. No sooner had something promising occurred on the world research horizon then it could be in place in an experimental protocol in an adjacent foreign country.

Along the way, and from a patient load that reached 100 by late 1989, we had come across some of the observations and contradictions other researchers have noted:

--   Some individuals with Kaposi's sarcoma had little or no meaningful immune distortion. (And KS, at least in the early stage, did not *look* like cancer in the HLB Blood Test.)

--   At least one patient (KS without other opportunistic infections) had had a probable KS lesion on the leg for *at least* 15 years. This Dutch patient had only light immune distortion and was not ill when he first visited the BRI.

--   Some of the ARC or pre-ARC patients had low T-cell "ratios" only because they had very elevated T8 ("suppressor") levels, which, together with their basic vitality, lack of symptoms and opportunistic infections, suggested (despite HIV seropositivity) some protective or other benign effect from T8s.

--   Some individuals with several hundred T4 cells had many symptoms and were truly "sick."

--   Some patients with T4 levels well below 100 remained relatively healthy in terms of signs, symptoms and general energy. This led us to question, with others, the relevance of the T4/T8 panels as any more than occasional indicators.

--   In general, however, as clinical signs and symptoms diminished, absolute T4 numbers increased.

--   By far the majority of our patients had a prior history of substance abuse. The few who did not had another element in common: recently diagnosed secondary syphilis a little before or close to the time they were found to be "HIV seropositive."

Such programs, of course, cannot fit well into the allopathic paradigm:

They are individualized, they are ever varying, they are not "randomized," "double-blinded" or "placebo-controlled," and therefore are not "scientific" in the allopathically tinged semantics of the word. We admit that followup is spotty, and also that we lost control of many patients after they left us, as they understandably grasped for one straw (be it herbal, drug, meditative technique, vitamin) after another in their desperate struggle to stay alive.

Some died within a year or two of initial therapy, yet others continued to flourish in generally good heatlh.

In a crisis management program of short duration, only the physical aspects of the disease could be dealt with. Only indirect efforts were made to foster the winning attitude which numbers of AIDS researchers suggest may be the key to overall survival.

However, the determination of HIV/AIDS patients to change lifestyle, eating habits and sexual practices indicated in most (but not all) of our patients a readiness to participate in the healing process from all angles.

The frustration in the program, of course, is its essential flaw: why should patients (usually Americans) have to leave their own country for an experimental, multifactorial protocol whose followup at home would be difficult at best?

But the answer to this question involves the politics--not the science -- of HIV/AIDS.

(NOTE: *As per arrangement with Mexican officials, the 6-year experimental program ended in November 1989 although BRI continued tracing the 100-plus patients seen since 1983. Early results confirmed that, in the main, stage I patients did not advance to stage II, nor stage II to stage III. Stages IIIs could expect considerable life extensions.*)

REFERENCES

(1)   Bradford, R.W., et al., Oxidology. Los Altos, CA: The Bradford Foundation, 1985.

(2)   Bradford, R.W., et al., Hydrogen Peroxide: the Misunderstood Oxidant. Chula Vista CA: The Bradford Foundation, 1987.

(3)   Bradford, R.W., et al., Exogenous Oxidative Mechanisms in Combating Infectious Diseases. Chula Vista CA: The Bradford Foundation, 1986.

(4)   Bradford, R.W., et al., The Biochemistry of Live-Cell Therapy. Chula Vista CA: The Bradford Foundation, 1986.

(5)   Kuhnau, W.W., Live-cell Therapy: My Life with a Medical Breakthrough. Tijuana, Mexico: Artes Graficas, 1983.

(6)   Heikkila, R.E., and F.S. Cabbat, "The prevention of Alloxan-induced diabetes by amygdalin." Life Sciences, 27:8, 1980.

(7)   Culbert, M.L., "The AIDS paradigm." Townsend Letter for Doctors, October 1988.

(8)   Brown, Raymond K., AIDS, Cancer and the Medical Establishment. New York: Speller, 1986.

Chapter Seventeen

A RATIONAL PROGRAM
FOR THE PREVENTION OF HIV/AIDS

In the foregoing, we have demonstrated that a single thread runs through the multifarious aspects of HIV/AIDS, be they causation, epidemiology, or even management:

No AIDS-related illness seems able to occur other than in people who are already "sick" -- sick at least in terms of a compromised immune system, or lowered overall host defense.

Whether drug users, homosexuals, hemophiliacs, infants, the elderly or persons receiving blood transfusions and blood products, promiscuous heterosexuals, prostitutes, or combinations of any of these, AIDS patients have in common signs of earlier immunological or host-defense deterioration.

At least, this is the clear picture up to now. The proponents of HIV-as-inevitably-leading-to-death believe they are still right -- that, over time, all HIV-infected people will eventually succumb to AIDS-related diseases. Not gifted with prescience, we cannot claim this conclusion is totally wrong -- but so far death is simply not inevitable. There will continue to be many deaths from AIDS-related illness, but we would argue strongly that many of these deaths need not occur.

The first and foremost logical extrapolation of the data is that the best defense against mankind's latest killer disease is that which holds true for virtually any pathology or condition: a strong immune system or overall host defense.

We have attempted to show that numerous factors may be involved in setting the stage for overt HIV/AIDS through depressing the immune system -- among them earlier viral and bacteriological infections,interreactions with other viruses, drug use, parasites, antibiotics and corticosteroid treatments, toxic drugs, possibly anal lubricants, possibly vaccinations, poor sanitation and hygiene, even fluoridated water and mental stress -- and nutritional deficiencies, excesses and alterations in the food chain caused by processing.

The second logical extrapolation of the data -- and, we believe, *markedly* secondary in importance -- is that, given the undeniable semen and blood connection in AIDS epidemiology, lifestyle changes in terms of sexual habits are called for, yet these may be relatively simple and imply neither total frustration nor celibacy.

We have further sought to show that the dominance in American medicine of the allopathic model, so intertwined with pharmaceutical interests, has largely blinded much of Western medical orthodoxy to acceptance either of the multifactorial concept of HIV/AIDS causation or of a multifactorial, holistic and eclectic treatment approach.

Indeed, if any "goods" can be said to be harvestable from the current crisis, surely they lie within the fields of greatly enhancing the concepts of immunology, preventive medicine and, more than ever, *promotive health* -- and the profound relevance of nutrition and mental aspects to promotive health.

One of the most startling realities in global health, as we have seen, is that it is the Western world, particularly the U.S.A. and industrialized western European nations (together with Australia and New Zealand) where the major impact of AIDS/ARC occurs despite widespread viral infection in the poor countries of central Africa and to some extent the Caribbean.

The generally held point of view that American society is well-fed and healthy founders on the stark reality that it is the Western -- not the Third -- World in which chronic, systemic degenerative diseases and an epidemic of actual man-made or iatrogenic illnesses and conditions abound.

We have indicated that it is entirely possible (and in much of the industrialized Western world it actually occurs) that whole populations can be both over-fed and undernourished at the same time. We have shown that a profound alteration in and chemical tampering with the food chain wrought by the exigencies of modern civilization have led to subtle, but very real, nutritional deficiencies.

We have also shown that some of these deficiencies (such as adequate essential fatty acids, zinc, Vitamin C, etc.) may be involved with immune dysregulation, and that further insult may be added by common, socially sanctioned drugs (caffeine and nicotine being suspect) and greatly added by the so-called "recreational" or "street" drugs (be they ingested, injected, smoked or sniffed).

The hydrogenation processing of polyunsaturated fatty acids may play far more of a role in immune damage than hitherto suspected, through the blocking of prostaglandin E1 synthesis -- a condition enhanced by further dietary deprivation caused by or related to drug use and/or the ingestion of nutritionless refined "junk foods."

It would seem reasonable, therefore, to suggest that the "prudent diet" already advanced by broad areas of Western medical orthodoxy (at the original behest, let the record show, of "unorthodox" researchers and doctors) for heart disease and cancer prevention also be in effect for AIDS prevention: that is, less animal fat, somewhat less animal protein, fewer refined carbohydrates, fewer canned and frozen foods, and fewer stimulants, and consumption of more fresh, raw, natural fruits and vegetables.

To a considerable extent, spring and mineral water are preferable to fluoridated water, herbal teas are preferable to tea itself, and coffee intake, at the very least, could well be reduced if not eliminated. Avoidance of refined sugars and starches and less intake of salt and/or sodium in general are important in such diets, and they make sense in a prudent anti-AIDS/ARC eating plan. And cigarette smoking, the maximum addiction, may be absolutely lethal to an otherwise "good" eating program. In terms of HIV/AIDS, the continual irritation of the lung's delicate tissues is a flirtation with disaster.

Since strict adherence to even a generalized dietary program may be considerably difficult in a mobile urban society, nutritional replenishment through supplements seems to make eminently good sense for most people most of the time.

Supplements may include essential vitamins and minerals as well as the EFAs (essential fatty acids). Of direct bearing on AIDS and ARC, immune enhancement with Vitamin C and zinc alone, as has been suggested, is worthwhile. Other nutrients with some kind of evidence of immune enhancement include the amino acids L-cysteine and L-methionine, beta-carotene (and Vitamin A itself), Vitamins E and B6, folic acid, and the minerals (aside from zinc) including germanium, selenium, manganese, and possibly iron.

Antioxidant enzyme combinations including super-oxide dismutase (SOD) and catalase, which may also help modulate immunity, other natural substances, including L-glutathione, and even natural laetrile or amygdalin in the form of black, bitter fruit seeds (particularly of apricots, pears, peaches, plums, prunes and apples) may be useful as scavengers of reactive oxygen toxic species (ROTS) for over-all health.

The continuing importance of aerobic exercise prac-ticed in even minimal amounts daily is of demonstrated benefit in a program of promotive health and preventive medicine and normally forms a part of holistic therapy for the management of degenerative disease.

Avoidance of "street" and "recreational" drugs as well as of intravenous drugs (and certainly marijuana and cocaine) is an obvious adjunct to a healthy lifestyle.

There is a world of foods, food factors and herbs found useful in HIV/AIDS prevention as well as treatment (See Appendix III).

Herbs include garlic, an ancient and traditional medicine now found to have antibacterial, antimicrobial, antifungal, anticancer, antiviral, antiparasitical and other properties; ginseng (particularly eleuthero ginseng), for immune-enhancing properties; the Chinese herbs astragalus and ligustrum, now accepted even by American orthodoxy as potentially useful against cancer, and both of which have immune boosting characteristics; echinacea, na-tive to a wide area of North America and sufficiently studied to indicate, among many other things, immune stimulating potential; goldenseal, good for, among other things, anti-protozoal, anti-fungal and antimicrobial ac-tivity; certain mushrooms, particularly Shiitake, from which an experimental drug (Lentinan) has been extracted; licorice plant, extracts of which seem to be effective against HIV and the herpesvirus family; and many others.

Among foods and food factors there are spirulina (a kind of algae -- and attacked by the U.S. drug empire as "pond scum") which contains, among other things all the amino acids and a treasure trove of minerals and vitamins; chlorophyll, useful against infections, respiratory disorders, common colds and high blood pressure; wheat grass juice, which contains chlorophyll, fiber, many vitamins, minerals, carbohydrates and proteins -- virtually a whole food;

acidophilus and lactobacillus bifidus, for helping cleanse the gastrointestinal tract, restoring intestinal flora, and useful against *Candida albicans;* lecithin (active ingredient: choline), a fatty substance which may interfere with viral binding; Coenzyme Q, which may have immune-enhancing and antiviral properties; and bioflavonoids (companions of vitamin C), particularly quercitin, which may inhibit reverse transcriptase.

In the matter of sexual practices, the statistical correlations between HIV/AIDS and sex habits is noticeable in three areas: multiplicity of sexual partners, receptive and insertive anal sex and penile-vaginal sex.

Despite the howlings of moralists exhorting to abstinence and celibacy (excellent suggestions for candidates for the sainthood and altogether admirable) or at the very least long-standing monogamous relationships, it is biologically unreasonable and even socially unsound to campaign against sex itself, however collectively purgative such thinking may be.

The sexual correlation with HIV/AIDS in effect means that ultimately the entire sexually active population of the planet is ostensibly and potentially "at risk", and if societal norms were changed to act on this possibility there would be a mass decrease in human population.

Therefore, logic and prudence suggest constraints on promiscuity, great concern for hygiene and, at the very least, the use of condoms and spermicides in penile-vaginal intercourse, and avoidance of anal intercourse altogether.

With years of research now apparent, there simply statistically are no meaningful correlations between oral-genital sex and "deep kissing" and HIV/AIDS, but because modes of transmission are absolutely *not* fully specific and the possibility that other routes of infection may occur, simple prudence and caution are dictated in the latter two areas.

The avoidance of drug use, particularly when adjunctive to sexual activity, and, when all else fails, non-sharing and/or sterilization of needles, are also clearly imperative.

A return to courtship, to marital and relationship fidelity and a constant awareness that one should truly know the life and habits of a sex partner are reasonable approaches to dealing with HIV/AIDS.

Eight years from the naming of the syndrome and

six years from the "discovery" of its unlikely single cause, in the "age of AIDS" prudence in diet, prudence in lifestyle, prudence in sex, and implementation of the Golden Rule remain the rational approaches to prevention.

APPENDIX I

THE HIV/LAS/ARC/AIDS INFECTION CURVE

Presumably, the entire curve of infection whose end stage is "full-blown" AIDS (See *Revision of CDC Surveillance Case Definition for Acquired Immunodeficiency Syndrome*) begins with exposure, or exposures, to the Human Immunodeficiency Virus (HIV). Symptoms of this exposure may be noticeable as early as 6 days (flu-like symptoms persisting days or weeks), or there may be no symptoms for months, years -- or ever. It is not certain when antibodies form to HIV (this may be months to years). Blood may turn "seropositive" for HIV antibodies in the absence of physical symptoms; there may be symptoms suggestive of the HIV/AIDS infection curve without "seropositivity" for HIV antibodies.

Following exposure or exposures to HIV (or the factors causing the infection curve) there may be a period of months to years in which pathological complaints are relatively minor. They may include but not be limited to occasional generalized fatigue, occasional night sweats, spiking fevers, other flu-like symptoms, dermatological features, structural pains, possible Herpes zoster (shingles). Any or all of these may suggest immune impairment. An immune panel ("T-cell test") may indicate the classical immunological disturbance common in HIV/AIDS -- inversion of the T4/T8 cellular ratio -- and declining T4s. This test alone does not confirm HIV/AIDS.

For some patients, a lengthy period (several weeks to several months) of hardened lymph glands (lymphadenopathy syndrome -- LAS) with or without flu-like symptoms may mark the first clinical presence of HIV/AIDS, with the blood usually (but not always) "seropositive" for HIV antibodies. The vaguely defined AIDS-Related Complex (ARC) phase, parts of which now overlap with the revised case definition for AIDS, may include persistent chronic fatigue, persistent chronic flu-like symptoms, fevers, swollen glands, generalized *Candida albicans* infection, night sweats, suspicious weight loss, chronic diarrhea, possibly mood swings, joint, muscle and bone pain, dermatological involvements and sleep disturbances. Both "seropositivity" for HIV antibodies and characteristic immune panel distortions are usually apparent at this level. ARC-level symptoms have been known to persist for months to years without advancing to "full-blown" AIDS; some people have died of conditions related to ARC.

NOTE: There are several experimental tests for isolating or culturing HIV or parts of it from blood. These assays may detect HIV infection well before the appearance of antibodies. It is possible that neither antibodies nor virus will be found at the terminal stage of AIDS; there also are cases of appearing and disappearing antibodies and viral particles during the infection curve.

There are other immunological signs which may be associated with HIV/AIDS. The more prominent are reactions to delayed hypersensitivity tests.

THE WALTER REED CLASSIFICATION SYSTEM, which charts the course of patients from apparent exposure to HIV up to and including "full-blown" AIDS, utilizes a level of 400 T4 ("helper") cells per cubic millimeter of blood as an immunological break-even point, and the presence of chronic lymphadenopathy, yeast infection ("thrush"), delayed hypersensitivity tests and HIV antibody or virus positivity as markers (abstracted from *Scientific American,* October 1988.)

WR Stage 1 -- HIV positivity only.

WR Stage 2 -- HIV positivity, chronic lymphadenopathy only.

WR Stage 3 -- HIV positivity, with or without chronic lymphadenopathy, T4 cells below 400.

WR Stage 4 -- HIV positivity, with or without chronic lymphadenopathy, T4 cells below 400, partial defect in delayed hypersensitivity.

WR Stage 5 -- HIV positivity, with or without chronic lymphadenopathy, T4 cells below 400, complete failure to respond to delayed hypersensitivity tests, and/or thrush.

WR Stage 6 -- HIV positivity, with or without chronic lymphadenopathy, T4 cells below 400, partial or complete failure on delayed hypersensitivity tests, with or without thrush, and with opportunistic infections.

Actual AIDS (see following) consists of a varying number of "opportunistic" infections and, usually, blood tests to confirm HIV antibodies or active virus, and immunological disturbances.

Revision of the CDC Surveillance Case Definition for Acquired Immunodeficiency Syndrome

Reported by
Council of State and Territorial Epidemiologists;
AIDS Program, Center for Infectious Diseases, CDC

INTRODUCTION

The following revised case definition for surveillance of acquired immunodeficiency syndrome (AIDS) was developed by CDC in collaboration with public health and clinical specialists. The Council of State and Territorial Epidemiologists (CSTE) has officially recommended adoption of the revised definition for national reporting of AIDS. The objectives of the revision are a) to track more effectively the severe disabling morbidity associated with infection with human immunodeficiency virus (HIV) (including HIV-1 and HIV-2); b) to simplify reporting of AIDS cases; c) to increase the sensitivity and specificity of the definition through greater diagnostic application of laboratory evidence for HIV infection; and d) to be consistent with current diagnostic practice, which in some cases includes presumptive, i.e., without confirmatory laboratory evidence, diagnosis of AIDS-indicative diseases (e.g., *Pneumocystis carinii* pneumonia, Kaposi's sarcoma).

The definition is organized into three sections that depend on the status of laboratory evidence of HIV infection (e.g., HIV antibody) (Figure 1). The major proposed changes apply to patients with laboratory evidence for HIV infection: a) inclusion of HIV encephalopathy, HIV wasting syndrome, and a broader range of specific AIDS-indicative diseases (Section II.A); b) inclusion of AIDS patients whose indicator diseases are diagnosed presumptively (Section II.B); and c) elimination of exclusions due to other causes of immunodeficiency (Section I.A).

Application of the definition for children differs from that for adults in two ways. First, multiple or recurrent serious bacterial infections and lymphoid interstitial pneumonia/pulmonary lymphoid hyperplasia are accepted as indicative of AIDS among children but not among adults. Second, for children<15 months of age whose mothers are thought to have had HIV infection during the child's perinatal period, the laboratory criteria for HIV infection are more stringent, since the presence of HIV antibody in the child is, by itself, insufficient evidence for HIV infection because of the persistence of passively acquired maternal antibodies < 15 months after birth.

The new definition is effective immediately. State and local health departments are requested to apply the new definition henceforth to patients reported to them. The initiation of the actual reporting of cases that meet the new definition is targeted for September 1, 1987, when modified computer software and report forms should be in place to accommodate the changes. CSTE has recommended retrospective application of the revised definition to patients already reported to health departments. The new definition follows:

1987 REVISION OF CASE DEFINITION FOR AIDS FOR SURVEILLANCE PURPOSES

For national reporting, a case of AIDS is defined as an illness characterized by one or more of the following "indicator" diseases, depending on the status of laboratory evidence of HIV infection, as shown below.

I. Without Laboratory Evidence Regarding HIV Infection

If laboratory tests for HIV were not performed or gave inconclusive results (See Appendix I) and the patient had no other cause of immunodeficiency listed in Section I.A below, then any disease listed in Section I.B indicates AIDS if it was diagnosed by a definitive method (See Appendix II).

A. Causes of immunodeficiency that disqualify diseases as indicators of AIDS in the absence of laboratory evidence for HIV infection

1. high-dose or long-term systemic corticosteroid therapy or other immuno-suppressive/cytotoxic therapy ≤3 months before the onset of the indicator disease

2. any of the following diseases diagnosed ≤3 months after diagnosis of the indicator disease: Hodgkin's disease, non-Hodgkin's lymphoma (other than primary brain lymphoma), lymphocytic leukemia, multiple myeloma, any other cancer of lymphoreticular or histiocytic tissue, or angioimmu-noblastic lymphadenopathy

3. a genetic (congenital) immunodeficiency syndrome or an acquired immu-nodeficiency syndrome atypical of HIV infection, such as one involving hypogammaglobulinemia

B. Indicator diseases diagnosed definitively (See Appendix II)

1. candidiasis of the esophagus, trachea, bronchi, or lungs
2. cryptococcosis, extrapulmonary
3. cryptosporidiosis with diarrhea persisting >1 month
4. cytomegalovirus disease of an organ other than liver, spleen, or lymph nodes in a patient >1 month of age
5. herpes simplex virus infection causing a mucocutaneous ulcer that persists longer than 1 month; or bronchitis, pneumonitis, or esophagitis for any duration affecting a patient >1 month of age
6. Kaposi's sarcoma affecting a patient < 60 years of age
7. lymphoma of the brain (primary) affecting a patient < 60 years of age
8. lymphoid interstitial pneumonia and/or pulmonary lymphoid hyperplasia (LIP/PLH complex) affecting a child <13 years of age
9. *Mycobacterium avium* complex or *M. kansasii* disease, disseminated (at a site other than or in addition to lungs, skin, or cervical or hilar lymph nodes)
10. *Pneumocystis carinii* pneumonia
11. progressive multifocal leukoencephalopathy
12. toxoplasmosis of the brain affecting a patient >1 month of age

II. With Laboratory Evidence for HIV Infection

Regardless of the presence of other causes of immunodeficiency (I.A), in the presence of laboratory evidence for HIV infection (See Appendix I), any disease listed above (I.B) or below (II.A or II.B) indicates a diagnosis of AIDS.

A. Indicator diseases diagnosed definitively (*See* Appendix II)

1. bacterial infections, multiple or recurrent (any combination of at least two within a 2-year period), of the following types affecting a child < 13 years of age:

   septicemia, pneumonia, meningitis, bone or joint infection, or abscess of an internal organ or body cavity (excluding otitis media or superficial skin or mucosal abscesses), caused by *Haemophilus*, *Streptococcus* (including pneumococcus), or other pyogenic bacteria

2. coccidioidomycosis, disseminated (at a site other than or in addition to lungs or cervical or hilar lymph nodes)

3. HIV encephalopathy (also called "HIV dementia," "AIDS dementia," or "subacute encephalitis due to HIV") (*See* Appendix II for description)

4. histoplasmosis, disseminated (at a site other than or in addition to lungs or cervical or hilar lymph nodes)

5. isosporiasis with diarrhea persisting >1 month

6. Kaposi's sarcoma at any age

7. lymphoma of the brain (primary) at any age

8. other non-Hodgkin's lymphoma of B-cell or unknown immunologic phenotype and the following histologic types:

   a. small noncleaved lymphoma (either Burkitt or non-Burkitt type) (*See* Appendix IV for equivalent terms and numeric codes used in the *International Classification of Diseases*, Ninth Revision, Clinical Modification)

   b. immunoblastic sarcoma (equivalent to any of the following, although not necessarily all in combination: immunoblastic lymphoma, large-cell lymphoma, diffuse histiocytic lymphoma, diffuse undifferentiated lymphoma, or high-grade lymphoma) (*See* Appendix IV for equivalent terms and numeric codes used in the *International Classification of Diseases*, Ninth Revision, Clinical Modification)

   Note: Lymphomas are not included here if they are of T-cell immunologic phenotype or their histologic type is not described or is described as "lymphocytic," "lymphoblastic," "small cleaved," or "plasmacytoid lymphocytic"

9. any mycobacterial disease caused by mycobacteria other than *M. tuberculosis*, disseminated (at a site other than or in addition to lungs, skin, or cervical or hilar lymph nodes)

10. disease caused by *M. tuberculosis*, extrapulmonary (involving at least one site outside the lungs, regardless of whether there is concurrent pulmonary involvement)

11. *Salmonella* (nontyphoid) septicemia, recurrent

12. HIV wasting syndrome (emaciation, "slim disease") (*See* Appendix II for description)

B. Indicator diseases diagnosed presumptively (by a method other than those in Appendix II)

Note: Given the seriousness of diseases indicative of AIDS, it is generally important to diagnose them definitively, especially when therapy that would be used may have serious side effects or when definitive diagnosis is needed for eligibility for antiretroviral therapy. Nonetheless, in some situations, a patient's condition will not permit the performance of definitive tests. In other situations, accepted clinical practice may be to diagnose presumptively based on the presence of characteristic clinical and laboratory abnormalities. Guidelines for presumptive diagnoses are suggested in Appendix III.

1. candidiasis of the esophagus
2. cytomegalovirus retinitis with loss of vision
3. Kaposi's sarcoma
4. lymphoid interstitial pneumonia and/or pulmonary lymphoid hyperplasia (LIP/PLH complex) affecting a child <13 years of age
5. mycobacterial disease (acid-fast bacilli with species not identified by culture), disseminated (involving at least one site other than or in addition to lungs, skin, or cervical or hilar lymph nodes)
6. *Pneumocystis carinii* pneumonia
7. toxoplasmosis of the brain affecting a patient >1 month of age

III. With Laboratory Evidence Against HIV Infection

With laboratory test results negative for HIV infection (*See* Appendix I), a diagnosis of AIDS for surveillance purposes is ruled out *unless*:

A. all the other causes of immunodeficiency listed above in Section I.A are excluded; AND
B. the patient has had either:
   1. *Pneumocystis carinii* pneumonia diagnosed by a definitive method (*See* Appendix II); OR
   2. a. any of the other diseases indicative of AIDS listed above in Section I.B diagnosed by a definitive method (*See* Appendix II); AND
      b. a T-helper/inducer (CD4) lymphocyte count <400/mm^3.

COMMENTARY

The surveillance of severe disease associated with HIV infection remains an essential, though not the only, indicator of the course of the HIV epidemic. The number of AIDS cases and the relative distribution of cases by demographic, geographic, and behavioral risk variables are the oldest indices of the epidemic, which began in 1981 and for which data are available retrospectively back to 1978. The original surveillance case definition, based on then-available knowledge, provided useful epidemiologic data on severe HIV disease (*1*). To ensure a reasonable predictive value for underlying immunodeficiency caused by what was then an unknown agent, the indicators of AIDS in the old case definition were restricted to particular opportunistic diseases diagnosed by reliable methods in patients without specific known causes of immunodeficiency. After HIV was discovered to be the cause of AIDS, however, and highly sensitive and specific HIV-antibody tests became available, the spectrum of manifestations of HIV infection became better defined, and classification systems for HIV infection were developed (*2-5*). It became apparent that some progressive, seriously disabling, and even fatal conditions (e.g., encephalopathy, wasting syndrome) affecting a substantial number of HIV-infected patients were not subject to epidemiologic surveillance, as they were not included in the AIDS case definition. For reporting purposes, the revision adds to the definition most of those severe non-infectious, non-cancerous HIV-associated conditions that are categorized in the CDC clinical classification systems for HIV infection among adults and children (4,5).

Another limitation of the old definition was that AIDS-indicative diseases are diagnosed presumptively (i.e., without confirmation by methods required by the old definition) in 10%-15% of patients diagnosed with such diseases; thus, an appreciable proportion of AIDS cases were missed for reporting purposes (6,7). This proportion may be increasing, which would compromise the old case definition's usefulness as a tool for monitoring trends. The revised case definition permits the reporting of these clinically diagnosed cases as long as there is laboratory evidence of HIV infection.

The effectiveness of the revision will depend on how extensively HIV-antibody tests are used. Approximately one third of AIDS patients in the United States have been from New York City and San Francisco, where, since 1985, < 7% have been reported with HIV-antibody test results, compared with > 60% in other areas. The impact of the revision on the reported numbers of AIDS cases will also depend on the proportion of AIDS patients in whom indicator diseases are diagnosed presumptively rather than definitively. The use of presumptive diagnostic criteria varies geographically, being more common in certain rural areas and in urban areas with many indigent AIDS patients.

To avoid confusion about what should be reported to health departments, the term "AIDS" should refer only to conditions meeting the surveillance definition. This definition is intended only to provide consistent statistical data for public health purposes. Clinicians will not rely on this definition alone to diagnose serious disease caused by HIV infection in individual patients because there may be additional information that would lead to a more accurate diagnosis. For example, patients who are not reportable under the definition because they have either a negative HIV-antibody test or, in the presence of HIV antibody, an opportunistic disease not listed in the definition as an indicator of AIDS nonetheless may be diagnosed as having serious HIV disease on consideration of other clinical or laboratory characteristics of HIV infection or a history of exposure to HIV.

Conversely, the AIDS surveillance definition may rarely misclassify other patients as having serious HIV disease if they have no HIV-antibody test but have an AIDS-indicative disease with a background incidence unrelated to HIV infection, such as cryptococcal meningitis.

The diagnostic criteria accepted by the AIDS surveillance case definition should not be interpreted as the standard of good medical practice. Presumptive diagnoses are accepted in the definition because not to count them would be to ignore substantial morbidity resulting from HIV infection. Likewise, the definition accepts a reactive screening test for HIV antibody without confirmation by a supplemental test because a repeatedly reactive screening test result, in combination with an indicator disease, is highly indicative of true HIV disease. For national surveillance purposes, the tiny proportion of possibly false-positive screening tests in persons with AIDS-indicative diseases is of little consequence. For the individual patient, however, a correct diagnosis is critically important. The use of supplemental tests is, therefore, strongly endorsed. An increase in the diagnostic use of HIV-antibody tests could improve both the quality of medical care and the function of the new case definition, as well as assist in providing counselling to prevent transmission of HIV.

FIGURE I. Flow diagram for revised CDC case definition of AIDS, September 1, 1987

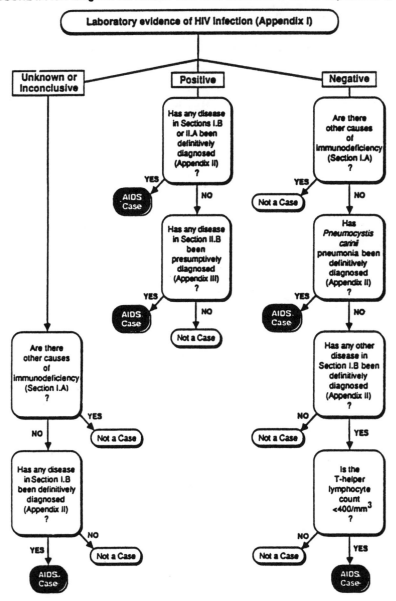

References

1. World Health Organization. Acquired immunodeficiency syndrome (AIDS): WHO/CDC case definition for AIDS. WHO Wkly Epidemiol Rec 1986;61:69-72.
2. Haverkos HW, Gottlieb MS, Killen JY, Edelman R. Classification of HTLV-III/LAV-related diseases [Letter]. J Infect Dis 1985;152:1095.
3. Redfield RR, Wright DC, Tramont EC. The Walter Reed staging classification of HTLV-III infection. N Engl J Med 1986;314:131-2.
4. CDC. Classification system for human T-lymphotropic virus type III/lymphadenopathy-associated virus infections. MMWR 1986;35:334-9.
5. CDC. Classification system for human immunodeficiency virus (HIV) infection in children under 13 years of age. MMWR 1987;36:225-30,235.
6. Hardy AM, Starcher ET, Morgan WM, et al. Review of death certificates to assess completeness of AIDS case reporting. Pub Hlth Rep 1987;102(4):386-91.
7. Starcher ET, Biel JK, Rivera-Castano R, Day JM, Hopkins SG, Miller JW. The impact of presumptively diagnosed opportunistic infections and cancers on national reporting of AIDS [Abstract]. Washington, DC : III International Conference on AIDS, June 1-5, 1987.

APPENDIX I

Laboratory Evidence For or Against HIV Infection

1. **For Infection:**
   When a patient has disease consistent with AIDS:
   a. a serum specimen from a patient ≥15 months of age, or from a child <15 months of age whose mother is not thought to have had HIV infection during the child's perinatal period, that is repeatedly reactive for HIV antibody by a screening test (e.g., enzyme-linked immunosorbent assay [ELISA]), as long as subsequent HIV-antibody tests (e.g., Western blot, immunofluorescence assay), if done, are positive; **OR**
   b. a serum specimen from a child < 15 months of age, whose mother is thought to have had HIV infection during the child's perinatal period, that is repeatedly reactive for HIV antibody by a screening test (e.g., ELISA), plus increased serum immunoglobulin levels and at least one of the following abnormal immunologic test results: reduced absolute lymphocyte count, depressed CD4 (T-helper) lymphocyte count, or decreased CD4/CD8 (helper/suppressor) ratio, as long as subsequent antibody tests (e.g., Western blot, immunofluorescence assay), if done, are positive; **OR**
   c. a positive test for HIV serum antigen; **OR**
   d. a positive HIV culture confirmed by both reverse transcriptase detection and a specific HIV-antigen test or in situ hybridization using a nucleic acid probe; **OR**
   e. a positive result on any other highly specific test for HIV (e.g., nucleic acid probe of peripheral blood lymphocytes).

2. **Against Infection:**
   A nonreactive screening test for serum antibody to HIV (e.g., ELISA) without a reactive or positive result on any other test for HIV infection (e.g., antibody, antigen, culture), if done.

3. **Inconclusive (Neither For nor Against Infection):**
   a. a repeatedly reactive screening test for serum antibody to HIV (e.g., ELISA) followed by a negative or inconclusive supplemental test (e.g., Western blot, immunofluorescence assay) without a positive HIV culture or serum antigen test, if done; **OR**
   b. a serum specimen from a child < 15 months of age, whose mother is thought to have had HIV infection during the child's perinatal period, that is repeatedly reactive for HIV antibody by a screening test, even if positive by a supplemental test, without additional evidence for immunodeficiency as described above (in 1.b) and without a positive HIV culture or serum antigen test, if done.

APPENDIX II

Definitive Diagnostic Methods for Diseases Indicative of AIDS

Diseases	Definitive Diagnostic Methods

cryptosporidiosis
cytomegalovirus
isosporiasis
Kaposi's sarcoma
lymphoma
lymphoid pneumonia
  or hyperplasia
Pneumocystis carinii
  pneumonia
progressive multifocal
  leukoencephalopathy
toxoplasmosis
	microscopy (histology or cytology).

candidiasis	gross inspection by endoscopy or autopsy or by microscopy (histology or cytology) on a specimen obtained directly from the tissues affected (including scrapings from the mucosal surface), not from a culture.
coccidioidomycosis cryptococcosis herpes simplex virus histoplasmosis	microscopy (histology or cytology), culture, or detection of antigen in a specimen obtained directly from the tissues affected or a fluid from those tissues.
tuberculosis other mycobacteriosis salmonellosis other bacterial infection	culture.

HIV encephalopathy*
(dementia)

clinical findings of disabling cognitive and/or motor dysfunction interfering with occupation or activities of daily living, or loss of behavioral developmental milestones affecting a child, progressing over weeks to months, in the absence of a concurrent illness or condition other than HIV infection that could explain the findings. Methods to rule out such concurrent illnesses and conditions must include cerebrospinal fluid examination and either brain imaging (computed tomography or magnetic resonance) or autopsy.

HIV wasting syndrome*

findings of profound involuntary weight loss >10% of baseline body weight plus either chronic diarrhea (at least two loose stools per day for ≥ 30 days) or chronic weakness and documented fever (for ≥ 30 days, intermittent or constant) in the absence of a concurrent illness or condition other than HIV infection that could explain the findings (e.g., cancer, tuberculosis, cryptosporidiosis, or other specific enteritis).

*For HIV encephalopathy and HIV wasting syndrome, the methods of diagnosis described here are not truly definitive, but are sufficiently rigorous for surveillance purposes.

APPENDIX III

Suggested Guidelines for Presumptive Diagnosis of Diseases Indicative of AIDS

Diseases	Presumptive Diagnostic Criteria
candidiasis of esophagus	a. recent onset of retrosternal pain on swallowing; AND b. oral candidiasis diagnosed by the gross appearance of white patches or plaques on an erythematous base or by the microscopic appearance of fungal mycelial filaments in an uncultured specimen scraped from the oral mucosa.
cytomegalovirus retinitis	a characteristic appearance on serial ophthalmoscopic examinations (e.g., discrete patches of retinal whitening with distinct borders, spreading in a centrifugal manner, following blood vessels, progressing over several months, frequently associated with retinal vasculitis, hemorrhage, and necrosis). Resolution of active disease leaves retinal scarring and atrophy with retinal pigment epithelial mottling.
mycobacteriosis	microscopy of a specimen from stool or normally sterile body fluids or tissue from a site other than lungs, skin, or cervical or hilar lymph nodes, showing acid-fast bacilli of a species not identified by culture.
Kaposi's sarcoma	a characteristic gross appearance of an erythematous or violaceous plaque-like lesion on skin or mucous membrane. (Note: Presumptive diagnosis of Kaposi's sarcoma should not be made by clinicians who have seen few cases of it.)
lymphoid interstitial pneumonia	bilateral reticulonodular interstitial pulmonary infiltrates present on chest X ray for ≥2 months with no pathogen identified and no response to antibiotic treatment.
Pneumocystis carinii pneumonia	a. a history of dyspnea on exertion or nonproductive cough of recent onset (within the past 3 months); AND b. chest X-ray evidence of diffuse bilateral interstitial infiltrates or gallium scan evidence of diffuse bilateral pulmonary disease; AND c. arterial blood gas analysis showing an arterial pO_2 of <70 mm Hg or a low respiratory diffusing capacity (<80% of predicted values) or an increase in the alveolar-arterial oxygen tension gradient; AND d. no evidence of a bacterial pneumonia.

toxoplasmosis of the brain	a. recent onset of a focal neurologic abnormality consistent with intracranial disease or a reduced level of consciousness; **AND**
	b. brain imaging evidence of a lesion having a mass effect (on computed tomography or nuclear magnetic resonance) or the radiographic appearance of which is enhanced by injection of contrast medium; **AND**
	c. serum antibody to toxoplasmosis or successful response to therapy for toxoplasmosis.

APPENDIX II

DRUG INDUSTRY AND GENETIC ENGINEERING-DERIVED SUBSTANCES AND TECHNIQUES IN USE OR INVESTIGATION IN THE HIV/AIDS INFECTION CURVE. (Some of these are listed as "alternatives" in Appendix III.) Not included here are various medications long authorized for use in various bacterial, parasite, and fungal infections and as anti-cancer treatments or anti-dementia medications. Some "old drugs" found particularly useful in some expressions of AIDS are included. "U.S. Status" refers to the approximate legal status of these medications as of 1990 in the U.S., if known.

COMPOUND	POSSIBLE MODE OF ACTION/STATUS
ACTIVATED CD8 CELLS	Removal, separation, treatment with interleukin-2 and other genetically engineered material of CD8 ("suppressor") cells may booster a natural defense mechanism against HIV/AIDS. **U.S. STATUS** -- investigation
ACYCLOVIR (a/k/a/ Zovirax)	antiviral useful against herpesvirus and possibly other viruses. **U.S. STATUS** -- experimentally legal in U.S. ; authorized for herpes therapy
AEROSOL PENTAMIDINE	aerosol form of Pentamidine, used for over 40 years as an anti-parasite drug; particularly useful against **Pneumocystis carinii**. **U.S. STATUS** -- authorized
AME(AMPHOTERICIN METHYL ESTER)	water-soluble derivative of amphotericin-B, an anti-fungal; some suggestion of anti-HIV activity. **U.S. STATUS** -- investigation
AMPLIGEN (mismatched, double-stranded RNA)	possible antiviral, immune-boosting effects with no toxicity and clinical improvement, but earlier research not confirmed. **U.S. STATUS** -- investigation

278

COMPOUND	POSSIBLE MODE OF ACTION/STATUS
ANSAMYCIN (a/k/a Rifabutin, Rifabutine)	experimental drug possibly useful against M.A.I., with other drugs and may have anti-HIV effects. **U.S. STATUS** -- investigation
ANTABUSE (a/k/a Disulfiram)	a prescription drug used to treat alcoholism, Antabuse is said by some to be an alternative to Imuthiol (DTC). **U.S. STATUS** -- investigation
AS-101	potential immune-modulating agent. **U.S. STATUS** -- investigation
AVAROL, AVARONE	antimitotic, antimutagenic agents from the marine sponge **Dysidea avara**. **U.S. STATUS** -- investigation
AZIDOURIDINE (AzdU, CS-87)	a drug found to be non-toxic in animals and active against HIV in vitro. **U.S. STATUS** -- investigation
AZITHROMYCIN	Yugoslavia-approved antibiotic effective in toxoplasmosis in mice; may have human application.
AZT (a/k/a azidothymidine, zidovudine, Retrovir)	reverse transcriptase inhibitor useful against HIV, probably synergistic with several other drugs. **U.S. STATUS** -- authorized
BHT	food preservative shown to have some antiviral effects, may inhibit or inactivate lipid-coated viruses. **U.S. STATUS** -- investigation
BILE SALTS	inactivated HIV in vitro and destroyed persistently HIV-infected cells. **U.S. STATUS** -- investigation
BLUE-GREEN ALGAE	U.S. National Cancer Institute research has confirmed that compounds in two strains of blue-green algae protect human T-cells from HIV; chemicals derived therefrom said active against HIV in vitro. **U.S. STATUS** -- investigation
BONE MARROW GRAFTS	technique for immune system reconstitution; some evidence of improvement in HIV/AIDS. **U.S. STATUS** -- investigation

279

COMPOUND	POSSIBLE MODE OF ACTION/STATUS
CARRISYN	a stable acetylated sugar derived from Aloe Vera may have antiviral properties. **U.S. STATUS** -- investigation
CASTANOSPERMINE	substance found in an Australian chestnut inhibits HIV <u>in vitro</u>. **U.S. STATUS** -- investigation
CD4 (SOLUBLE CD4)	a genetically altered protein found on helper cell receptor sites, Soluble CD4 may provide a bogus target for HIV. **U.S. STATUS** -- investigation
CIPROFLOXACIN	new drug may be useful in combination with anti-tuberculosis drugs against M.A.I. infection. **U.S. STATUS** -- investigation
CLINDAMYCIN/ PRIMAQUINE combination	Canadian research shows this is an effective combination against Pneumocystis pneumonia, with the major side effect being a maculopapular rash; Clindamycin has also been found useful against staphylococcal skin infections in AIDS. **U.S. STATUS** -- investigation
COMPOUND Q (GLQ-223, Tricosanthin)	a highly purified extract of a protein from a Chinese cucumber root; <u>in</u> <u>vitro</u> studies showed macrophage-killing capability; human trials began in 1989. **U.S. STATUS** -- cleared for human trials
D4T	a nucleoside analog, animal and laboratory tests find this drug less toxic than AZT and effective against HIV. **U.S. STATUS** -- investigation
D-PENICILLAMINE	antiviral drug, found possibly useful in LAS, ARC and as HIV suppressor but has side effects. **U.S. STATUS** -- investigation
DAPSONE	drug authorized for use in leprosy; mixed results against HIV. **U.S. STATUS** -- investigation
DDA (DIDEOXYADENOSINE)	experimental antiviral drug may work synergistically with AZT or DDC against HIV. **U.S. STATUS** -- investigation

COMPOUND	POSSIBLE MODE OF ACTION/STATUS
DDC **(DIDEOXYCYTIDINE)**	antiviral which provides false building bloc for HIV, may be synergistic with AZT, seems to reduce toxicity of latter. <u>**U.S. STATUS**</u> -- investigation
DDI **(DIDEOXYINOSINE)**	originally thought less toxic than AZT, fatal pancreatitis developed in several patients given experimental doses of this nucleoside analog. Has antiviral properties. <u>**U.S. STATUS**</u> -- investigation
DEXTRAN SULFATE	anti-arteriosclerotic drug used as antiviral; inhibits reverse transcriptase, blocks formation of syncytial cells, useful with AZT, widely used in several countries but not yet authorized in U.S.A. 1989 research said not promising in HIV/AIDS. <u>**U.S. STATUS**</u> -- investigation
DHEA **(DEHYDROEPIANDROSTERONE)**	adrenal hormone or manufactured version thereof, apparently useful in immune modulation. <u>**U.S. STATUS**</u> -- investigation
DHPG (a/k/a **Ganciclovir,** **Cytovene)** **(DIHYDROXYPROPOXYMETHYL-GUANINE)**	may have antiviral properties, may be useful in CMV retinitis, CMV colitis. <u>**U.S. STATUS**</u> -- authorized
DICLAZURIL	Zairian research indicates effectiveness against AIDS-related diarrhea caused by <u>Isopora</u> <u>belli</u>; may be effective against several parasites and for use in cryptosporidiosis.
DIPYRIDAMOLE (DPM) **(Persantine)**	anti-clotting drug may be useful in enhancing activity of AZT and DDC; U.S. research. <u>**U.S. STATUS**</u> -- investigation
DNCB **(DINITROCHLOROBENZENE)**	industrial chemical possibly useful in immune modulation. <u>**U.S. STATUS**</u> -- investigation
FANSIDAR	anti-malarial drug useful against pneumocystis, though with side effects. <u>**U.S. STATUS**</u> -- investigation
FLT **(Fluorodeoxythymidine)**	Swedish research claims this failed anti-cancer drug is more effective than AZT (laboratory cultures) and is active against a simian AIDS virus.

COMPOUND	POSSIBLE MODE OF ACTION/STATUS

FLUCONAZOLE experimental drug for systemic fungal infections, esp. cryptococcal meningitis, though may have broader uses. **U.S. STATUS** -- authorized

FOSCARNET (TRISODIUM PHOSPHONOFORMATE) Swedish antiviral shown effective in CMV infections, indication of HIV efficacy, useful in acyclovir-resistant herpes. **U.S. STATUS** -- investigation

FUSIDIN (FUSIDIC ACID) antibiotic marketed since 1962, seems to protect cells from HIV, may be toxic to uninfected cells; foreign research. **U.S. STATUS** -- investigation

GM CSF (GRANULOCYTE-MACROPHAGE COLONY STIMULATING FACTOR) genetically engineered booster has increased white blood cell counts. **U.S. STATUS** -- investigation

HEPT (hydroxyethoxymethyl-phenylthiothymine) Japanese antiviral seems to work against HIV in T-cells and macrophages.

HOE/BAY 964 German research reported this (hydrogensulfate) disodium salt as possible HIV inhibitor.

HPA 23 French antiviral drug with side effects; some success in HIV inhibition; reverse transcriptase inhibitor. **U.S. STATUS** -- investigation

HPMC(a/k/a/ (S)-HPMC) Belgian research suggests in vitro efficacy against cytomegalovirus

HYBRIDONS reported "designer drug" said to inhibit HIV in laboratory tests. **U.S. STATUS** -- investigation

IMMUNE-GLOBULIN IG-IV potential immune modulating agent. **U.S. STATUS** -- investigation

IMREG 1 extract of human white blood cells; may help increase T4 cells. **U.S. STATUS** -- investigation

COMPOUND	POSSIBLE MODE OF ACTION/STATUS

IMUTHIOL (a/k/a/ DTC, Ditiocarb) (DIETHYLDITHI- OCARBAMATE)

chemical long used in agriculture, this French product shows immune modulating and antiviral properties with little toxicity. **U.S. STATUS** -- investigation

INTERFERONS

alpha-interferon seen to have antiviral, possible anticancer effects, may work well with AZT, particularly in Kaposi's sarcoma. **U.S. STATUS** -- authorized

BETA-INTERFERON **U.S. STATUS** -- investigation

GAMMA-INTERFERON **U.S. STATUS** -- investigation **(highly toxic)**

INTERLEUKIN-2

high-tech immune modulator, possibly useful in combination therapy, thought too toxic for long-term use. **U.S. STATUS** -- investigation

ISOPRINOSINE (Methisoprinol)

manufactured immune-modulator, drug has shown considerable immune-boosting benefits in foreign research but remains unauthorized in U.S.A.. **U.S. STATUS** -- investigation

LEVAMISOL

an immunotropic experimental antiviral drug, esp. against herpes. **U.S. STATUS** -- investigation

MEGACE (Megestrol Acetate)

anti-cancer drug apparently helps in stimulating appetite and weight gain and may contribute to patient longevity. **U.S. STATUS** -- investigation

METHIONINE- ENKEPALIN

potential immune modulating agent. **U.S. STATUS** -- investigation

MM-1

"secret" antiviral drug tested in Egypt and Zaire; origin unknown; no side effects reported

MONOCLONAL ANTIBODIES

manmade antibodies to fight infections. **U.S. STATUS** -- investigation

COMPOUND	POSSIBLE MODE OF ACTION/STATUS
MONOPHOSPHORYL LIPID (MPL)	some research suggests this product may selectively reduce the activity of T8 cells. **U.S. STATUS** -- investigation
NAC (n-acetylcysteine)	European bronchitis drug, a potent antioxidant, inhibits HIV in vitro, seems to be a mild immune modulator. **U.S. STATUS** -- investigation
NALTREXONE	drug already authorized as opiate addiction blocker in drug users; may have immune modulating, anti-infective capability. **U.S. STATUS** -- investigation
PAP (pokeweed antiviral protein)	Fused with a monoclonal antibody, PAP slows down HIV reproduction, spares most unifected cells. **U.S. STATUS** -- investigation
PASSIVE IMMUNOTHERAPY	infusing of plasma from otherwise healthy HIV antibody-positive donors into advanced HIV/AIDS patients has led to transient improvements in antibody tests, reduction in symptoms, increase in T-lymphocytes, decrease in culturable HIV. **U.S. STATUS** -- investigation
PENICILLIN	broad-spectrum antibiotic may be useful in various manifestations of HIV/AIDS; some assume certain if not all manifestations of HIV/AIDS are syphilis. **U.S. STATUS** -- investigation (recommended as adjuvant therapy)
PEPTIDE T	an amino acid combination version of a natural brain hormone, Peptide T may hinder HIV cell binding, has been associated with reduced infection of T4 cells, improvement in full-blown AIDS patients, improved memory, no toxicity. **U.S. STATUS** -- investigation
PHOSPHOROTHIOATE ANALOGS OF OLIGODEOXYNUCLEOTIDES	refers to a new class of antiviral agents said to be effective in different degrees against HIV. **U.S. STATUS** -- investigation
PSEUDOMONAS EXOTOXIN A	a "redesigned" very potent poison complexed with CD4 protein and E.coli kills HIV-infected white blood cells in vitro. **U.S. STATUS** -- investigation

COMPOUND	POSSIBLE MODE OF ACTION/STATUS
R82150	Belgian/U.S. research suggests antiviral activity in animals with no appreciable toxicity. **U.S. STATUS** -- investigation
RECOMBINANT ERYTHROPOIETIN	genetically engineered version of a natural hormone stimulates red blood cell production; useful against AZT-induced anemia. **U.S. STATUS** -- authorized
RIBAVIRIN (a/k/a/ Virazole, Vilona)	considerable research indicates antiviral activity; may be reverse transcriptase or viral mRNA inhibitor; still unauthorized in U.S.A.; little toxicity particularly in multiphase programs. **U.S. STATUS** -- investigation
ROXITHROMYCIN	this French antibiotic shows anti-toxoplasmosis activity in test animals and crosses the blood-brain barrier in humans.
SALK HIV VACCINE	Clinical trials underway in U.S. of HIV vaccine for persons already infected. **U.S. STATUS** -- clinical trials
TAGAMET	this anti-ulcer drug has shown immune-enhancing, anti-herpervirus family activity. **U.S. STATUS** -- investigation
THYMIC HUMORAL FACTOR	thymus-derived agent may be immune modulator. **U.S. STATUS** -- investigation
THYMOPENTIN	potential immunomodulating agent. **U.S. STATUS** -- investigation
THYMOSTIMULINE	potential immunomodulating agent. **U.S. STATUS** -- investigation
TRIMETHOPRIM/ SULFAMETHOXAZOLE (a/k/a Bactrim, Septra)	combination antibiotic treatment for acute infections particularly pneumocystis; side effects. **U.S. STATUS** -- authorized
TRIMETREXATE	experimental anticancer drug found useful against pneumocystis, esp. with leucovorin as a "rescue"; potentially very toxic. **U.S. STATUS** -- authorized
TUMOR NECROSIS FACTOR	developed from cancer research, this agent might work synergistically with alpha-interferon against HIV. **U.S. STATUS** -- investigation

COMPOUND	POSSIBLE MODE OF ACTION/STATUS

TYPHOID VACCINE   a number of U.S. doctors now use typhoid vaccine as an immune-enhancer under a U.S. Patent arrangement; is often used in combination with antibiotic therapy under the view that much of AIDS is syphilis.   **U.S. STATUS** -- investigation

UA-001   possible antiviral agent.   **U.S. STATUS** -- investigation

U-81749   One of a class of experimental compounds being developed to inhibit activity of the enzyme protease, said vital to HIV's ability to grow and mature inside cells. Laboratory research only at this point.   **U.S. STATUS** -- investigation

APPENDIX III

"Alternative" methods and substances (usually developed outside the synthetic drug industry) being found useful in HIV/AIDS though not officially authorized for use in the U.S.A. for the syndrome. Some of these are under active scientific investigation by U.S. authorities. Some, while manufactured drugs of American origin (EDTA and DMSO, for example), are recognized for limited conditions and otherwise regarded as unproven in others, including HIV/AIDS. Some of these substances are part of, or work in combination with, other compounds or products. Among the food factors and herbs are several with many properties (typical herbs are "pharmacological nightmares" with many useful -- and not so useful -- ingredients.) All the substances, compounds and products mentioned here have been reported in the literature or anecdotally as useful in the HIV/AIDS infection curve. They may be any of the following: "adaptogenic" (helping the body deal with non-specific stress), "antioxidant" (helping block toxic oxygen products), "immune-modulating" (helping balance the immune system), "immune-enhancing" (helping stimulate the immune system), "anticarcinogenic" (blocking cancer), "anti-inflammatory", "antiseptic", "antibiotic", "antimicrobial", "antibacterial", "antiviral", and "antifungal." (**WARNING:** A number of herbs and natural substances, including mushrooms, may be poisonous, and elevated doses or levels of various compounds may have side effects. Inclusion of any substance, product or method in this list is not a statement of guaranteed benefit in HIV/AIDS. Self-treatment with experimental medicines and many other substances is extremely risky, particularly in life-threatening conditions.)

SUBSTANCE, PRODUCT OR METHOD	PRESUMED USE OR THEORY OF ACTION, COMMENTS
ACIDOPHILUS	food combination of beneficial microorganisms; helps cleanse gastrointestinal tract, has anti-parasite, antifungal properties

287

SUBSTANCE, PRODUCT OR METHOD	PRESUMED USE OR THEORY OF ACTION, COMMENTS
ACUPUNCTURE, ACUPRESSURE	Oriental techniques (needle and touch) to interrupt or stimulate energy flows and block or reduce pain
AL-721 (and several "workalikes")	egg yolk extract, similar to lecithin; an Israeli-research combination of neutral lipids, phosphatidylcholine and phosphatidylethanilamine in a 7:2:1 ratio. Seems to inhibit binding by lipid-coated viruses
ALOE VERA	broad-spectrum herb apparently is antifungal and immune-enhancing; a useful chemical, <u>carrisyn</u>, has been extracted from it
AMINO ACIDS	useful for a wide variety of conditions, amino acids (22 by recent count) are used in various combinations in many metabolic treatment protocols. A balanced formulation is usually a worthwhile supplement, though some suggest the exclusion of arginine if herpes is present. L-cysteine and L- methionine are thought to have immune enhancement potential. The tripeptide (3-member chain) glutathione is a useful antioxidant
BACH BOWEL NOSODES	homeopathic version of vaccines developed by Dr. Edward Bach, London, from a patient's own bowel bacteria. Reportedly useful in many disease conditions
BEE PROPOLIS	the resinous substance gathered by bees from trees (used as cement in hives) may be of benefit against thrush and fungal infections in general and leukoplakia. Extensive anecdotal reports from East Bloc

288

SUBSTANCE, PRODUCT OR METHOD	PRESUMED USE OR THEORY OF ACTION, COMMENTS
BIOELECTRICITY	several methods are being experimentally used to deal with HIV/AIDS through interference in, or adjustment of, electromagnetic fields; these range from topical application of magnets to various wave- and energy- emitting devices (see also FREQUENCY MACHINES)
CHAPARRAL, CHAPARRAL TEA	this extensively studied North American herb has been used as a folk medicine for many years. It has immune-stimulating polysaccharides and has antiseptic, antibiotic, antioxidant and anticarcinogenic properties. Its powerful antioxidant/anticarcinogenic is NDGA. Used as capsules or tea
CHINESE HERBS	from the extensive herbal pharmacopeia of China and the Orient has come a wide selection of herbs with many properties useful in HIV/AIDS. U.S. orthodoxy accepts the anticarcinogenic use of Astragalus membranaceus and Lugustrum lucidum. Anti-HIV activity has been reported in a combination of Lonicera japonica, Lithospermum erythrorhizon, Prunella vulgaris, Viola yedoensis, Epimedium grandiflorum, and licorice root; U.S.-Hong Kong research has suggested this combination in laboratory effectivity against HIV: Viola yedoensis, Arctium lappa, Andrographis paniculata, Lithospermum erythrorhizon, Alternanthera philoxeroides. Schizandra may be antiviral (hepatitis); Ganoderma (Rei-shi mushroom) is immune-enhancing. Many Chinese herbs are currently under study singly or as combinations (e.g., Fu Zheng.)

SUBSTANCE, PRODUCT OR METHOD	PRESUMED USE OR THEORY OF ACTION, COMMENTS
CHIROPRACTIC	spinal manipulations to treat "subluxations" also may help pain relief, stimulate energy
CHLOROPHYLL	chlorophyll, which carries oxygen through living organisms, has been observed to be of benefit in skin, head, respiratory and oral infections and in peptic ulcers, colon disorders and ulcerative colitis. May help immune modulation
CO-ENZYME Q (CO-ENZYME Q10)	discovered in 1957, this natural substance, found in many foods, is used as prescription medicine in Japan for heart disease. Animal studies suggest it may be an immune modulator and may restore balance between different kinds of T-cells
COLONICS	various techniques to cleanse the gastrointestinal tract range from herbal and coffee enemas to the use of machines and boards for deep-bowel cleaning. All are aimed at detoxifying the G.I. tract and helping restore intestinal flora as a major segment of promotive health
CORTISOL ANTAGONISTS	based on the theory that certain drug treatments and processed foods upset the "stress hormone" balance leading to an excess of cortisol (adrenal hormone) which in turn is immunosuppressive and may be a co-factor in HIV/AIDS, some research suggests the use of various "antagonists" to cortisol, including Vitamin C, Dilantin, salicylates, procaine, Lidocaine, DHEA, somatotrophic hormone; hormone imbalance is a target for live-cell therapy, q.v.

SUBSTANCE, PRODUCT OR METHOD	PRESUMED USE OR THEORY OF ACTION, COMMENTS
DIETS	dietary manipulation is a vital part of virtually every multifactorial metabolic therapy. It may range from the restrictive (ma- crobiotic; Gerson) to the generalized meta- program (less animal fats and proteins, more unrefined natural grains, fewer or no refined carbohydrates, fewer or no stimulants, more natural fresh fruits and vegetables, their juices, roots, sprouts) to certain specialized combination foods ("energy soup", for example.) Yeast-free diets are advised for persons in whom yeast infection with **Candida albicans** is a major problem. Regard for biochemical individuality in lieu of food faddism is suggested
DIOXYCHLOR	an oxidative agent researched/developed by American Biologics has antiviral, antibacterial, antifungal properties as an intravenous infusion, topical gel or homeopathic drops. Essentially non-toxic; releases nascent atomic oxygen
DMSO(dimethyl sulfoxide)	this incredible compound, technically authorized only for treatment of a bladder disease, is a carrier agent and has immune-modulating, immune-enhancing, "free radical"-scavenging, anti-inflammatory, analgesic, anticarcinogenic and possibly antiviral properties
ECHINACEA	the best-known immune-enhancing herb in North America, echinacea also has antiviral, antibiotic and wound-healing properties though should not be taken in large quantities

SUBSTANCE, PRODUCT OR METHOD	PRESUMED USE OR THEORY OF ACTION, COMMENTS
EDTA(ethylene-diamine-tetraacetic acid)	the primary synthetic chemical used in chelation therapy (hence greatly improving peripheral vascular conditions and removing toxic minerals and metals from the body), "man's miracle molecule" may also have antiretroviral effects and "potentiates" live-cell therapy
ENZYMES	enzyme administration is often given for "free radical"-scavenging, antiinflammatory and protein-digesting enhancement and for possible anticarcinogenic uses. The antioxidant enzymes include superoxide dismutase (SOD) and catalase. Therapeutic proteolytic enzymes include bromelain, papain, trypsin, chymotrypsin. These may be complexed with amylase, L-glutathione and/or specific vitamins and minerals. Some combinations of proteolytic enzymes are regarded as particularly useful in HIV/AIDS
EVENING PRIMROSE OIL	a natural source of essential fatty acids
FATTY ACIDS (including Essential Fatty Acids -- EFA)	this broad spectrum of natural substances has curative, cleansing effects. Some may help modulate immune response, others have antifungal, antiviral effects. Included in HIV/AIDS use are eicosapentaenoic acid (EPA), arachidonic acid (AA), linoleic acid (LA), gamma-linolenic acid (GLA), lauric acid (whose derivative monolaurin has antiviral effects), butyric acid (useful especially in lymphomas). Certain herbs and food factors such as evening primrose oil have high concentrations of EFAs

292

SUBSTANCE, PRODUCT OR METHOD	PRESUMED USE OR THEORY OF ACTION, COMMENTS
FOLIC ACID	the B vitamin most commonly found to be deficient in the U.S., folic acid is vital to immune function. With Vitamin E and B6, it is involved in protein synthesis and nucleic acid production as well as proper digestion
FREQUENCY MACHINES	Electronic devices, some said based on the theories of the late Royal Rife, said to demolish HIV "bio-electrically" by tuning to appropriate frequency
GARLIC	the most studied and best known of the multipurpose herbs, garlic (containing a potent package of useful vitamins, minerals, bioflavonoids, etc.) has antimicrobial, antibacterial, anticarcinogenic, antifungal, blood-normalizing, blood pressure-lowering, antiviral, antiparasitical and other effects, and some of its ingredients are immune-modulating
GERMANIUM	information on this mineral, particularly the organic variety, indicates immune-modulating, anticarcinogenic, natural interferon-stimulating capabilities
GINSENG	the various kinds of ginseng are the best known of the "adaptogens" (substances helping the body deal with non-specific stress.) Panax and Eleuthero are the more important varieties. Ginseng has drug antidote, blood pressure-normalizing, energy-enhancing properties, among many others
GLUTATHIONE	Current research, finding AIDS patients deficient in glutathione, suggests use of this tripeptide as an immune stimulator; frequently used as part of antioxidant enzyme combinations

293

SUBSTANCE, PRODUCT OR METHOD	PRESUMED USE OR THEORY OF ACTION, COMMENTS
GOLDENSEAL	this widely used North American herb has immune-modulating as well as antimicrobial and antifungal properties, has been used against intestinal parasites common in HIV/AIDS and is of benefit against diarrhea
HOMEOPATHIC REMEDIES	an extensive group of homeopathic dilutions has been anecdotally reported useful in managing many HIV/AIDS symptoms. The products include, but are not limited to: Agaricus, Aranea didema, Arsenicum, Bacillinum, Badiaga, Baptista, Belladonna, Byronia, Carcinosin, Cyclosporine, Dulcamara, Influenzium, Kali carb., Lachesis, Lycopodium, Merculiris, Muriatic acid, Natrum mur., Nitric acid, Phosphorus, Phosphoric acid, Rhus tox., Sulphur, Typhoidinum, Trifolium prat., Thuya
HYDRAZINE SULFATE	this controversial anti-cancer compound appears useful in combating the wasting syndrome and enhancing appetite
HYDROGEN PEROXIDE	an oxidative agent and antiseptic, hydrogen peroxide may be useful at lower concentrations against Candida; theoretically it should be antiviral, antifungal and antibacterial, but some research strongly suggests it is dangerous at high doses because of triggering the deleterious "free radical cascade"
HYPERICUM (St. John's Wort)	this herb has shown strong anti-retroviral activity in animal tests; its extract, hypericin, has been used as an antidepressant (large doses reportedly poisoned grazing animals)

294

SUBSTANCE, PRODUCT OR METHOD	PRESUMED USE OR THEORY OF ACTION, COMMENTS
HYPERIMMUNE MILK	antibody extracts of the milk of cows exposed to Crytosporidiosis, hyperimmune milk is under study for particular use in this HIV/AIDS condition
IMAGING, MEDITATION, etc.	probably a majority of long-term HIV/AIDS patients involved in various metabolic/eclectic programs are using some form of guided imagery, meditation or other mind-control techniques as part of treatment
ISCADOR (Viscum album)	Mistletoe extract used for more than 6 decades in Europe as an anti-cancer agent blocks cell clumping (syncytia) in cells in vitro and seems to enhance immune systems several ways in humans; subcutaneous injections
LAETRILE (amygdalin)	an unapproved anticarcinogenic, laetrile has free radical-scavenging and energy-boosting properties; its oral forms may give rise to thiocyanate, involved in many vital metabolic functions
LECITHIN	this naturally occurring fatty substance may make it more difficult for viruses to attach to T-4 cells (among many other uses)
LENTINAN	extracted from the Japanese Shiitake mushroom, this medication has long been used in cancer therapy (Japan) without toxicity, and apparently increases T cells. Not yet available as a U.S. treatment
LEPTOTAENIA (Lomatium dissectum)	Herb seems to inhibit bacteria, viruses, fungi, stimulate immunity, decrease inflammation

SUBSTANCE, PRODUCT OR METHOD	PRESUMED USE OR THEORY OF ACTION, COMMENTS
LICORICE (glycyrrhizin)	extracts of the licorice plant have been shown to be useful against cancer and certain viruses, including HIV, EBV and hepatitis B. The primary chemical is glycyrrhizin. Licorice root has been used for years in China and is available in heatlh food stores. Care in administration is advised
LITHIUM	this metallic element may have several immune-modulating and antiviral features, with part of its activity involved in blocking the synthesis of prostaglandin E1
LIVE-CELL THERAPY	not legally available in the U.S.A., this 50-year-old European technique is the subcutaneous injection of suspensions of cellular material from embryonic or fetal tissues, usually of the endocrine (but also other) organs. Live-cell therapy primarily harmonizes hormones by balancing the endocrine system and has immune-modulating effects. In HIV/AIDS, thymic material is thought to be of great benefit in modulating the immune system. Some injections (primarily of the umbilicus) are directed against cancer
MONOLAURIN	the monoglycerol ester of lauric acid (of the fatty acids), this derivative of mother's milk is a recognized food additive and is known to be effective against various lipid-coated viruses and bacteria, and is not toxic. Approved in U.S. as a food additive for more than 20 years

296

SUBSTANCE, PRODUCT OR METHOD	PRESUMED USE OR THEORY OF ACTION, COMMENTS
MUSHROOMS	long used as medicinal plants, many mushrooms have been studied for antiviral and anticarcinogenic properties. Lentinan is extracted from Shiitake. Extracts from the following species apparently have antiviral properties: Lentinus edodes, Flammulina velutipes, Calvatis gigantes, Poria obliqua, Agaricus bisporus. Some mushrooms are poisonous, and unidentifiable mushrooms should never be regarded as safe for consumption
OZONE	ozone infusions into the blood by Dr. Horst Keif in West Germany have reportedly helped many patients. Substances which release nascent atomic oxygen have antiviral, antibacterial, antifungal properties. A U.S. patent has been granted to one company for research with ozone in "inactivating lipid envelope viruses" and thus use against EBV, hepatitis and herpes
PAU D'ARCO (lapacho, ipe roxo, tajibo, tajebo)	the tea from the bark of this South American tree has been found to be an adaptogen and immune modulator and is of benefit in many facets of HIV/AIDS and many other conditions
QUERCITIN	one of the bioflavonoids, or near-vitamins, quercitin seems to inhibit reverse transcriptase activity, is active against herpes and is an antioxidant
RETICULOSE	developed in 1934 and later modified, Reticulose is an antiviral agent comprised of peptones, peptides, lipoprotein and nucleic acid. Before its removal from U.S. commerce when new FDA statutes were implemented in 1962, extensive research

297

SUBSTANCE, PRODUCT OR METHOD	PRESUMED USE OR THEORY OF ACTION, COMMENTS
	established the product's antiviral, immune-modulating properties. As a bearer of octapeptides it may inhibit HIV receptor binding and T-cell infectivity. Used abroad against many viral infections; foreign distributor involved in studies seeking FDA approval
REVICI METHODS	the "guided lipid" therapies of Emanuel Revici, M.D., New York, utilize lipid combinations with minerals (especially selenium) in metabolic protocols for many conditions, including HIV/AIDS. These methods modulate immunity and produce antiviral effects, among others
SARSAPARILLA	the old-time folk remedy herbal medicine is an easily obtainable adaptogen
SELENIUM	a recognized immune enhancer, this mineral is also a free radical scavenger and provides protection against toxic metals. It is associated with anticancer properties as well. Dose levels should be closely monitored
SOLUTEIN	the result of decades of U.S.-based research, this combination of protein fractions from several snake venoms has been shown to enhance immune responses and eliminate certain opportunistic infections in HIV/AIDS patients. Zenith Corporation maintains an ongoing research program in Mexico with collaboration by major U.S. research centers
SPIRULINA (food algae)	spirulina has a broad array of uses since it contains almost all the amino acids (including nine "essentials"), protein, B

298

SUBSTANCE, PRODUCT OR METHOD	PRESUMED USE OR THEORY OF ACTION, COMMENTS
	vitamins, Vitamin E and Vitamin A precursors. Spirulina-Dumaliella preparation has been shown to improve immune systems in cancer-stricken animals
STAPHAGE LYSATE	this "germ's germ" is a useful artificial immune enhancer and is also antibacterial
THYMUS GLANDULAR	in lieu of live-cell therapy, not available in the U.S., some HIV/AIDS patients take injections, tablets or capsules of thymus glandular material for possible immune modulation
URINE THERAPY	U.S./European experimental treatments based on ancient medicine suggest the oral consumption of one's own urine in small amounts has been of considerable value in several cases of HIV/AIDS
VITAMIN A (beta-carotene)	beta-carotene is the precursor of Vitamin A. These substances have immune-enhancing, immune-modulating, antioxidant and possibly, in therapeutic megadoses, antiviral properties, and also are used in the metabolic management of cancer. Megadoses of Vitamin A may be given in emulsified form. Vitamin A toxicity should be carefully monitored. Beta carotene is essentially non-toxic
VITAMIN B1 (thiamine)	helps modulate immune function
VITAMIN B2 (riboflavin)	helps modulate immune function
VITAMIN B5 (pantothenic acid)	this B vitamin is a recognized immune-enhancer through several routes of action and an antioxidant and is a primary supporting nutrient for adrenal cortical insufficiency

299

SUBSTANCE, PRODUCT OR METHOD	PRESUMED USE OR THEORY OF ACTION, COMMENTS
VITAMIN B6 (pyridoxine)	immune enhancer, antioxidant and possibly the most protective of the B vitamins
VITAMIN B12 (cyanocobalamin)	helps modulate immune function and especially influences T-cell function
VITAMIN C (ascorbic acid, ascorbate)	possibly the premiere vitamin, Vitamin C is a potent antioxidant, has chelating properties, is antiviral and immune-enhancing. It also plays an important role in strengthening collagen, or cellular cement. Megadoses of intravenous Vitamin C have been observed to bring full-blown AIDS symptoms under control for long periods of time
VITAMIN E (tocopherols)	a demonstrated antioxidant, immune enhancer and natural chelating agent, Vitamin E has many uses at virtually every stage of the HIV/AIDS infection curve
WHEAT GRASS, WHEAT GRASS JUICE	containing chlorophyll, many B Vitamins, fiber, proteins, carbohydrates and natural laetrile (anticarcinogenic), this food product is a favorite adjunctive therapy in many HIV/AIDS cases
ZINC	zinc, as an immune modulator, plays many roles in immune function, is part of more than 100 enzymes, and is involved in the healing process. It is probably the single most important mineral in HIV/AIDS therapy

APPENDIX IV

THE HIV-POSITIVE, AIDS/ARC BRADFORD RESEARCH INSTITUTE-MEXICO PROGRAM: AN OVERVIEW

(C) 1988, The Bradford Research Institute (M. L. Culbert)

(NOTE: The experimental program concluded in November 1989. Followup of patients continues).

The Bradford Research Institute-Mexico division treatment program for AIDS/ARC is based on the following assumptions:

1. Immune systems are susceptible of being either rebuilt or repaired or at the very least substantially aided by intervening therapies.

2. It is extremely doubtful that HIV virus is the single cause of the immune deficit common to the span of infection variously --- and changeably --- described as "acquired immune deficiency syndrome" (AIDS) and/or its predecessor or parallel state, "AIDS-related complex" (ARC).

3. For the immune deficit (and infection of other cells) attributable to HIV to occur, there almost certainly are inductive co-factors; and for even the synergism between HIV and the inductive co-factors to bring about infection, there almost certainly is the need for prior immune (or related) damage due to a host of predisposing factors.

4. The probable inductive co-factors to HIV include the herpesvirus family, most importantly Epstein-Barr Virus (EBV), cytomegalovirus (CMV) and herpes I and/or II.

5. As set forth in my 1986 monograph[1], and additional research, the predisposing factors to AIDS/ARC infection, in no particular sequence of importance, are: prior venereal infections, most importantly syphilis; substance abuse, whether the substances be injected, eaten, drunk, smoked or snorted; abuse of antibiotics and steroids; several elements common to processed food, particularly altered fatty acids and inadequate amounts of natural fatty acids, and excess refined carbohydrates; fluoridated water; gastrointestinal and other parasites; certain lubricants in-

301

volved in sexplay; yeast infection, primarily Candida albicans; poor hygiene in general; prior viral infections; vaccinations; environmental poisoning; specific sex acts (in the latter category is the overwhelming statistical correlation between unprotected insertive anal sex and multiplicity of sexual partners; secondarily, unprotected insertive vaginal sex, though the risk for both passive and active partners in this act seems more equally shared than in the matter of active and passive partners in unprotected insertive anal sex); blood transfusion; blood transfer between mother and fetus; sharing of needles in intravenous drug abuse; ritual tattooing, circumcision (male and female) with common instruments, as in Africa, and other scarification practices; multiple use of syringes, as in parts of the Third World.

(The extreme mutability of HIV does not preclude other routes of transmission, but there is no statistical reason -- at least as of summer 1988 -- to assume that AIDS/ARC infection is transmitted other than by blood to blood, blood to semen, semen to blood, even though HIV has been shown to appear in every body fluid. It is doubtful, though obviously possible, that a single sexual exposure to HIV is sufficient to lead to AIDS/ARC.[2])

6. Victims of AIDS/ARC are not succumbing to HIV but to well-known pathologies whose sudden lethality occurs after immune systems are already severely crippled -- a crippling due either to HIV and its co-factors, or possibly due to HIV alone, or due to the co-factors alone. Therefore, therapeutic strategies in full-blown AIDS directed primarily at HIV are the military equivalent of bombs dropped on the wrong target. The drug approach to prophylaxis of HIV, if indeed it is the putative "AIDS virus", is obviously more effective in the *early* phase of the course of infection than later.

7. The earlier an immune deficit is detected, the earlier a prophylactic intervention to modulate the immune system (and indeed all systems comprising vaguely what may be called "host defense") is called for, and the more effective it will be. Despite "establishment" doubts as to there being any real way to enhance immunity substantial information suggests that a broad range of vitamins, minerals, enzymes, amino acids and other natural substances helps to modulate or stimulate immunity, and these substances should be part of any multifactorial program for what is,

after all, a multifactorial condition.

8. Because various viruses, including those not presently identified, are presumptively involved at every stage of AIDS/ ARC, then a broad pattern of anti-viral substances is necessary. Certain agents which are immunomodulating are also anti-viral. Since pathologic bacteria and fungi are also involved in various of the diseases associated with AIDS/ARC, prophylactic anti-bacterial, anti-fungal weapons are called for, as is treatment of parasites.

9. The outcome of actual HIV exposure is simply *not known*, and the insistence on a "positive blood test" corresponding to 100% mortality from AIDS/ARC is a thought, not a fact. Moreover, a strategy based solely on HIV inhibition in what is a multifactorial condition is a central error in the "establishment's" so far vain efforts to "cure" the syndrome. Patients who are HIV-positive must be counseled that positivity is not necessarily a death sentence, and that early intervention to enhance host defense, alter lifestyle, eat properly, and think properly is a must to rebuilding or at least improving host defense.

10. The biologically reasonable approach to managing AIDS/ARC is (a) enhancing overall host defense while (b) aggressively attacking viruses, bacteria and fungi while (c) maintaining a metabolically sound eating program, (d) exercising and (e) inculcating a "winning" attitude in the thought process -- for example, insisting that one is not "dying from" but rather "living with" immune depression.

The BRI worldwide has pioneered what it calls "individualized, integrated metabolic programs (IIMP)" for virtually all major chronic disease. What we may call, imperfectly, "HIV Disease" (in lieu of AIDS/ARC) is no exception. That is, the specific substances, amounts and routes of administration may vary from patient to patient: an IIMP for HIV Disease is not cookbook medicine.

Elements of such programs which we have now utilized on about 5 dozen HIV Disease patients over approximately 5 years include the following:

Non-specific immune enhancers (which, at some levels, are also anti-virals); Vitamins A,C,E, beta-carotene, vitamins B1, B6 and folic acid, essential fatty acids in various combinations (AL-721 being one of them), zinc, selenium, iron, chlorophyll, garlic and amino acids

303

L-cysteine and L-methionine, together with aerobic exercise.

Synthetic immune-stimulating drugs: isoprinosine, levamisol.

Immune modulation, endocrine balancing, regeneration or rejuvenation of damaged tissues: live-cell therapy (embryonic or fetal animal cell suspensions given subcutaneously).

Synthetic anti-viral experimental drugs: acyclovir, ribavirin, staphage lysate. (AL-721 and dextran sulfate have recently been added.)

Synthetic multipurpose anti-viral, anti-bacterial, anti-fungal: Dioxychlor (BRI propietary forms of an industrial oxidative agent for topical, oral, intravenous use).

Check for and treatment of parasites.

Broad-spectrum antibiotic: aqueous penicillin.[3]

Dietary recommendations: detoxifying and energy-enhancing through fruit and vegetable juices; mostly vegetarian diet, banning of refined carbohydrates, stimulants; banning or restricting animal fats and proteins; herbals teas; restricting vinegars, sugar-containing or yeast-connected foods.

GI tract cleansing: herbal teas, herbal enemas, coffee enemas, lactobacillus bifidus, acidophilus.

Antioxidant enzymes and other substances: SOD, catalase, DMSO, OXY-5000 combination, anti-inflammatory enzymes. Certain vitamins, minerals, and amino acids also have antioxidant action. Antioxidant enzymes may also help modulate immunity.

Possible anti-viral as well as enhancer of live-cell activity: EDTA (chelating agent).

Broad-spectrum herbals.

AN OVERVIEW OF THE MULTIFACTORIAL TREATMENT PROGRAM FOR IMMUNE DEPRESSION AT BRI-MEXICO

Beginning in late 1983, BRI-Mexico began accepting patients diagnosed as "full-blown" AIDS. The first few patients were of stretcher-case advanced Kaposi's sarcoma with other opportunistic infections, and of ambulatory KS with opportunistic infections. ARC-level and asymptomatic AIDS cases did not begin treatment with us until about 1985/86. Some general observations as to patients and results:

1. As of summer 1988, 60 HIV-related patients have been seen by BRI-Mexico. Due to inadequate records, or followup, or the fact some patients stayed too little time for meaningful evaluation, and given the deaths of a few initial stretcher patients, we have records and followup on 49 patients.

2. In no case of "full-blown" AIDS has the BRI protocol been the *only* protocol followed. Full-blown AIDS patients, possibly a third of the total (depending on the varying definitions by the Centers of Disease Control of just what constitutes "full-blown" AIDS), usually came to us following failure on other therapies and have frequently mixed other therapies when leaving us.

3. HIV-related patients have in the majority been treated by an intensive, 10-day program. About a dozen have been treated with a limited, mostly-oral program.

4. All patients have been males, ranging in age from 20 to mid-50s. All but two have been professed homosexuals, and all but two have reported some form of substance abuse.

5. In the last three years, we are aware of five deaths, all of full-blown AIDS, from our patient load. In every case, significant improvement (enhancement of absolute T4 cells, decrease in clinical symptoms) has been noted. Most others whom we can trace are either stable or improving.

6. At least three dozen ARC or early-AIDS cases have shown transient to consistent signs of improvement in overall immune function, most noticeably normalization or near-normalization of T4 counts, as well as decrease in clinical signs and symptoms, overall energy and weight gain. Some of these are at the three-year level.

7. In terms of full-blown AIDS, one of the earliest KS patients went through the full course of treatment twice over $4^1/2$ years, and succumbed only after a return to toxic chemotherapy and heavy antibiotics following a relapse.

8. Currently, at least six full-blown AIDS cases are

stable.

9. In two ARC-level cases and one AIDS-level case HIV virus can no longer be cultured from blood, and all three patients are not only stable but working and feeling well. The three HIV-free (that is, from blood) patients were so diagnosed in 1988.

10. In one AIDS-level patient, immunoblastic lymphoma vanished within a month of treatment and he remains stable.

11. In one AIDS-level patient, cryptococcal meningitis has disappeared completely.

12. One full-blown AIDS patient (primarily PCP pneumonia) survived 21 months on a mixed BRI and "orthodox" protocol. During this time he was able to take oral AZT for a full year without the need for blood transfusions, worked a normal shift and ultimately relapsed for a third time following the use of aerosol pentamidine and several other drugs. At one point during his BRI therapy a case of "walking pneumonia" he suffered was eradicated in three days simply with infusions of Dioxychlor and Vitamin C.

13. We have seen rapid, if sometimes transient, destruction of KS lesions with Dioxychlor topically applied alone.

14. In one ARC patient, the T4 cell count doubled in a week's time and tripled within a month as overall symptoms subsided.

15. In several patients T4 cells normalized but the T4:T8 ratio remains low because T8's remain high, suggestive of a protective or other benign effect from elevated T8 cells. In these patients there are no signs or symptoms of immune dysfunction.

16. Despite these relatively remarkable results on a small but growing patient population the BRI protocols do not claim "cure" nor can we predict how long the stabilized patients will remain stable.

Our general conclusions:

1. The advance to overt pathology in immune-compromised or HIV-positive patients is halted or slowed.

2. The advance to worse pathology in ARC-level

patients is halted or slowed.

3. Improved longevity and quality of life are the norm in full-blown AIDS cases. The advance of disease has been at least slowed in several.

4. We believe a substantial number of HIV-positive, ARC-level or early AIDS patients can survive in ordinarily good health for an unquantifiable period of time, with most of them likely to remain in a lifelong "carrier state" of generally good health as long as they take adequate dietary, exercise and lifestyle precautions.

5. AIDS/ARC should not be seen as a necessarily fatal syndrome.

6. Results in overall improvement and halting (and even reversing) disease are better the earlier this kind of intervention is performed.

A NOTE ON DIOXYCHLOR
(PREPARATIONS OF EXOGENOUS
OXIDATIVE COMPOUNDS)

BRI worldwide research on oxidology --- the study of reactive toxic species in health and disease --- led BRI to the consideration of a family of industrial oxidative compounds as the premiere among the oxidative agents. Dioxychlor, our name for these compounds, is essentially free of the metabolically damaging side effects of the "natural" endogenous oxidative agent, hydrogen peroxide, and of the major "natural" exogenous oxidative agent, ozone, in that it does not initiate the potentially disruptive free-radical cascade or other biological side effects of these species. Dioxychlor's primary benefit is the release of atomic oxygen, a natural way to directly inhibit or destroy viruses, bacteria and fungi without producing significant, if any, toxic effects along the way. *In vitro* research[4] has demonstrated the efficacy of these compounds against HIV, EBV, CMV, hepatitis, polio and a number of other pathological organisms and structures.

PATIENT FOLLOWUP

AIDS/ARC patients are monitored following their release from the 10-day program, usually by telephone or letter. We are interested in ongoing T-cell tests and/or any viral assays (antigen P24, PCR, etc.) indicative of viral inhibition. AIDS/ARC patients are usually asked to return occasionally for "booster" live-cell injections, or occasional "drips" of Dioxychlor. It is not yet established for how lengthy a period of time they will remain on oral drugs (ribavirin) although they will be asked to adhere to a program of host defense-enhancing supplements and dietary constraints for the foreseeable future.

(1)   Culbert, Michael L., AIDS: TERROR, TRUTH, TRIUMPH. Chula Vista, Ca.: The Bradford Research Institute, 1986

(2)   We will not deal here with the various theories as to the origin of HIV or similar viruses, including the strong possibility they may have been manufactured. HIV itself is so aberrant from other such structures that no firm conclusions as to how/where/ when it may mutate or in what form can be arrived at.

(3)   Since virtually every major pathology or sign in "full-blown AIDS" has historically been found in advanced third-stage or neurosyphilis, and because a number of researchers treat AIDS as if it were syphilis, and because aqueous penicillin --- rather than the more common benzathine penicillin --- apparently crosses the "blood/brain barrier", it has been used in some cases.

(4)   Bradford, R.W.; Allen, H.W.; Culbert, M.L., EXOGENOUS OXIDATIVE MECHANISMS IN COMBATING INFECTIOUS AGENTS. Chula Vista, Ca.: Bradford Research Institute, 1986.

INDEX

(Roman numerals denote Appendices)

A

309

310

312

316

progressive multifocal leukoencephalopathy 59,98
prostaglandin El 148,149,
150,152-153,154,213
Pryor, William 244
pseudomonas exotoxin A **II**
psychoneuroimmunology (PNI)
235-237

Q

quercitin 261, **III**

R

R82150 **II**
R-HEV test 66
Radding, Wilson 35
radionics 224-225,226
Ramos, Elizabeth 207
Randolph, Theron 126
recombinant erythropoieten 27
Redfield, Robert R. 67
refined carbohydrates 149
Reich, Wilhelm 75,225,226
Renner, John 199-200
respiratory syncytial virus 201
Reticulose **III**
reverse transcriptase
28,56,65,74,200
Revici, Emmanuel 214
Revici methods **III**
Reyes Syndrome 131
rheumatoid arthritis 129
ribavirin (Virazole, Vilona)
26,201,251, **II**
Rife, Royal 75,225,226
"Rife instrument" 226
Rio de Janeiro 22,162
RIPA test 66
Robert-Guroff, M. 70

Robilotti, J.C. 137
Robinson, William 68
Rodriguez, Luis 61
Roger's Recovery from AIDS 207
Rothschild, Jonathan 213
Rothschild, Peter R. 213,237
ROTS ("reactive oxygen toxic
species") 128,163,244-245
Roxithromycin **II**
Rozenbaum, W. 92
"Rush" 119
Rutgers University 250
Rwanda 93,121,133

S

SAIDS (simian AIDS) 40
Salk, Jonas 41
Salk HIV Vaccine **II**
saliva 91,94
Salmonella 138
San Francisco, AIDS cases
decline in, 91; "cohort"
study, 33-34,62,171-172;
fluoridation in, 160-161
San Francisco Chronicle 43
San Francisco Department of
Public Health 114,137
Sao Paolo 162
Saper, Clifford R. 237
sarsaparilla **III**
Saturn V Moon Vehicle Project 227
Schmidt, Casper S. 237-238
Schnittman, Steven M. 55
Schrauzer, Gerhard 244
scurvy 49
Seale, John 167-168,170
Seattle 121,197
Seibert, Florence 75
selenium 213,214,216,250,259, **III**
semen, 87
Septra **II**

320

visna virus
Vitamin A 213,214,215,250,259, **III**
Vitamin B complex 214
Vitamin B1 (thiamin) **III**
Vitamin B2 (riboflavin) **III**
Vitamin B5 (pantothenic acid)
213, **III**
Vitamin B6 (pyridoxine)
149,213,216,250, **III**
Vitamin B12 (cyanocobalamin)
III
Vitamin B17 see laetrile
Vitamin C 49,149,155,205,210-212,
213,214,215,250, **III**
Vitamin E 213,214,215,250,259, **III**

Witkin, Steven S. 89
Wong-Stahl, Flossie 57
World Health Organization (WHO)
1,13,39,42,43,168
Wright, Pearce 168

Y

yaws 190
yeast infection 128-129
Yiamouyiannis, John 159-160,
162-163
yoga 218,238
Young, Frank 199,209,210

W

Waldthaler, Urban 189
Wall Street Journal, The 57,69
Walter Reed Army Institute of
Research 56
Walter Reed Army Medical Center
93
Walter Reed Classification
System **I**
Washington Bureau of Intel-
ligence and Research 177
Washington Post, The 223
Washington Times, The 167
Weekly World News, 167
Weiss, Ted 11
Weissmann, Gerald 163
Western Blot test 36,66
Western Journal of Medicine 192
West Germany 162
wheat grass **III**
Whiteside, Mark 92,107,109,110,111,
112,141-142,147-148
Wierenga, Wendell 56
Wigmore, Ann 215
Wilson, Hank 120

Z

Zachar, Bruce 232
Zaire 32,93,111,133
Zambia 101
Ziegler, John L. 32
zidovudine see AZT
zinc 148,149,150,213,214,250, **III**

Information on the HIV/AIDS research treatment program at the Bradford
Research Institute—Mexico facility in Tijuana, B.C., Mexico, is available
from:

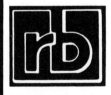